GROUNDING PSYCHOTHERAPY IN SELF-COMPASSION

Grounding Psychotherapy in Self-Compassion

EDITED BY

GALIA TYANO RONEN
SHARI GELLER

Foreword by Steven C. Hayes

THE GUILFORD PRESS
New York London

A Division of Guilford Publications, Inc.
www.guilford.com

Printed in the United States of America

This book is printed on acid-free paper.

Last digit is print number: 9 8 7 6 5 4 3 2 1

Library of Congress Cataloging-in-Publication Data

Names: Tyano Ronen, Galia, editor. | Geller, Shari M., editor.
Title: Grounding psychotherapy in self-compassion / edited by Galia Tyano Ronen, Shari Geller.
Description: New York : The Guilford Press, [2025] | Includes bibliographical references and index. |
Identifiers: LCCN 2024038840 | ISBN 9781462556731 (paperback) | ISBN 9781462556748 (cloth)
Subjects: LCSH: Sympathy. | Therapist and patient. | Compassion.
Classification: LCC BF575.S9 G76 2025 | DDC 177.7—dc23/eng/20241004
LC record available at *https://lccn.loc.gov/2024038840*

To my beloved mentors on earth, who taught me the essence of love, gentleness, fierceness, and compassion: Sam, Ginette, Lital, Liah, Noam, Yael, Roy, and Itay. I am grateful to all my loved ones who, by their enlightened presence, shined the path and warmed it gently so we could walk it together. To all of us, being our best to learn courageously to be compassionate to ourselves.

—G. T. R.

Deep appreciation and gratitude for all of those compassionate and loving beings who inspire me and ground me every day. I dedicate this book to all the special beings who teach me to be compassionate, including, but not limited to, Camilla, Rachel, Sarah, my family (Brown and Geller), Queenie, Dylan, and Zen. And to the memory of my mom and dad. With love and appreciation, I dedicate the merits of this book to them and to all sentient beings, the earth, therapists, and clients everywhere who may benefit from self-compassion.

—S. G.

About the Editors

Galia Tyano Ronen, MA, LCP, a licensed clinical psychologist in private practice in Israel, serves on the faculty of the Shiluv Mind Body Spirit Center, affiliated with the University of Haifa. She has specialized in mind–body–spirit mindfulness-based psychotherapy and supervision since the 1990s. Ms. Tyano Ronen is an artist, a certified focusing-oriented therapist, a certified mindfulness meditation teacher and mentor trained by Tara Brach and Jack Kornfield, and a certified mindful self-compassion (MSC) teacher. She is program developer and former director of the Self-Compassion in Psychotherapy Certificate Program offered by the Center for Mindful Self-Compassion. Ms. Tyano Ronen has pioneered MSC in Israel, has led worldwide workshops, and is responsible for the translation of the MSC program into Hebrew and for creating a bilingual MSC course for Arabs and Jews.

Shari Geller, PhD, a leader in the field of therapeutic presence, is founder and co-director of the Centre for MindBody Health in Toronto. A certified MSC teacher who has been weaving psychology and mindfulness since the 1990s, Dr. Geller teaches internationally and has published several books, as well as book chapters and articles. She serves on the teaching faculty in Health Psychology at York University and is Adjunct Professor in the Faculty of Music at the University of Toronto, in association with the Music and Health Research Collaboratory. Dr. Geller is a faculty member of the Self-Compassion in Psychotherapy Certificate Program offered by the Center for Mindful Self-Compassion and is chair of the Membership and Networking Committee of the International Society for Emotion Focused Therapy. She loves playing the handpan and drumming and founded the Therapeutic Rhythm and Mindfulness program.

Contributors

Shelby L. Alsup, PhD candidate, Department of Psychology, Pacific University, Forest Grove, Oregon

Michelle Becker, MA, LMFT, Center for Mindfulness, University of California San Diego, San Diego, California

José Ramón Yela Bernabé, PhD, Department of Psychology, Pontifical University of Salamanca, Salamanca, Spain

Gerson F. Borrero, MSc, Department of Psychology, Suffolk University, Boston, Massachusetts

Antonio Crego Díaz, PhD, Department of Psychology, Pontifical University of Salamanca, Salamanca, Spain

Shari Geller, PhD, CPsych, Centre for MindBody Health and Department of Psychology, York University, Toronto, Ontario, Canada

Christopher Germer, PhD, Department of Psychiatry, Harvard Medical School, Boston, Massachusetts

Paul Gilbert, PhD, Centre for Compassion Research and Training, College of Health, Psychology and Social Care, University of Derby, Derby, England

Steven Hickman, PsyD (retired), Centers for Integrative Health, University of California San Diego, La Jolla, California

Lorraine M. Hobbs, MA, Youth and Family Programs, Center for Mindfulness, University of California San Diego, San Diego, California

Jill Lillie, MA, School of Education and Counseling Psychology, Santa Clara University, Santa Clara, California

Jessica R. LoPresti, PhD, Department of Psychology, Suffolk University, Boston, Massachusetts

Tracy Ochester, PsyD, Midwest Alliance for Mindfulness, Leawood, Kansas

Susan M. Pollak, MTS, EdD, Center for Mindfulness and Compassion, Cambridge Health Alliance, Harvard Medical School, Cambridge, Massachusetts

Lizabeth Roemer, PhD, Department of Psychology, University of Massachusetts Boston, Boston, Massachusetts

Shayda Roohparvar, MA, School of Education and Counseling Psychology, Santa Clara University, Santa Clara, California

Ann Saffi Biasetti, PhD, LCSWR, An Embodied Life, Saratoga Springs, New York

Molly Sawdy, MS, Department of Psychology, Suffolk University, Boston, Massachusetts

Shauna Shapiro, PhD, School of Education and Counseling Psychology, Santa Clara University, Santa Clara, California

Lisa Shetler, MA, Embrace Psychology and Consulting, Gawler, South Australia, Australia

Daniel J. Siegel, MD, Mindsight Institute, Santa Monica, California

Ronald D. Siegel, PsyD, Department of Psychiatry, Harvard Medical School, Boston, Massachusetts

Sydney S. Spears, PhD, LSCSW (retired), School of Social Welfare, University of Kansas, Lawrence, Kansas; Center for Mindful Self-Compassion, Austin, Texas

Christian Stiglmayr, PhD, Working Group for Scientific Psychotherapy Berlin, Berlin, Germany

Galia Tyano Ronen, MA, LCP, Shiluv Mind Body Spirit Center, Kiryat Tivon, Israel

Benjamin Weinstein, PhD, Department of Psychology, Faculty of Social Sciences, Chiang Mai University, Chang Mai, Thailand

Elli Weisbaum, PhD, Faculty of Arts and Sciences and Department of Psychiatry, University of Toronto, Toronto, Ontario, Canada

Alfie Wishart, MRC, LPC, LCDC, Wishart Counseling, Dallas, Texas

Foreword

Compassionately Embracing the Moment

Self-compassion has been a growing empirical and practical force for progress in psychotherapy for many years. It is a radically transdiagnostic process that not only has been shown to have a profound impact on therapists, clients, and their relationship but also holds out hope for a kinder world that is more ready to step forward to meet the challenges of the day.

Self-compassion, self-kindness, and self-acceptance are more than just goals or techniques—they are a stance toward human experience itself. That stance can transform therapy from a hierarchical interaction to a cooperative one. It can transform the exploration of painful events from superficial strategies of problem solving into a deeper exploration of human consciousness, emotion, and intention. It is this change in agenda, stance, and practice that helps therapists become more present with their clients, enhancing their resilience and significantly reducing the risk of burnout while doing so.

Self-compassion is known to foster greater emotional and cognitive flexibility. This flexibility is crucial in psychotherapy, where rigid patterns of thinking and feeling often underlie the struggles our clients face. When practiced effectively, self-compassion helps reduce a sense of self that is overly ego based, allowing individuals to navigate life's challenges without the defense and pretense that a narrative sense of self can bring.

The impact of self-compassion is profoundly transdiagnostic. Unlike interventions that are built atop concepts of latent diseases, self-compassion is built atop our sense of common humanity, providing a framework that can be applied across various clinical contexts and concerns. That does not mean that self-compassion work should be vague or nonspecific. To the contrary, it requires an appreciation of the *particular* features of a client's experience—their anxiety, sadness, trauma, urges, and errors; their history, circumstances, relationships, memories, and values.

Understanding self-compassion also requires recognizing and fostering its link to compassion toward others. It's a mistake to think they automatically or mechanically go together—that is empirically untrue, and it flies in the face of the fact that everyone knows people who use the language of self-compassion or self-care in a selfish way. In wisdom traditions care is taken to avoid this—someone displaying selfish self-compassion at a mindfulness retreat may soon find themselves mindfully doing the dishes! Therapy needs that same sensitivity, driven by the knowledge that genuine self-compassion includes empathy and interconnectedness with others. That very interconnection is part of why self-compassion can enhance the therapeutic relationship and why this kind of work can help create a safe, supportive environment for clients. By fostering both sides of compassion, therapists can facilitate the integration of gains both socially and neurobiologically, creating more meaningful progress.

It helps in doing so to view self-compassion through the lens of evolutionary science. As social primates, we are wired for connection. Practices of self-compassion and compassion toward others are rooted in our evolutionary heritage. Understanding that heritage can help practitioners craft therapeutic relationships that foster safety and promote the integration of therapeutic gains, making those gains more sustainable over time. By connecting self-compassion with our evolutionary biology, therapists can intervene in ways that resonate on a deeper and more fundamentally human level.

In an analogous way, it is important that self-compassion not become an island unto itself in the politics of intervention science and practice. Maintaining the healthy interconnection between the now large family of mindfulness-, acceptance-, and compassion-based interventions is crucial as we advance psychological intervention itself. We have a lot to learn, and progress is best fostered by the needs and interests of the clients we serve, by empirical longitudinal data that illuminate the lives of each human being, and by cooperation and mutual respect among change agents themselves. The benefits of doing so will be felt in the consulting room in more openness to ideas, greater creativity, and reduced therapist burnout. Effective and empathetic caregivers and researchers treat themselves and others with kindness, fostering well-being while together we learn how to step up to the social challenges we face.

The need to improve psychotherapy is clear. Large gaps remain in how we address suffering and promote healing, and our rate of improvement is simply too low. The thoughtful chapters in this book offer guidance on plugging those gaps—in clinical practice and in our scholarship. We have clear signs that integrating self-compassion into psychotherapy will help advance our field if we are willing to take the long view and build community around the effort. As you will see reading the chapters to come, this is happening in the field on many fronts. Our profession is abuzz with ideas for how we can bring the promise of self-compassion into the consulting room. The editors and their chapter-author colleagues lay out what we know and what we don't and make concrete suggestions that can be integrated into our healing work and scientific efforts today. We, as researchers and practitioners, need to compassionately embrace the worldwide moment we are in. Just as climate change, immigration, economic disparities, war, and political division are impacting us all, inviting us into needless despair, putting more self-compassion and compassion into our work may be precisely what we and the world most need to persist and prosper.

STEVEN C. HAYES, PhD
Foundation Professor of Psychology Emeritus, University of Nevada, Reno
Initiator and Co-Developer of Acceptance and Commitment Therapy or Training

Acknowledgments

We bow in gratitude to Chris Germer and Kristin Neff, who created the mindful self-compassion program and have contributed to the growth of the field of self-compassion as well as our own cultivation of compassion. We are deeply appreciative of all the authors who contributed their lifetime knowledge and experience, and who generously shared it with us. Thank you for your patience and the good spirit of togetherness. We would like to thank Ann Saffi Biasetti for contributing to the initial proposal of this book.

We honor and thank all our teachers, mentors, and ancestors who supported us on this path; their beliefs and warmth were present and valuable to this process.

We are deeply grateful to our clients and colleagues who have taught us how to be present and compassionate, and who inspired and humbled us.

We are inspired by and thankful for the practice of self-compassion that brought us together, enabled this book to come into being, and supported us in the process.

Thank you, dear reader, for your curiosity and courage to take this journey with us all. May this book serve all sentient beings and be of use to alleviate suffering in the world.

Contents

PART II. A Self-Compassion-Based Clinician: What Shapes and Informs Practice

PART III. Applications of Self-Compassion in Psychotherapy

Purchasers of this book can download and print copies of the Appendix, which contains practices and scripts of many of the audio files, at *www.guilford.com/tyano-ronen-materials* for personal use or use with clients (see copyright page for details).

Introduction

Where Do We Begin Our Journey?

Galia Tyano Ronen
Shari Geller

Many times, we have been asked over the years, "Being a therapist, what allows you to listen and stay present when you are surrounded by so much pain and suffering?" Our answer would be summed up in one word: *compassion*. Compassion is a natural feeling arising in response to pain. It can include both inner (self) and outer compassion. Compassion toward others involves feeling and reverberating with clients' suffering while holding the intention to relieve it. To be present with clients' pain and suffering and navigate the challenges to doing so, including sustaining such a powerful state, we need self-compassion as well. Self-compassion focuses on bringing a kind and warm awareness to our pain and suffering and listening deeply to what we need. The focus of this book is on self-compassion as an important foundation for effective psychotherapy as well as a resource for clients and therapists alike.

The following case illustration highlights how the practice of self-compassion can benefit both therapists and clients in a session. (All names and identifying details have been changed to ensure confidentiality.)

> Dana recently started suffering from breathing difficulties and tightness in the chest and came to treatment for this reason. Dana is an energetic woman who has shared that she is not used to having physical sensations "stop her." She is an active woman, and these attacks disturbed her a lot. It was easy for me to like her. Her bursting liveliness, interest, and curiosity allowed her to have real and deep contact with life. Friends surround her; she also has a satisfying and benevolent marital relationship and a job she is satisfied with. Still, the physical limitation bothered her.

After several months of treatment, I (Galia) noted that there had been an improvement in Dana's physical symptoms, and it was possible to discuss in depth the mental and emotional layers related to this improvement.

During one of the sessions, I noticed myself having difficulty in stopping and postponing a response to what Dana was sharing. Something about Dana's energetic dash forward created a state of hyperarousal in the room, in both of us. I could feel it in my body as well as she could feel it in hers. The mutual discussion pace created a warm and close relationship for us. At the same time, the fast pace did not allow for pausing, staying, and observing or commenting on what was happening.

In that meeting, when I noticed what was happening inside of me, related to Dana's content of the meeting itself, I slowed down, placed a hand on my heart area, and took a deep breath noticing my ability to return to my center.

Dana noticed that and stopped her flow of speech.

We looked at each other.

"I'm running too fast, huh?" Dana asked.

"We both are," I answered. I breathed again and mostly exhaled a long breath.

Dana smiled and breathed deeply, too.

I smiled and said, "I invite you to take a deep breath, even a few, if it is appropriate and possible for you right now."

Dana took a few deep breaths.

"I invite you to check what is happening in your body now. What is your experience?"

Dana and I slowed down, and a space was created for observation, acceptance, and compassion toward what was present at that moment. Our ability to stay with what came up allowed for a compassionate intention toward both myself and her.

With compassion, we resonate with our clients' experience. The possibility we have as therapists to practice self-compassion enables us to then return to the center, as in this vignette, and be present for ourselves and our clients in a deep, loving, connected way. It is a privilege and honor to be able to transmit and share the practice with our clients, taking care of ourselves and the clients, as well as enhancing a deep sense of well-being.

The Nature of Inner and Outer Compassion

Compassion, whether it is turned inward toward ourselves or outward toward others, includes the reverberation we feel with pain as well as the want to alleviate it. It includes the nature of reality and the causes of suffering. It is a natural feeling arising in response to pain. In order for us to maintain this clear and inclusive mindset, it might be valuable to consider practicing attentive open awareness and self-compassion. How is compassion experienced? We understand it as having multiple facets:

- Attentiveness and a soft feeling of care for another
- A palpable sensation of sensitivity and resonance to pain along with a benevolent want to help
- A kind of deep embrace of the pain combined with a feeling of being alive
- Witnessing the occurrence of pain and a sense of warmth at its side
- Sorrow alongside a connection to a common human experience

What Is Self-Compassion?

Self-compassion is the sensitivity to the suffering we experience within ourselves, with a deep commitment to try to relieve it. It has been defined by Neff (2003) as including three components: mindfulness (nonjudgmental awareness of our experience), common humanity (feeling a part of the human global community; not alone in our suffering), and self-kindness (bringing kindness to our pain and experience). Self-compassion allows us to engage with suffering as opposed to turning away or dissociating from it. We may acquire the wisdom of learning how to do it by practicing it. It involves fierceness and courage to move over the obstacles that would make us pull back, to be compassionate to the parts in us that are frightening or we are ashamed of. The action aspect of compassion includes the ability to act decisively to reduce suffering out of warmth and softness.

How Is Self-Compassion Supportive?

Self-compassion is a powerful adjunct for clients in therapy to help them be with their pain and suffering, approaching it with warmth and kindness so that they can engage in the deeper work of therapy. It is also a beneficial resource for therapists, one that enables them to be present and stay in a deep, loving, connected way with clients in challenging moments, as well as for therapists' overall self-care. The benefits of self-compassion are transtheoretical—they can extend across therapy approaches and strengthen clients' and therapists' ability to be present with and work through issues and trauma with greater inner resources.

The action aspect of compassion includes a sense of common humanity, where we touch a place of humanness inside. We know that we too, at a different time, have felt pain and suffering, just as our clients do. We might also experience a resonance of our own pain during a session, hence it may call on us to lean toward our pain with compassion as well. Since the ability to feel compassion exists in us, we can learn to direct it inwardly.

Any daily practice of mindfulness is a foundation, a ground, a shelter, a space, a breath of fresh air. Practicing mindful self-compassion allows full breathing while diving underwater. In most types of therapy, we assume that the therapist's attitude toward the client's pain will be compassionate and they will do their best to relieve the client's pain in various ways.

However, at times it is challenging to maintain this state in the face of pain and trauma. The inner feeling is a lack of space. Therapists' survival aspect (physical, emotional, and mental) is activated like an internal alarm indicating a threat or danger. We may have moments where we feel shut down or self-critical in the face of the clients' intense and intimate experience of suffering. This is when the self-compassion system can be mobilized and helpful. The practice of self-compassion calms internal self-criticism and allows therapists to see the situation broadly, regaining presence and spaciousness that enables growth and support to the client and therapist.

If we practice with our clients' ways to arouse compassion, even if the evolutionary wiring to respond to a threat automatically is activated, the self-soothing system can also be activated. We are not just talking about awareness of self-criticism or repeating and memorizing positive affirmations for ourselves but about connecting to a calming internal belonging system. And not only by changing the content of things but also the emotional way in which we approach an internal dialogue.

If we practice self-compassion, then, when working with clients around their pain and trauma, even if the evolutionary wiring to respond to a threat automatically is activated in us, the self-soothing system can also be activated.

When we acknowledge pain (our own or our clients') by feeling and saying, "This is a moment of difficulty or suffering for me," we express self-compassion. We can then gently touch our body and wish ourselves well in a soft, calm, and empathetic tone. While encouraging ourselves and feeling a sense of belonging to common humanity, we can calm ourselves, feel protected, and take care of ourselves in the best way for us. This will enhance our capacity to serve our clients.

Why Implement Self-Compassion in Psychotherapy?

We (Galia and Shari) both were part of creating and implementing programs designed to teach therapists how to incorporate self-compassion in psychotherapy. After hearing the experiences of many therapists from around the world as well as clients, we were more convinced than ever that this is a powerful resource for both therapists and their clients. We were on a mission then to explore how we can further offer therapists this resource to implement into their psychotherapy practice and personal life. Here lie the seeds for this book to come to fruition.

Pain and suffering are at the heart of the human condition. The typical human reaction to pain is to feel overwhelmed, push it away, or deny its existence. Helping our clients to hold their pain with kindness, warmth, and courage helps them approach their pain with curiosity and build the resources to tolerate it so it can be worked through in therapy and transformed.

Therapists also need the resources deriving from self-compassion to be with the depth of pain they are witness to. Self-compassion helps them to recognize their own suffering in resonance with clients and to use it as a resource to be with this pain to help understand clients' experience more deeply or to let it go when it is not serving this purpose.

The practices of mindfulness and compassion meditation and the practice of psychotherapy are both responses to suffering—they address a profound level of conscious and nonconscious experience and rely on introspection. When we meditate, we can access our pain and open to it without reactivity. In therapy, we walk the path with clients, genuinely interested in listening and relieving suffering. We share the journey of witnessing and supporting them in working through their pain and finding a collective web of meaning from their experience. To feel healthier, healed, whole, and complete.

There is a tremendous benefit of self-compassion practice for the therapist in cultivating qualities of mind that support a healing therapeutic relationship. The core of the practice lies in the acceptance of the changing motion of all there is versus holding on to the self as static, which promotes added suffering. Practicing in this way helps us to connect with the beautiful parts of our everyday life, and to accept the flow of our life journey, and psychotherapy as part of it. When we meditate, we are interested in learning, and we love the wisdom that can be accessed when we observe the body and the mind.

Self-compassion allows us as therapists to take care of ourselves, to be attentive to our needs, and thereby to be better equipped to help ourselves and others. It can also significantly reduce burnout. Tanya Singer (Singer & Chierchia, 2016), who researched this topic, found that while empathy for suffering activates the insula region of the brain and an area in the posterior cortex associated with negative emotions, states of compassion activate central frontal parts of the cortex and the area of the brain called the ventral striatum associated with feelings of warmth, caring, and positive emotions. Practicing compassion allows for an increase in personal psychological well-being that enables a more regulated way of dealing with internal and external difficulties. It also affects interpersonal relationships and increases cooperation, trust, and endurance in complex situations. In this way, it helps us to care for ourselves when engaging in the difficult work of psychotherapy.

Self-Compassion for the Therapist: Caring for Ourselves and Our World

Sitting and practicing self-compassion together with our clients allows us to feel the pain that exists in our world, with tenderness, and to engage in a healthy and wise response to it. Compassion alleviates pain by allowing one, first, to recognize it, and second, to treat the part that feels the pain with gentleness and sensitivity. Lack of both awareness and compassionate treatment of pain (of the therapist or the client) adds additional stress and pressure and increases self-judgment. Self-criticism is a form of attacking ourselves. Our response is often an escape from ourselves, reflected in feeling stuck in repetitive thoughts or following repetitive emotional and behavioral patterns, such as taking on increased amounts of work, addictive substances, or food.

Self-compassion, on the other hand, allows a sense of belonging and connection to people and the world. A world where we are vulnerable to disease, old age, and death. Much of our path in life is determined by countless factors, not only by the choices we make, which are influenced by our personality. When we experience failure or lack of success, we tend to forget these factors and attribute the failure to our sole control. Even if it is due to factors beyond our control, we still attribute it to ourselves. This perception makes it difficult for us to escape from attributing the cause of difficult experiences to ourselves and hence the isolation and criticism. Our possibility to feel the environment around us, to observe what is happening in a wider perspective, in the space that exists between us and the experience happening, allows us to treat our problems with tenderness, with a sense of belonging, and to have the courage to look at the pain with compassion. We can, by practicing self-compassion, create that warm tender space to hold our difficult experiences. It is our responsibility as therapists to take care of our inner world, creating a softer direct way to access it and our clients as well.

How to Incorporate Self-Compassion into Psychotherapy

There are three levels of incorporating self-compassion into psychotherapy as a relationship-based process (Germer, 2023): compassionate therapeutic presence, relationship, and interventions.

Compassionate (Therapeutic) Presence

Bringing one's self fully to the other with compassion is the foundation for a strong therapeutic alliance and effective therapy (Geller & Greenberg, 2022). This includes therapists' embodied experience of presence, which includes simultaneously feeling grounded, immersed in the client's experience, and having an inner spaciousness and compassion. The therapist's compassion for themselves and their clients enables and fosters such presence. For therapists to cultivate therapeutic presence they must practice mindfulness and compassion to recognize and bring warmth and understanding to their own bodily felt emotional experience, including their pain and suffering. With self-compassion therapists can work through the challenges and barriers to being fully present with clients, while caring for themselves in and out of the therapy room.

Through the practice of mindfulness, we develop the possibility of staying with what is happening in the moment whether in emotion, thought, or feeling. This is how the ability to observe a complex event from a distance develops so that we can identify patterns and beliefs that govern us unconsciously, created as a result of traumatic and unresolved life events. With self-compassion, we can work through those experiences but meet our pain directly with warmth and kindness.

With inner and outer compassion, therapists can directly connect to their own and their client's experiences and stay steady and grounded in themselves, attuning both to the other, themselves, and the relationship between them. This allows therapists' presence to be sustained and to bloom. It also deepens the therapeutic relationship and alliance across therapeutic traditions (Geller et al., 2010; Geller & Greenberg, 2022).

Therapeutic Relationship

We know from psychotherapy research that the therapeutic relationship is the most essential aspect of effective therapy (Norcross & Lambert, 2019). When therapists bring their compassionate presence to their clients, clients feel seen, heard, felt, and safe, and the therapeutic relationships deepen (Geller & Greenberg, 2022). This sense of safety in relationships invites clients to engage in the difficult yet transformative work of therapy. The therapist needs to practice compassionate listening and compassionate speaking, reverberation, acceptance, and nonjudgment to provide this safety in the relationship. Often in Western society, clients and therapists tend to undervalue themselves (e.g., "feeling not good enough," "feeling not talented enough, "having insufficient knowledge or capability"). This criticism is experienced as an internal threat or danger and activates the sympathetic system to escape, fight, or freeze. To deal with these internal challenges, we can direct self-compassion toward the damaged/criticized area. In the same way, the client is learning to do it by practicing self-compassion, which further helps to deepen the relationship between them.

Self-compassion can mediate the experience of release from these critical mechanisms and allow a return to full presence for the client and an experience of personal well-being for the therapist. Hence, the very practice of self-compassion allows therapists to be open and present, which creates a benevolent, inclusive, and reassuring relationship with the client. To feel felt, to feel that you are feeling felt in therapy, means empathy, acceptance, and presence in addition to understanding and resonance. Two people who share a sacred and respectful space (Siegel, 2010). Both are in it together, without judgment and pressure, with compassion, and with a shared journey toward clients' growth and healing—curiosity, acceptance of what comes, shared discovery of the organically unfolding experience or meaning. In such moments, time slows down, wonder increases, and we can walk the path of healing together.

Therapeutic Interventions

This third aspect of bringing self-compassion into psychotherapy involves providing and practicing formal and informal self-compassion exercises for clients to practice during and after the sessions. In session, practicing together with our clients allows us to feel their pain and our collective pain with compassion and strengthens the resource of compassion as a wise response to it. Some therapists provide their clients with a recording of a practice or a task to do during the week to help them be with their pain with compassion in order to work through and cultivate a deeper sense of inner compassion. Practicing outside of the session builds the neural muscles for natural compassion to be felt and experienced when pain arises.

Self-compassion-based therapy is expressed in these three ways. Therapists practice self-compassion for themselves to cultivate *therapeutic presence* and to work through barriers to being present and more open. In session, they practice with their clients, which models compassion, expresses compassion, and deepens the relationship. The *compassionate therapeutic relationship* then becomes the vehicle for self-compassion to be felt and strengthened in clients.

Intention and Organization of This Book

This book dives deeply into the importance and influence of self-compassion for the therapist, for the client, and for the therapeutic relationship. The core process of self-compassion has great potential to ease a wide variety of challenges, such as depression, anxiety, trauma, disordered eating, and emotional dysregulation. It can be incorporated naturally into just about any treatment approach. In this way we see self-compassion as transtheoretical, offering a beneficial resource across most therapy approaches.

While the authors provide valuable insights into how self-compassion can be incorporated into therapy, many chapters also include case examples, interventions, or practices. We have collected many of the practices in an appendix for easy access for the reader to listen to and utilize for their personal and clinical practice. The practices and exercises in the Appendix are also available online, along with audio recordings of many of them. Readers can find these online materials at *www.guilford.com/tyano-ronen-materials*.

Chapters in this book can be read sequentially or as stand-alone readings on particular topics of interest to the reader. Part I, Self-Compassion as a Change Process, establishes the pillars of self-compassion-informed psychotherapy. It includes a chapter on the history of self-compassion (Chapter 1) by Christopher Germer; Paul Gilbert (Chapter 2) describes the evolutionary and biopsychosocial approach to the development of self-compassion; Elli Weisbaum, Shelby L. Alsup, and Daniel J. Siegel (Chapter 3) discuss the neurophysiology of self-compassion in psychotherapy and interpersonal neurobiology; Sydney Spears and Tracy Ochester (Chapter 4) explore working with challenges of cross-cultural identity with self-compassion; and José Ramón Yela Bernabé and Antonio Crego Díaz (Chapter 5) explore the research on the mechanisms of therapeutic change due to mindful self-compassion practice.

Part II, A Self-Compassion-Based Clinician, focuses on what shapes and informs therapists' practice. These chapters include practice for the clinician to develop the skills necessary for a self-compassionate clinical practice focusing on the growth and development a psychotherapist needs to engage in to embody a self-compassionate way of delivering psychotherapy. It includes how self-compassion shapes and influences a clinician and their personal development, as well as their delivery of self-compassion.

Shari Geller (Chapter 6) explores the important basic role of developing therapeutic presence, as well as the interplay of presence and self-compassion in psychotherapy; Shauna Shapiro, Shayda Roohparvar, and Jill Lillie (Chapter 7) open a conversation about the power of a self-compassionate mindset that supports them personally and professionally; Galia Tyano Ronen (Chapter 8) exposes ways that therapists can cultivate the practice of self-compassion that will support their work; Susan M. Pollak (Chapter 9) discusses how self-compassion is a powerful addition to trauma therapy; and Steven Hickman (Chapter 10) describes the inner process of inquiry in psychotherapy.

Part III, Applications of Self-Compassion in Psychotherapy, explores self-compassion within various clinical frameworks, populations, and diagnostic categories. Christopher Germer (Chapter 11) highlights how self-compassion helps work with shame; Alfie Wishart (Chapter 12) examines self-compassion as it applies to substance use disorders; Paul Gilbert (Chapter 13) discusses compassion and self-compassion as a therapeutic element in the treatment of depression; Christian Stiglmayr (Chapter 14) describes the contribution of self-compassion to the dialectical behavior therapy model of psychotherapy for clients with borderline personality disorder; Lizabeth Roemer, Gerson F. Borrero, Molly Sawdy, and Jessica R. LoPresti (Chapter 15) address cultivating self-compassion for anxiety; Ann Saffi Biasetti (Chapter 16) explores the process of self-compassion in eating disorder recovery; Michelle Becker (Chapter 17) focuses on self-compassion training for couples and relationship distress; Lisa Shetler and Lorraine M. Hobbs (Chapter 18) inform us how self-compassion can help in working with teens in psychotherapy; Ronald D. Siegel (Chapter 19) shares his wisdom about chronic pain; and Benjamin Weinstein (Chapter 20) explores the integration of self-compassion into acceptance and commitment therapy. In the final chapter, Concluding Reflections, we (Galia and Shari) integrate all of this wisdom by extracting themes from various chapters and offering suggestions for incorporating self-compassion into psychotherapy.

We encourage you to walk slowly through these chapters as there is much wisdom to receive to help strengthen yourself and your psychotherapy practice with self-compassion. We also encourage you to courageously try the practices offered, generating or strengthening your self-compassion practice, as a foundation for offering it to your clients.

We wish you a fruitful reading and hope you find this book useful and eye- and heart-opening.

REFERENCES

Geller, S. M., & Greenberg, L. S. (2022). *Therapeutic presence: A mindful approach to effective therapeutic relationships* (2nd ed.). American Psychological Association.

Geller, S. M., Greenberg, L. S., & Watson, J. C. (2010). Therapist and client perceptions of therapeutic presence: The development of a measure. *Journal of Psychotherapy Research, 20*(5), 599–610.

Germer, C. (2023). Self-compassion in psychotherapy: Clinical integration, evidence base and mechanisms of change. In A. Finlay-Jones, K. Bluth, & K. Neff (Eds.), *Handbook of self-compassion* (pp. 379–416). Springer.

Neff, K. (2003). Self-compassion: An alternative conceptualization of a healthy attitude toward oneself. *Self and Identity, 2*(2), 85–101.

Norcross, J. C., & Lambert, M. J. (Eds.). (2019). *Psychotherapy relationships that work: Vol. 1. Evidence-based therapist contributions.* Oxford University Press.

Siegel, D. J. (2010). *The mindful therapist: A clinician's guide to mindsight and neural integration.* Norton.

Singer, T., & Chierchia, G. (2016). *The neuroscience of compassion and empathy and their link to prosocial motivation and behavior.* Max Planck Institute for Human Cognitive and Brain Science.

PART I

Self-Compassion as a Change Process

1

A Model of Self-Compassion-Based Therapy

Christopher Germer

Compassion is a resource that has alleviated human suffering since time immemorial. The word is derived from its Latin roots: *com* (with) and *passion* (suffering). Our ability to *be* with a person's suffering, without denying, amplifying, or avoiding it, is fundamentally healing. Just recall the last time that you were struggling and someone took the time to listen deeply and speak compassionately with you. Chances are that you felt better, even though the circumstances of your life had not changed.

Compassion has been defined as "the feeling that arises when witnessing another's suffering and that motivates a subsequent desire to help" (Goetz et al., 2010, p. 351). From the Buddhist perspective, compassion can be directed outward toward others or inward toward oneself. Self-compassion is inner compassion. Research shows that people are generally more compassionate toward others than themselves (López et al., 2018). An informal definition of self-compassion is treating ourselves with the same kindness and understanding as we would treat a good friend. It's a compassionate U-turn.

In 2003, Kristin Neff (2003b) operationally defined self-compassion and created the Self-Compassion Scale (SCS; Neff, 2003a), which has been used in most self-compassion research. There are currently over 7,000 articles on self-compassion in the academic literature. The research clearly shows that self-compassion is good for mental health and well-being. Self-compassion is closely associated with happiness and life satisfaction, emotional resilience and coping, healthy habits such as diet and exercise, and more satisfying personal relationships (Neff, 2023). Self-compassion also appears to alleviate a wide range of psychological disorders, including anxiety, depression, eating disorders, addiction, personality disorders, and psychosis (Germer, 2023). In light of the empirical evidence, more and more clinicians are becoming interested in helping their clients cultivate the resource of self-compassion.

This makes sense. Imagine that you have a client who suffers from anxiety or depression. Over the course of therapy, your client learns to recognize and validate how they feel rather than getting caught in useless rumination (mindfulness). Your client begins to feel less alone and more connected to others in the midst of their struggles (common humanity). Your client's inner dialogue is reassuring and supportive rather than dismissive or self-critical (self-kindness). Taken together, your client has become more self-compassionate and might even be able to manage life more on their own.

The purpose of this chapter is to outline a model of therapy called *self-compassion-based therapy*. First, I review the definition of self-compassion and the history of self-compassion in therapy. Then I explore the research on self-compassion as a transtheoretical and transdiagnostic process in therapy, identify three levels that self-compassion can be integrated into therapy, and consider putative mechanisms by which self-compassion creates positive change in therapy. Two practices are included in this chapter to give readers a direct experience of self-compassion.

What's in a Model?

The value of a therapy model lies in its ability to guide treatment. A model of therapy contains four main elements: (1) how symptoms are caused and maintained, (2) treatment techniques, (3) putative mechanisms of change, and (4) empirical support (Boswell et al., 2010). At present, the theory, research, and practice of self-compassion-based therapy appears robust enough to consider it a distinct model of therapy.

Therapy models are constructed out of converging theoretical, empirical, and clinical trends. The lens of the investigator inevitably influences how a model is described. The self-compassion-based therapy model described in this chapter is primarily informed by the mindful self-compassion (MSC) program (Germer & Neff, 2019; Neff & Germer, 2018), as I, along with Kristin Neff, developed the MSC program. Furthermore, most of the research on self-compassion uses Neff's SCS (Neff, 2003a), which has had a significant impact on how self-compassion is conceptualized and studied (Cha et al., 2023). MSC was originally designed as a training for the general public, not a therapy, but as you can see in this book, many clinicians are integrating the concepts and practices of MSC into their therapeutic work.

Another major influence on the current model is compassion-focused therapy (CFT; Gilbert, 2009, 2010), developed by Paul Gilbert and colleagues to help clients cultivate compassion for themselves and others. Most research on self-compassion-based therapy has investigated CFT. Other empirically supported, self-compassion-based therapies that influenced the current model are acceptance and commitment therapy (Hayes et al., 2011), internal family systems (IFS; Schwartz & Sweezy, 2019), and emotion-focused therapy (EFT; Greenberg, 2006). The founders and practitioners of each self-compassion-based therapy would probably articulate the self-compassion-based therapy model in their own terms, but hopefully, the current effort is spacious enough to inspire therapists of all stripes to integrate self-compassion more deliberately into how they are doing therapy already.

What's Self-Compassion?

Let's start by reviewing what we mean by self-compassion. According to Neff's (2003b) model, self-compassion has three components: (1) mindfulness versus overidentification, (2) common humanity versus isolation, and (3) self-kindness versus self-criticism. These components are overlapping yet conceptually distinct.

Mindfulness refers to spacious, balanced, friendly awareness of moment-to-moment experience. The opposite quality, overidentification, means that we get entangled in our thoughts and feelings and lose perspective. A depressed client who spends hours ruminating about being a "bad person" is overly identified with that particular narrative of their life. Mindfulness allows the same person to see their thoughts and feelings as just that—temporary and incomplete constructions of reality. This perspective opens new possibilities, including the possibility of a compassionate response.

Self-compassion includes a sense of *common humanity*. When we struggle with emotional pain, we tend to blame ourselves for it and feel isolated and alone. Feeling alone only amplifies our suffering. However, when we're mindful and stop resisting our pain, or we connect with another person (like a therapist) amidst our pain, we're more likely to understand that suffering is part of life and our pain becomes more tolerable.

The third component is *self-kindness*. When things go wrong, we tend to be patient, understanding, and supportive of others and relatively harsh and critical of ourselves. Self-kindness refers to actively caring for ourselves when we suffer, fail, or feel inadequate. It's a benevolent attitude, despite our mistakes and imperfections, which allows us to learn and grow.

Many therapists equate self-compassion with self-kindness alone. However, without the components of common humanity and mindfulness, self-kindness can devolve into self-pity or sugarcoating reality, respectively.

On the other hand, some mindfulness-based therapists assume that self-compassion is nothing new—that it's part and parcel of mindfulness. We often see in clinical practice, however, that it is difficult to be mindful when we're in the grip of intense and disturbing emotions like shame, grief, rage, or despair unless we first hold *ourselves* in a warm and kind embrace. That's self-compassion. Finally, the component of common humanity helps us respond wisely to our challenges by making it possible to look beyond ourselves at the many causes and conditions that contribute to our suffering and to find a path forward. The three components of self-compassion work synergistically to help our clients heal and thrive.

Clinicians also tend to equate compassion and self-compassion with tender qualities like nurturing—qualities that are especially important when a client needs to be comforted, soothed, reassured, or validated. However, sometimes our clients need to protect themselves by creating safe boundaries, or by providing for their deepest needs, or encouraging themselves to overcome difficult challenges. That's when self-compassion needs to take a tough, even fierce turn (Neff, 2021). Both tender and fierce self-compassion can be taught and learned in psychotherapy.

To have a direct experience of the three components of self-compassion, try Practice A, "Self-Compassion Break," in the Appendix.

History of Self-Compassion in Psychotherapy

Although self-compassion is a relatively recent empirical construct, it has been embedded in psychotherapy for over a century under the umbrella of "self-acceptance." William James, Sigmund Freud, and B. F. Skinner all considered acceptance (self and others) to be a beneficial quality (Williams & Lynn, 2010). Carl Rogers (1951) specifically emphasized *self*-acceptance as a core change process in therapy. In the 1990s, with the introduction of mindfulness- and acceptance-based therapies (Hayes et al., 2011; Linehan, 1993; Segal et al., 2018), the focus of acceptance shifted away from the *person* to the person's *experience*. Mindfulness is loving awareness of moment-to-moment *experience* and compassion is loving awareness of the *experiencer*. Currently, the pendulum is swinging back to acceptance of the person with therapies such as CFT, and IFS, and secular compassion training programs like MSC and compassion cultivation training (CCT; Goldin & Jazaieri, 2017). CFT was the first empirically supported, explicitly compassion-based therapy. Paul Gilbert had the revolutionary insight, back in 2000, that the *tone* of a client's inner dialogue was more important than the *content* of thinking to alleviate depression. The main agenda of CFT is to "warm up the conversation" (P. Gilbert, personal communication, July 28, 2014).

Historically, the term *compassion* has been relatively absent from psychotherapy, perhaps because of its association with religion. However, compassion has not been absent from therapy itself—it has been embraced as therapeutic empathy. Empathy is experiencing the world of another as one's own. When we resonate with a client's experience, we are empathic. Nowadays, compassion is defined as empathy *plus* the wish and effort to alleviate suffering (Jinpa, 2010, in Jazaieri et al., 2014; Singer & Klimecki, 2014). Since the sole purpose of therapy is to alleviate suffering, therapeutic empathy has always been about compassion. From a research perspective, empathy is a strong predictor of therapy outcomes (Elliott et al., 2018).

At the present time, self-compassion is nestled comfortably in the emerging school of *mindfulness-*, *acceptance-*, and *compassion-based psychotherapy* (Germer & Siegel, 2012; Germer et al., 2016). The unifying principle of this school is helping clients to cultivate an accepting, nonadversarial relationship with their experience or with themselves. Mindfulness-based therapies regulate emotions by regulating attention and awareness—*what* we pay attention to and *how* we pay attention (Segal et al., 2018). Acceptance-based therapies focus more on nonavoidance and acceptance of moment-to-moment experiences (Hayes et al., 2011). Compassion-based therapies regulate emotion by activating qualities of warmth, care, and connection (Gilbert, 2009). Self-compassion-based therapy is a model *within* the model of mindfulness-, acceptance-, and compassion-based therapy because it contains elements of the other therapies but focuses primarily on changing our relationship to suffering through the cultivation of self-compassion.

Transdiagnostic and Transtheoretical Change Process

Although the research base still has some important gaps, empirical studies indicate that self-compassion is an underlying change process in therapy.

Transdiagnostic Process

Self-compassion-based therapy has been shown to alleviate a broad range of clinical conditions, suggesting that self-compassion is a *transdiagnostic* change process (Cuppage et al., 2018). For example, clinical diagnoses that improved with compassion-based treatment include anxiety, depression, trauma, eating disorders, addictions, personality disorders, and psychosis (see Germer, 2023). A meta-analysis of compassion-based interventions for different diagnoses found that treatment significantly relieved psychological distress and increased self-compassion even when the studies used active control groups (Kirby et al., 2017). Meta-analyses specifically on *self*-compassion-based interventions found strong effect sizes for eating behavior and rumination (Ferrari et al., 2019), and small to medium effects for stress, anxiety, depression, and posttraumatic stress (Han & Kim, 2023).

Most of the outcome research showing positive change across diagnoses has been conducted using CFT (Millard et al., 2023). Although CFT cultivates compassion for self *and* others, it may be considered a self-compassion-based therapy because it primarily helps clients to be less harsh and more compassionate with themselves (see Chapters 2 and 13 for more about CFT). More randomized controlled trials are needed because the existing research contains many pilot or feasibility studies (Craig et al., 2020).

Self-compassion training for the general public has also demonstrated improvements in mental health. For example, MSC reduced anxiety and depression among adults in the community (Neff & Germer, 2013), as well as depressive symptoms among patients with diabetes (Friis et al., 2016). CCT has two self-compassion modules, decreased worry and emotional suppression (Jazaieri et al., 2014). Stand-alone compassion imagery training also produced psychological improvement in nonclinical populations (Maner et al., 2023).

There is a wealth of correlational data showing that self-compassion is associated with reduced psychopathology in adults (MacBeth & Gumley, 2012) and adolescents (Marsh et al., 2018), as well as adaptive coping (Ewert et al., 2021). Self-compassion correlates with fewer eating disorders (Braun et al., 2016) and decreased symptoms of obsessive–compulsive disorder (Wetterneck et al., 2013) and schizophrenia (Eicher et al., 2013). Self-compassion is consistently associated with less severe posttraumatic stress disorder (Winders et al., 2020). On the other hand, *low* self-compassion levels are found among people with bipolar disorder (Døssing et al., 2015), depression (Krieger et al., 2013), generalized anxiety disorder (Hoge et al., 2013), and substance use disorder (Phelps et al., 2018). Taken together, intervention and correlational studies clearly indicate that self-compassion is good for mental health.

Transtheoretical Process

Self-compassion has also been linked to successful outcomes in different kinds of therapies, suggesting that self-compassion is a *transtheoretical* change process. For example, both psychodynamic and cognitive therapy for Cluster C personality disorders (avoidant, dependent, obsessive–compulsive) increased self-compassion, and those increases predicted decreases in psychiatric symptoms, interpersonal problems, and personality pathology (Schanche et al., 2011). Neff and colleagues (2007) conducted a study with the two-chair technique from EFT, a form of humanistic therapy, and found that it increased self-compassion and decreased self-criticism along with fewer experiences of depression, rumination, thought suppression, and anxiety. Recently, clinicians have begun integrating self-compassion training into cognitive and behavior therapies (Baumgardner & Benoit, 2024; Javidi et al., 2023).

Mindfulness- and acceptance-based treatments also increase self-compassion. Wadsworth and colleagues (2018) treated patients with dialectical behavior therapy and cognitive-behavioral therapy and found that improvements in anxiety and depression were related to increases in self-compassion. Participation in mindfulness-based cognitive therapy (MBCT) increased self-compassion even though self-compassion is not usually taught implicitly in MBCT (Birnie et al., 2010) and mediation analysis showed that self-compassion is responsible for many of the positive effects of MBCT (Kuyken et al., 2010). A meta-analysis of mindfulness programs with nonclinical populations showed a significant medium effect of pre–post changes in self-compassion (Golden et al., 2021).

In summary, the current research evidence on self-compassion as a transdiagnostic and transtheoretical change process is encouraging and growing rapidly.

Integrating Self-Compassion into Therapy

Self-compassion can be integrated into psychotherapy at three levels: (1) *compassionate presence*—how therapists relate to their own experience in therapy, (2) *compassionate alliance*—how therapists engage with their clients, and (3) *compassionate interventions*—how clients relate to themselves, especially during home practice. If a therapist brings all three levels into their clinical work, they are practicing self-compassion-based therapy. (See Chapter 11 for a case vignette of self-compassion-based treatment of shame.)

Level 1: Compassionate Presence

Compassionate presence refers to the clinician being with their own moment-to-moment experience in a compassionate way during therapy. Clinicians can be present while listening quietly or speaking with a client. According to Shari Geller (2017), therapeutic (or compassionate) presence entails being open to the client's moment-to-moment experience, attuning inwardly to how the clinician is resonating with the client while staying in contact with the relationship between them (see Chapter 6 for more on presence).

Although compassionate presence is not easily observable, it can have a meaningful impact on our clients. How does this work? We have specialized neurons in our brains—mirror neurons—that allow us to directly experience in our own bodies what other people are experiencing (Kilner & Lemon, 2013). Furthermore, people synchronize with one another on many levels—neural, perceptual, affective, physiological, verbal, and behavioral—which is a critical survival skill for human beings (Hu et al., 2022; Koole & Tschacher, 2016) and enhances the experience of compassion (Valdesolo & DeSteno, 2011). Interpersonal synchronization also allows us to regulate the emotional experience of others, such as when a therapist remains unruffled while a client relates a traumatic experience that has the effect of calming the client.

Compassionate presence can be practiced and learned. Bourgault and Dionne (2019) found that self-compassion practice is linked to therapeutic presence. Clinical psychology trainees who took the MSC training raised their self-compassion levels, but only when they were committed to the training (Yela et al., 2020). Personal practice, such as loving-kindness and compassion meditation, can help a clinician become more self-compassionate (Lv et al., 2023; Reilly & Stuyvenberg, 2023).

Level 2: Compassionate Alliance

The *compassionate alliance*, variously called the therapeutic alliance, therapeutic relationship, working relationship, or therapeutic bond, is considered a common factor in effective therapy. In a meta-analysis, Elliot and colleagues (2011) found that empathy is a relatively strong predictor of therapy outcome across different theoretical orientations. In another meta-analysis, Lambert and Ogles (2004) found that successful therapists tended to be warmer, more empathic, understanding, and supportive of their clients, and were less likely to blame, ignore, neglect, or reject their clients.

It appears that personal practice can also enhance the therapeutic alliance. Bibeau and colleagues (2016) found that loving-kindness and compassion meditation can have a positive impact on numerous therapeutic variables related to empathy, such as altruism, positive regard, prosocial behavior, affective empathy, and empathic accuracy.

There is a rule of thumb in the MSC program: "The best way to *teach* self-compassion is to *be* compassionate." In the therapeutic relationship, that means sustaining compassion for oneself and for the client while doing therapy. This can be difficult when clinicians feel the distress of their clients as their own (empathic distress). Self-compassion can help therapists disentangle and make room for compassionate responding. A practice that can be applied in the midst of challenging moments of therapy is giving and receiving compassion (see Practice B, "Giving and Receiving Compassion," in the Appendix).

Key Elements in a Compassionate Therapeutic Relationship

What does a compassionate therapeutic relationship look like? It has three key elements (three *R*'s): radical acceptance, resonance, and resource building. *Radical acceptance* is the overall attitude of the treatment process, *resonance* is the primary mode of engagement, and *resource building* is the desired outcome of the therapy relationship. The three *R*'s are based on the "inquiry" method used by teachers of the MSC training to help their participants cultivate self-compassion (Germer & Neff, 2019).

Radical acceptance was first defined by Marsha Linehan as "the fully open experience of what is, entering into reality just as it is, at this moment . . . acceptance without the haze of what one wants and does not want it to be" (Robins et al., 2004, pp. 39–40). From a self-compassion point of view, radical acceptance means accepting *ourselves* just as we are. The invitation is to temporarily suspend the change agenda and allow kindness to flow naturally in response to suffering. As Carl Rogers (1961/1995) wrote, "the curious paradox is that when I accept myself as I am . . . change seems to come about almost unnoticed" (p. 17).

Resonance refers to affective attunement between the therapist and client—a sense of "feeling felt" (Siegel, 2010, p. 136). Interpersonal synchrony is a way of measuring resonance. Synchronous body movements between the therapist and client predicted the quality of the alliance as rated by the client at the end of therapy (Ramseyer & Tschacher, 2011). Neural synchrony, using dual electroencephalography, also correlated with the strength of the alliance (Lecchi et al., 2019). Skin conductance synchrony between therapist and client even predicted therapy *success*—namely, reduced symptom severity (Gernert et al., 2023).

Resource building is the third aspect of a compassionate alliance. How can a therapist help a client cultivate self-compassion through conversation? In the MSC training, the "inquiry" method serves this purpose. Inquiry is a self-to-other dialogue that mirrors the self-to-self relationship that teachers wish to cultivate in their students (see Chapter 10 for more on inquiry). In therapy, the first step is for the clinician to remain connected and aware of their own moment-to-moment experience—*listening with the heart*. Then, when it is the therapist's turn to speak, the therapist can share what touched or moved them while the client was talking (rather than their *thoughts* about what touched them)—*speaking from the heart*. For example, if the therapist was moved by a strength they saw in the client—such as courage, curiosity, mindfulness, or self-compassion—that can be named as an invitation to further discussion. If the therapist was touched by a client's suffering—such as grief, sadness, or confusion—such moments of resonance can also be shared with clients, followed by self-compassion questions like "What do you need right now?," "What do you need to hear in a moment like this?," or "How would you treat a friend in the same situation as you?"

Level 3: Compassionate Interventions

Most clinicians think of interventions, especially home practices like meditation, when they think of self-compassion in therapy. However, interventions need to be grounded on the first two levels of integration: a compassionate presence and a compassionate relationship. Clients are more likely to do home practices if they feel connected with their therapists and the home practices arise out of relevant issues that were discussed in therapy. Not all clients are willing to do home practices, and if they don't, they can still learn self-compassion from the other two levels of treatment. Home practices are important because 1 hour of therapy per week is not much time to learn new habits of thinking and behaving. Studies on neuroplasticity show that mental practices like meditation can lead to changes in the structure and function of the brain (Lazar et al., 2005; Valk et al., 2017).

There is a wealth of self-compassion practices that clinicians can adapt for individual clients, especially from the MSC training and CFT (Irons & Beaumont, 2017; Neff & Germer, 2018). Clinicians can also modify traditional cognitive-behavioral exercises to cultivate self-compassion, such as adding compassionate self-talk to exposure therapy or behavioral activation. The self-compassion questions "What do you need right now?" and "How would you treat a friend?" also lead naturally to customizable home practices.

Mechanisms of Change

How does self-compassion work in therapy? An empirical argument has yet to be made that increases in mindfulness, common humanity, and self-kindness, and reductions in rumination, isolation, and self-criticism, are what lead to improvement in self-compassion-based therapy. Different self-compassion interventions are also likely to activate different components of self-compassion to varying degrees (Dreisoerner, Junker, & Van Dick, 2021).

Emotion regulation is a mechanism of change that is closely associated with self-compassion and therapy in general (Inwood & Ferrari, 2018; Paucsik et al., 2023). Neurophysiologically, self-compassion seems to improve emotion regulation by decreasing fear, especially by reducing activity in the sympathetic nervous system (Breines et al., 2015; Dreisoerner, Junker, Schlotz, et al., 2021). Self-compassion also increases a sense of safety by enhancing vagally mediated heart rate variability (Petrocchi et al., 2017). Activity in the prefrontal cortex of the brain, an area commonly associated with emotion regulation, seems to be involved in self-compassionate responding as well (Guan et al., 2021; Parrish et al., 2018).

There are also a number of psychological mechanisms that may explain how self-compassion works. *Secure attachment* is associated with self-compassion (Joeng et al., 2017) and self-compassion mediates the relationship between insecure attachment and emotional distress (Mackintosh et al., 2018). *Reduced shame* is another putative mechanism. Shame is a predisposing factor in a wide variety of clinical conditions and many studies show that when self-compassion increases in therapy, shame tends to decrease (Kelly et al., 2014; Proeve et al., 2018). *Nonavoidance* may also explain how self-compassion works in therapy. For example, posttraumatic stress disorder is maintained by avoiding traumatic memories (Marx & Sloan, 2005) and self-compassion helps people acknowledge and accept their traumatic memories (Thompson & Waltz, 2008). At the simplest level, self-compassion may work by *classical counterconditioning.* When we pair a distress state with a compassion state (such as writing a compassionate letter to oneself), the distress state becomes more tolerable (Shaw & Kelly, 2024). Overall, the research on mechanisms of change suggests that when a client feels safe and supported, positive change can occur. This view overlaps with the research on the importance of empathy and positive regard in successful therapy.

Conclusion

In conclusion, current research demonstrates that self-compassion is good for mental health and self-compassion can be learned in therapy. The self-compassion-based psychotherapy model is embedded in the mindfulness-, acceptance-, and compassion-based model of therapy, but it is uniquely focused on helping clients cultivate a kind and supportive relationship with *themselves* in the midst of psychological suffering. Clients can learn self-compassion from the therapist's compassionate presence, the therapy relationship, and home practices, depending on the client's needs and the orientation of the therapist. An important foundation for doing this type of clinical work is a personal self-compassion practice. Self-compassion appears to work by enhancing emotion regulation through a variety of psychological and neurophysiological processes. Important areas for future research include (1) well-controlled studies of therapies specifically designed to enhance self-compassion in clients, (2) outcome research on individual self-compassion practices, and (3) mechanisms of change in specific psychological conditions and populations. Although there is still much to be learned, therapists should feel emboldened by our current level of understanding to explore innovative ways of integrating self-compassion into therapy.

REFERENCES

Baumgardner, M., & Benoit, A. (2024). Integrating cognitive-behavioral therapy with compassion-focused therapy for the treatment of social anxiety disorder: An evidence-based case study. *Clinical Case Studies, 23*(2), 127–145.

Bibeau, M., Dionne, F., & Leblanc, J. (2016). Can compassion meditation contribute to the development of psychotherapists' empathy? A review. *Mindfulness, 7*(1), 255–263.

Birnie, K., Speca, M., & Carlson, L. E. (2010). Exploring self-compassion and empathy in the context of mindfulness-based stress reduction (MBSR). *Stress and Health, 26*(5), 359–371.

Boswell, J. F., Sharpless, B. A., Greenberg, L. S., Heatherington, L., Huppert, J. D., Barber, J. P., et al. (2010). Schools of psychotherapy and the beginnings of a scientific approach. In D. H. Barlow (Ed.), *The Oxford handbook of clinical psychology* (pp. 98–127). Oxford Academic.

Bourgault, M., & Dionne, F. (2019). Therapeutic presence and mindfulness: Mediating role of self-compassion and psychological distress among psychologists. *Mindfulness, 10*(4), 650–656.

Braun, T. D., Park, C. L., & Gorin, A. (2016). Self-compassion, body image, and disordered eating: A review of the literature. *Body Image, 17*, 117–131.

Breines, J. G., McInnis, C. M., Kuras, Y. I., Thoma, M. V., Gianferante, D., Hanlin, L., et al. (2015). Self-compassionate young adults show lower salivary alpha-amylase responses to repeated psychosocial stress. *Self and Identity, 14*(4), 390–402.

Cha, J. E., Serlachius, A. S., Kirby, J. N., & Consedine, N. S. (2023). What do (and don't) we know about self-compassion? Trends and issues in theory, mechanisms, and outcomes. *Mindfulness, 14*(11), 2657–2669.

Craig, C., Hiskey, S., & Spector, A. (2020). Compassion focused therapy: A systematic review of its effectiveness and acceptability in clinical populations. *Expert Review of Neurotherapeutics, 20*(4), 385–400.

Cuppage, J., Baird, K., Gibson, J., Booth, R., & Hevey, D. (2018). Compassion focused therapy: Exploring the effectiveness with a transdiagnostic group and potential processes of change. *British Journal of Clinical Psychology, 57*(2), 240–254.

Døssing, M., Nilsson, K. K., Svejstrup, S. R., Sørensen, V. V., Straarup, K. N., & Hansen, T. B. (2015). Low self-compassion in patients with bipolar disorder. *Comprehensive Psychiatry, 60*, 53–58.

Dreisoerner, A., Junker, N. M., Schlotz, W., Heimrich, J., Bloemeke, S., Ditzen, B., & van Dick, R. (2021). Self-soothing touch and being hugged reduce cortisol responses to stress: A randomized controlled trial on stress, physical touch, and social identity. *Comprehensive Psychoneuroendocrinology, 8*, 100091.

Dreisoerner, A., Junker, N. M., & van Dick, R. (2021). The relationship among the components of self-compassion: A pilot study using a compassionate writing intervention to enhance self-kindness, common humanity, and mindfulness. *Journal of Happiness Studies, 22*, 21–47.

Eicher, A. C., Davis, L. W., & Lysaker, P. H. (2013). Self-compassion: A novel link with symptoms in schizophrenia? *Journal of Nervous and Mental Disease, 201*(5), 389–393.

Elliott, R., Bohart, A. C., Watson, J. C., & Greenberg, L. S. (2011). Empathy. *Psychotherapy, 48*(1), 43–49.

Elliott, R., Bohart, A. C., Watson, J. C., & Murphy, D. (2018). Therapist empathy and client outcome: An updated meta-analysis. *Psychotherapy, 55*(4), 399–410.

Ewert, C., Vater, A., & Schröder-Abé, M. (2021). Self-compassion and coping: A meta-analysis. *Mindfulness, 12*, 1063–1077.

Ferrari, M., Hunt, C., Harrysunker, A., Abbott, M. J., Beath, A. P., & Einstein, D. A. (2019). Self-compassion interventions and psychosocial outcomes: A meta-analysis of RCTs. *Mindfulness, 10*(8), 1455–1473.

Friis, A. M., Johnson, M. H., Cutfield, R. G., & Consedine, N. S. (2016). Kindness matters: A randomized controlled trial of a mindful self-compassion intervention improves depression, distress, and HbA1c among patients with diabetes. *Diabetes Care, 39*(11), 1963–1971.

Geller, S. M. (2017). *A practical guide to cultivating therapeutic presence.* American Psychological Association.

Germer, C. (2023). Self-compassion in psychotherapy: Clinical integration, evidence base, and mechanisms of change. In A. Finlay-Jones, K. Bluth, & K. Neff (Eds.), *Handbook of self-compassion* (pp. 379–415). Springer International.

Germer, C., & Neff, K. (2019). *Teaching the mindful self-compassion program: A guide for professionals.* Guilford Press.

Germer, C., Siegel, R. D., & Fulton, P. R. (Eds.). (2016). *Mindfulness and psychotherapy.* Guilford Press.

Germer, C. K., & Siegel, R. D. (Eds.). (2012). *Wisdom and compassion in psychotherapy: Deepening mindfulness in clinical practice.* Guilford Press.

Gernert, C. C., Nelson, A., Falkai, P., & Falter-Wagner, C. M. (2023). Synchrony in psychotherapy: High physiological positive concordance predicts symptom reduction and negative concordance predicts symptom aggravation. *International Journal of Methods in Psychiatric Research, 33*(1), e1978.

Gilbert, P. (2009). Introducing compassion-focused therapy. *Advances in Psychiatric Treatment, 15*(3), 199.

Gilbert, P. (2010). *Compassion focused therapy: Distinctive features.* Routledge.

Goetz, J. L., Keltner, D., & Simon-Thomas, E. (2010). Compassion: An evolutionary analysis and empirical review. *Psychological Bulletin, 136*(3), 351–374.

Golden, H. L., Vosper, J., Kingston, J., & Ellett, L. (2021). The impact of mindfulness-based programmes on self-compassion in nonclinical populations: A systematic review and meta-analysis. *Mindfulness, 12*, 29–52.

Goldin, P. R., & Jazaieri, H. (2017). The compassion cultivation training (CCT) program. In E. M. Seppala, S. Simon-Thomas, S. L. Brown, M. C. Worline, C. D. Cameron, & J. R. Doty (Eds.), *The Oxford handbook of compassion science* (pp. 237–246). Oxford University Press.

Greenberg, L. (2006). Emotion-focused therapy: A synopsis. *Journal of Contemporary Psychotherapy, 36*(2), 87–93.

Guan, F., Liu, G., Pedersen, W. S., Chen, O., Zhao, S., Sui, J., & Peng, K. (2021). Neurostructural correlates of dispositional self-compassion. *Neuropsychologia, 160*, 107978.

Han, A., & Kim, T. H. (2023). Effects of self-compassion interventions on reducing depressive symptoms, anxiety, and stress: A meta-analysis. *Mindfulness, 5*, 1–29.

Hayes, S. C., Strosahl, K. D., & Wilson, K. G. (2011). *Acceptance and commitment therapy: The process and practice of mindful change.* Guilford Press.

Hoge, E. A., Hölzel, B. K., Marques, L., Metcalf, C. A., Brach, N., Lazar, S. W., & Simon, N. M. (2013). Mindfulness and self-compassion in generalized anxiety disorder: Examining predictors of disability. *Evidence-Based Complementary and Alternative Medicine, 576258.*

Hu, Y., Cheng, X., Pan, Y., & Hu, Y. (2022). The intrapersonal and interpersonal consequences of interpersonal synchrony. *Acta Psychologica, 224*, 103513.

Inwood, E., & Ferrari, M. (2018). Mechanisms of change in the relationship between self-compassion, emotion regulation, and mental health: A systematic review. *Applied Psychology: Health and Well-Being, 10*(2), 215–235.

Irons, C., & Beaumont, E. (2017). *The compassionate mind workbook: A step-by-step guide to developing your compassionate self.* Robinson.

Javidi, Z., Prior, K. N., Sloan, T. L., & Bond, M. J. (2023). A randomized controlled trial of self-compassion versus cognitive therapy for complex psychopathologies. *Current Psychology, 42*(2), 946–954.

Jazaieri, H., McGonigal, K., Jinpa, T., Doty, J. R., Gross, J. J., & Goldin, P. R. (2014). A randomized controlled trial of compassion cultivation training: Effects on mindfulness, affect, and emotion regulation. *Motivation and Emotion, 38*(1), 23–35.

Joeng, J. R., Turner, S. L., Kim, E. Y., Choi, S. A., Lee, Y. J., & Kim, J. K. (2017). Insecure attachment and emotional distress: Fear of self-compassion and self-compassion as mediators. *Personality and Individual Differences, 112*, 6–11.

Kelly, A. C., Carter, J. C., & Borairi, S. (2014). Are improvements in shame and self-compassion early in eating disorders treatment associated with better patient outcomes? *International Journal of Eating Disorders, 47*(1), 54–64.

Kilner, J. M., & Lemon, R. N. (2013). What we know currently about mirror neurons. *Current Biology, 23*(23), R1057–R1062.

Kirby, J. N., Tellegen, C. L., & Steindl, S. R. (2017). A meta-analysis of compassion-based interventions: Current state of knowledge and future directions. *Behavior Therapy, 48*(6), 778–792.

Koole, S. L., & Tschacher, W. (2016). Synchrony in psychotherapy: A review and an integrative framework for the therapeutic alliance. *Frontiers in Psychology, 7*, 862.

Krieger, T., Altenstein, D., Baettig, I., Doerig, N., & Holtforth, M. G. (2013). Self-compassion in depression: Associations with depressive symptoms, rumination, and avoidance in depressed outpatients. *Behavior Therapy, 44*(3), 501–513.

Kuyken, W., Watkins, E., Holden, E., White, K., Taylor, R. S., Byford, S., et al. (2010). How does mindfulness-based cognitive therapy work? *Behaviour Research and Therapy, 48*(11), 1105–1112.

Lambert, M., & Ogles, B. (2004). The efficacy and effectiveness of psychotherapy. In A. E. Bergin & S. L. Garfield (Eds.), *Handbook of psychotherapy and behavior change* (pp. 139–193). Wiley.

Lazar, S. W., Kerr, C. E., Wasserman, R. H., Gray, J. R., Greve, D. N., Treadway, M. T., et al. (2005). Meditation experience is associated with increased cortical thickness. *Neuroreport, 16*(17), 1893–1897.

Lecchi, T., da Silva, K., Giommi, F., & Leong, V. (2019). Using dual-EEG to explore therapist–client interpersonal neural synchrony. *Frontiers in Psychiatry,* 1–15.

Linehan, M. M. (1993). *Skills training manual for treating borderline personality disorder.* Guilford Press.

López, A., Sanderman, R., Ranchor, A. V., & Schroevers, M. J. (2018). Compassion for others and self-compassion: Levels, correlates, and relationship with psychological well-being. *Mindfulness, 9,* 325–331.

Lv, J., Jiang, Y., Li, R., Chen, Y., Gu, X., Zhou, J., et al. (2023). Effects of loving-kindness and compassion meditations on self-compassion: A systematic review and meta-analysis. *Clinical Psychology: Science and Practice, 31*(1), 19–35.

MacBeth, A., & Gumley, A. (2012). Exploring compassion: A meta-analysis of the association between self-compassion and psychopathology. *Clinical Psychology Review, 32*(6), 545–552.

Mackintosh, K., Power, K., Schwannauer, M., & Chan, S. W. (2018). The relationships between self-compassion, attachment, and interpersonal problems in clinical patients with mixed anxiety and depression, and emotional distress. *Mindfulness, 9*(3), 961–971.

Maner, S., Morris, P. G., & Flewitt, B. I. (2023). A systematic review of the effectiveness of compassion focused imagery in improving psychological outcomes in clinical and non-clinical adult populations. *Clinical Psychology and Psychotherapy, 30*(2), 250–269.

Marsh, I. C., Chan, S. W., & MacBeth, A. (2018). Self-compassion and psychological distress in adolescents—a meta-analysis. *Mindfulness, 9,* 1011–1027.

Marx, B. P., & Sloan, D. M. (2005). Peritraumatic dissociation and experiential avoidance as predictors of posttraumatic stress symptomatology. *Behaviour Research and Therapy, 43*(5), 569–583.

Millard, L. A., Wan, M. W., Smith, D. M., & Wittkowski, A. (2023). The effectiveness of compassion focused therapy with clinical populations: A systematic review and meta-analysis. *Journal of Affective Disorders, 326,* 168–192.

Neff, K. D. (2003a). The development and validation of a scale to measure self-compassion. *Self and Identity,* 2(3), 223–250.

Neff, K. (2003b). Self-compassion: An alternative conceptualization of a healthy attitude toward oneself. *Self and Identity,* 2(2), 85–101.

Neff, K. D. (2023). Self-compassion: Theory, method, research, and intervention. *Annual Review of Psychology, 74*, 193–218.

Neff, K. D., & Germer, C. K. (2013). A pilot study and randomized controlled trial of the mindful self-compassion program. *Journal of Clinical Psychology, 69*(1), 28–44.

Neff, K., & Germer, C. (2018). *The mindful self-compassion workbook: A proven way to accept yourself, build inner strength, and thrive.* Guilford Press.

Neff, K. D., Kirkpatrick, K. L., & Rude, S. S. (2007). Self-compassion and adaptive psychological functioning. *Journal of Research in Personality, 41*(1), 139–154.

Parrish, M. H., Inagaki, T. K., Muscatell, K. A., Haltom, K. E., Leary, M. R., & Eisenberger, N. I. (2018). Self-compassion and responses to negative social feedback: The role of fronto-amygdala circuit connectivity. *Self and Identity, 17*(6), 723–738.

Paucsik, M., Nardelli, C., Bortolon, C., Shankland, R., Leys, C., & Baeyens, C. (2023). Self-compassion and emotion regulation: Testing a mediation model. *Cognition and Emotion, 37*(1), 49–61.

Petrocchi, N., Ottaviani, C., & Couyoumdjian, A. (2017). Compassion at the mirror: Exposure to a mirror increases the efficacy of a self-compassion manipulation in enhancing soothing positive affect and heart rate variability. *Journal of Positive Psychology, 12*(6), 525–536.

Phelps, C. L., Paniagua, S. M., Willcockson, I. U., & Potter, J. S. (2018). The relationship between self-compassion and the risk for substance use disorder. *Drug and Alcohol Dependence, 183*, 78–81.

Proeve, M., Anton, R., & Kenny, M. (2018). Effects of mindfulness-based cognitive therapy on shame, self-compassion and psychological distress in anxious and depressed patients: A pilot study. *Psychology and Psychotherapy: Theory, Research and Practice, 91*(4), 434–449.

Ramseyer, F., & Tschacher, W. (2011). Nonverbal synchrony in psychotherapy: Coordinated body movement reflects relationship quality and outcome. *Journal of Consulting and Clinical Psychology, 79*(3), 284–295.

Reilly, E. B., & Stuyvenberg, C. L. (2023). A meta-analysis of loving-kindness meditations on self-compassion. *Mindfulness, 14*(10), 2299–2310.

Robins, C. J., Schmidt, H., III, & Linehan, M. M. (2004). Dialectical behavior therapy: Synthesizing radical acceptance with skillful means. In S. Hayes, V. Follette, & M. Linehan (Eds.), *Mindfulness and acceptance* (pp. 30–44). Guilford Press.

Rogers, C. R. (1951). *Client-centered therapy: Its current practice, implications, and theory, with chapters.* Houghton Mifflin.

Rogers, C. (1995). *On becoming a person: A therapist's view of psychotherapy.* Houghton Mifflin. (Original work published 1961)

Schanche, E., Stiles, T. C., McCullough, L., Svartberg, M., & Nielsen, G. H. (2011). The relationship between activating affects, inhibitory affects, and self-compassion in patients with Cluster C personality disorders. *Psychotherapy, 48*(3), 293–303.

Schwartz, R. C., & Sweezy, M. (2019). *Internal family systems therapy* (2nd ed.). Guilford Press.

Segal, Z., Williams, M., & Teasdale, J. (2018). *Mindfulness-based cognitive therapy for depression*. Guilford Press.

Shaw, J., & Kelly, A. (2024). How exposure to personal distress with and without self-compassion affects distress tolerance: Results from a two-sample randomized trial. *Mindfulness, 15*, 570–585.

Siegel, D. J. (2010). *Mindsight: The new science of personal transformation*. Bantam.

Singer, T., & Klimecki, O. M. (2014). Empathy and compassion. *Current Biology, 24*(18), R875–R878.

Thompson, B. L., & Waltz, J. (2008). Self-compassion and PTSD symptom severity. *Journal of Traumatic Stress, 21*(6), 556–558.

Valdesolo, P., & DeSteno, D. (2011). Synchrony and the social tuning of compassion. *Emotion, 11*(2), 262–266.

Valk, S. L., Bernhardt, B. C., Trautwein, F.-M., Böckler, A., Kanske, P., Guizard, N., et al. (2017). Structural plasticity of the social brain: Differential change after socio-affective and cognitive mental training. *Science Advances, 3*(10), e1700489.

Wadsworth, L. P., Forgeard, M., Hsu, K. J., Kertz, S., Treadway, M., & Björgvinsson, T. (2018). Examining the role of repetitive negative thinking in relations between positive and negative aspects of self-compassion and symptom improvement during intensive treatment. *Cognitive Therapy and Research, 42*(3), 236–249.

Wetterneck, C. T., Lee, E. B., Smith, A. H., & Hart, J. M. (2013). Courage, self-compassion, and values in obsessive–compulsive disorder. *Journal of Contextual Behavioral Science, 2*(3–4), 68–73.

Williams, J. C., & Lynn, S. J. (2010). Acceptance: An historical and conceptual review. *Imagination, Cognition and Personality, 30*(1), 5–56.

Winders, S. J., Murphy, O., Looney, K., & O'Reilly, G. (2020). Self-compassion, trauma, and posttraumatic stress disorder: A systematic review. *Clinical Psychology and Psychotherapy, 27*(3), 300–329.

Yela, J. R., Gómez-Martínez, M. Á., Crego, A., & Jiménez, L. (2020). Effects of the mindful self-compassion programme on clinical and health psychology trainees' well-being: A pilot study. *Clinical Psychologist, 24*(1), 41–54.

2

Compassion and Self-Compassion

A Biopsychosocial and Evolutionary Approach

Paul Gilbert

Compassion: The Two Approaches

Although the word *compassion* does not always translate across languages, in most cultures there is general agreement that humans can be motivated to be caring. One aspect of caring is compassion, which can be defined as *being sensitive to suffering in self and others and with a commitment to try to alleviate and prevent it* (Gilbert, 2009, 2014, 2022a). Self-compassion is applying this motive to the self (Gilbert, 2000, 2009; Neff, 2011). Hence, given that compassion is a motive, with an "If *A*, then do *B*" algorithm, this means that for all forms of compassion we need to be able to identify two different processes underpinning our abilities to *A*: detect, notice, and be sensitive and empathic to distress, and move toward it, not away from it (called *engagement*); and then *B*: be guided toward appropriate helpful *actions*. Di Bello and colleagues (2021) have shown that engagement and action are underpinned by different psychophysiological systems. In Buddhist traditions, compassion motivation manifests as a wish: *the wish that all sentient beings be free of suffering and the causes of suffering* (Dalai Lama, 1995). Hence, in pursuing the *causes* of suffering we are also pursuing the *prevention* of suffering, meaning that prevention must be part of the definition and guide our orientation in the world (Gilbert & Choden, 2013).

The cultivation of compassion has long been a central focus within the contemplative traditions to promote well-being and moral behavior (Condon & Makransky, 2020) with various forms of training now established (Ferrari et al., 2019; Neff, 2011; Weng et al., 2018), including addressing mental health difficulties (Gilbert & Simos, 2022). To explore the effectiveness of compassion-focused therapy (CFT) that was specifically developed with and for people with mental health difficulties, Petrocchi and colleagues (2024) conducted a meta-analysis of CFT from 47 studies (7,875 participants) conducted over a 14-year period. In regard to mental health symptoms, CFT was superior to control conditions (passive) with a large effect size (g = 0.72). For studies with active control conditions (cognitive-behavioral therapy, mindfulness, or treatment as usual), a smaller but moderate to large effect size was reported (g = 0.49). Hence, the psychophysiolgical impact of helping people shift into a compassionate state of mind has been demonstrated, in this and other studies, to have powerful therapeutic effects.

This chapter outlines an evolutionary and biopsychosocial approach to compassion that highlights the importance of understanding compassion as an evolved contextually shaped motive. Like all motives, it evolves with the capacity to (1) detect information/stimuli relevant to the motive, stimulate the appropriate physiological systems needed to analyze that information, and then (2) activate the needed psychophysiological systems to work out and then take appropriate action relevant to the motive. Whether the motive is the need to eat, compete for resources, engage in sexual relationships, or care for offspring, each motive works in the same way. Understanding these different processes in compassion motives enables us to then explore the subskills and processes that underpin each. In addition, we can understand how different motives can be in conflict with each other and suppress each other. For example, at times, the cost of compassion suppresses empathy for suffering (Scheffer et al., 2022). Two very different resource distribution strategies are called control and hold versus care and share (Gilbert, 2021). Control and hold are the typical resource acquiring strategies in most nonhuman primates where access is dependent on power and threat. In contrast, the evolution of egalitarian human hunter-gatherers moved away from such resource regulation into care and share where contribution became a status mediator. It was in this environment where caring for, sharing with, and helping others flourished as a strategy that compassion really got going (Gilbert, 2021). Different cultures, however, can overstimulate control and hold strategies in people, leading to vast inequalities of resources as we now experience in capitalistic societies. The salient point is that compassion is a motive that can be in conflict with other motives.

Skills of Engagement

The skills of engagement can involve paying attention/noticing suffering, moving toward it, not turning away or closing down, tolerating the distress of engaging with suffering, and developing empathic insight into the nature and causes of suffering. This requires certain forms of wisdom, courage, and commitment. However, these are insufficient because we must switch attention from engagement to empathic insight and reasoning on what will be helpful and with the courage to do it. Only being sensitive without some action component can lead to increased distress and burnout or what is sometimes called empathy fatigue (Klimecki & Singer, 2012). For example, a firefighter needs wisdom and insight into the nature of the fire they are facing (different fires have different causes and risks), which then links to their wisdom and courage of what to do and their committed action. Crucially, courage without wisdom can be reckless or even make things worse (rushing in impulsively), whereas wisdom without courage can be ineffective. And if we have both courage and wisdom but without commitment, compassion may again falter.

Understanding the nature of suffering, what is needed to be helpful, and how to build a commitment to live a compassionate identity requires different skills (Di Bello et al., 2020; Gilbert & Simos, 2022). Wisdom, courage, and commitment are the basis of compassion because moving toward suffering can be distressing, taking action can also be difficult, and staying committed to living compassionately over one's lifetime is not easy. Insight into the multiple and, at times, complex skills that underpin these three essential processes of compassion point to areas for specific cultivation, such as attention sensitivity, empathy, distress tolerance, and committed action. These in turn are rooted in evolved psychophysiological systems that also regulate and are regulated by more recently evolved cognitive competencies such as reasoning, empathy, mindfulness, and self-aware competencies (Gilbert, 2020, 2022a).

Compassion and Emotions

While compassion is a motive, compassion engagements, actions, and commitments stimulate different emotions. Emotions are in the service of motives. All life-forms have three basic life tasks underpinning motives:

1. The motives to avoid harm, identify threats, and protect the integrity of the self or others
2. The motives to seek out resources conducive to life and reproduction, such as food, shelter, sexual partners, and, for many species, to live in groups and have alliances
3. The motives to be safe, no need to be dealing with threats and seeking out resources that enable rest and digest functions

These three life task motives give rise to three types of emotion. Hence, we have emotions that are oriented to help us detect and deal with threat, such as anxiety, anger, and disgust; we have emotions that help us seek out resources and rewards, with a variety of positive emotions, such as excitement and joy; and we have emotions that are triggered when we feel safe and not pursuing safety or needed resources, such as contentment and peacefulness. These emotions texture compassion in different ways. For example, in taking risks to help somebody or ourselves, we might be in our threat system and have to regulate anxiety or anger in order to do what is helpful. Seeking out things we want and enjoy gives us pleasure, but if it's at the expense of others or a form of greed, then that is very noncompassionate. Sharing resources with those in need is a form of compassion. Helping others and relieving or preventing their suffering may be a source of great personal meaning, personal reward, joy, and eudaimonic happiness when we are successful. In learning how to regulate our emotions and ground ourselves, we might practice emotions associated with feeling safe and the rest and digest system. The emotions stimulated by compassion engagement, action, and commitment depend on the nature of suffering and the context.

Brain States and Compassion

CFT is rooted in an evolution-informed biopsychosocial brain state approach. Brain state theory has always been my background (Gilbert, 1984, 1989/2016; Gilbert & Simos, 2022). It is straightforward in that at any moment in time our brain is in a pattern and state of neuronal firing. This means that at any point in time our motives, emotions, thoughts, behavioral impulses, and memories are in specific patterns of activation with one another. As one moment flows into the next, that pattern of activation changes. Sometimes it is a smooth transition, sometimes events can cause sudden switches in brain state (Gilbert, 1984). Sometimes switches are intentional, sometimes not. For example, many states of suffering, such as anxiety, depression, hopelessness, and suicidality, are triggered against our will; they are not chosen or wanted and people can battle to try to get rid of them and to stop feeling them. CFT developed to change brain states—that is, change the *patterns* of our different functions in mind. This can be demonstrated quite easily. For example, if you sit down for a moment and bring to mind a worry that you have, you will stimulate a whole set of threat-linked processes (feelings, thoughts, behavioral impulses, memories, hopes, fears, psychophysiological patterns, etc.) within you. If, on the other hand, your mind focuses on someone you are irritated or angry with, a different pattern will emerge. If you focus on the fact that you are going on a long-planned holiday tomorrow, a different pattern will emerge, and if you focus on something erotic, then that will change blood flow to different organs of your body, generating feelings of arousal. So, different motives and emotions are linked with different brain state patterns. What you focus on can change a whole range of processes within you, that is, your brain and body state. Now, if you bring to mind a friend who has been very helpful to you with a sense of warmth and gratitude toward your friend, you will stimulate compassion brain states. If you remember a time when you helped your friend and they did well because of your help, you might stimulate a compassion feeling of joy that you could help.

Learning how to switch brain states is part of what compassion training is about (Gilbert & Simos, 2022). In other words, it seeks to pattern psychophysiological processes in particular ways. Indeed, we now know that compassion training can have major impacts on our brain and autonomic nervous system, empathic abilities, and values (Vrtička et al., 2017; Weng et al., 2018). Self-compassion is a way of stimulating particular brain states that organize multiple functions of the mind (how and to what we pay attention, how we empathize, how we reason, how we plan actions) that can help us with (for example) threat-based brain states (Kim et al., 2020). There are major differences between brain states linked to self-criticism and those linked to self-compassion (Kim et al., 2020; Longe et al., 2010).

The Evolution of Compassion

This leads us to the question of how care-based compassionate brain states came into being. Compassion evolved from the motive to care, which evolved to support the survival and flourishing of one's offspring (Cassidy & Shaver, 2016) and be supportive of others around us (e.g., friends; Camilleri et al., 2023). In addition to providing basic resources (e.g., food and shelter), attachment theory has identified two basic psychological processes of care. These are providing a secure base and a safe haven (Cassidy & Shaver, 2016). When the parent acts as a *secure base*, they provide an opportunity for the child to explore, learn, and grow in protected spaces, such that threat processing remains relatively low-key. In addition, a secure base offers opportunities to explore one's mind, be validated, feel empathically understood, and be encouraged to take risks and develop confidence. The cheerful (playful, warm, affectionate, and loving) emotions shared in such caring interactions help build inner confidence, a sense of self as being loved and *lovable*, and being valued and of value (can contribute). The second psychological function of caring is called a *safe haven*. This provides soothing, grounding, and stabilizing aspects of caring. CFT is rooted in these attachment functions (Gilbert, 1989/2016, 2022b). Hence, when we are being self-compassionate, we can pull on an internal sense of a secure base and haven in times of difficulty (Gilbert, 2022b) and we learn to self-validate, self-encourage, self-soothe, and so on. These different functions are depicted in Figure 2.1.

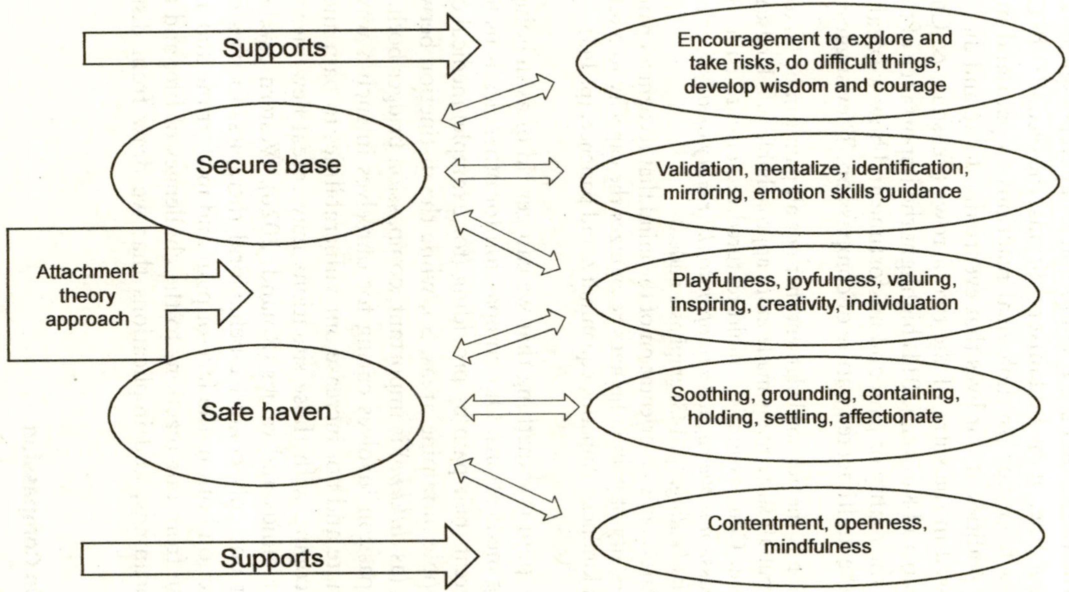

FIGURE 2.1. Outline of typical functions associated with a secure base and haven. From Gilbert (2022b). Copyright © Paul Gilbert.

Compassion and self-compassion are responses to suffering, so we also require an understanding of what we mean by suffering. The word *suffering* usually implies two different processes. The first is some form of pain and misfortune, and the second is our emotional and psychological reactions to pain and misfortune. In the Buddhist traditions, the second suffering, called *dukkha*, arises from our psychological reactions to pain and misfortune, including the realities of our lives that eventually decay and die. This principle is captured in the sutra of the two arrows (Teasdale & Chaskalson, 2013). Feldman and Kuyken (2011) highlight the importance of the interaction between the reality of pain and misfortune and how we deal with it by highlighting the multifaceted nature of compassion. They suggest that:

> Compassion is the acknowledgment that not all pain can be "fixed" or "solved" but all suffering is made more approachable in a landscape of compassion. Compassion is a multi-textured response to pain. *Above all, compassion is the capacity to open to the reality of suffering and to aspire to its healing.* (p. 143; emphasis added)
>
> Compassion is an orientation of the mind that recognizes pain and the universality of pain in humans recognizes the capacity to meet that pain with kindness, empathy, equanimity, and patience. (p. 145)

At times, pain is something that we can get rid of as in going for surgery or taking medications. Our compassion for others leads us to want to prevent and treat their pain by providing (for example) medical care to all or feeding people in famine areas. So, while the distinction between pain and suffering (as *dukkha*) is important, compassion bridges both.

Self-compassion involves caring for ourselves in such a way that we learn to alleviate and not increase our vulnerabilities to pain and disease. The path to coping with those situations may reveal new meanings and transform our minds and values (Roland, 2020). Western psychotherapy, especially but not only cognitive-behavioral therapies, focuses on taking appropriate action both in the face of pain and misfortune and also problems that arise from our reactions to the challenges of life, and the interpretations, meanings, and implications that we draw from distress and misfortune.

From Caring to Compassion

The evolution of caring behavior, particularly in attachment and in small-group contexts in many species, is many millions of years old. As such, it is a motivation that has genetic (Kucerova et al., 2023) and many psychophysiological systems underpinning it (Kim et al., 2020; Petrocchi et al., 2022; Vrtička et al., 2017). But basic care-focused motives are not compassion; crocodiles carrying their hatchlings to the water is not compassion.

What turns basic caring motivation into compassion is our recently evolved complex cognitive abilities that give rise to ways of (1) reasoning, (2) empathizing, and (3) knowing awareness. These support forms of self-awareness enable us to become "mindful," as observers and reflectors of our mind and its functioning and to discern helpful actions (Gilbert, 2009, 2022a). Indeed, the way recent cognitive competencies regulate motives and emotions is partly what distinguishes us from other species (LeDoux, 2020). Exploring the archaeological record, Spikins (2015) highlighted how humans have been caring for injured and diseased individuals for hundreds of thousands of years or more. It was the evolution of in-group caring behavior and the development of caring networks that helped contribute to our social intelligence (Camilleri et al., 2023). Behaving in ways that enable us to be part of caring networks is therefore also part of self-compassion; behaving in ways that result in being ridiculed, stigmatized, or rejected is not self-compassionate.

Human Compassion

Human compassion is not automatic caring but is rooted in the empathic insightful understanding of the need to be caring, insight into the causes of suffering, and empathic awareness of what is likely to be helpful or not. This can take careful reflection. While chimpanzees may pick up on the distress and needs of others and can engage in helpful behaviors, humans can work out what we (and others) are distressed about, for example, that we are lonely, have suffered major losses, are frightened about a recent diagnosis of cancer, or are suffering with a migraine. It is a mind that can have empathy and insight into the minds of self and others and wants to develop the wisdom for helpful responses and actions. Unfortunately, just as we can use our self-aware intelligence to promote compassion, we can also use it to promote the dark side of humanity in terms of wars, atrocities, torture, slavery, and gross social injustice. Humans are potentially a nasty, vicious, and dangerous species, including to other species and even our own selves (Gilbert, 2019). In addition, just as we can use our self-aware intelligence to be helpful to ourselves, we can also use it to judge and treat ourselves harshly, to generate a range of mood, anxiety, and paranoia problems. For these reasons, compassion has a major role to play in the *prevention of suffering, particularly* the suffering we cause ourselves and others because of our beliefs and attitudes that fuel our dark sides.

Addressing Self-Illusion

Around 590 B.C.E., a wealthy Indian prince, Siddhartha, was kept in a golden palace to protect him from seeing suffering (Anālayo, 2015; Yaden et al.,

2017). However, one day he managed to escape to the local village, where he discovered the three realities of disease, decay, and death. So distressed was he by these realities that he decided to set out on how to make sense of life and cope. He spent many years learning meditation and other practices and also became an ascetic, which meant he didn't eat much. Then, in an emaciated state and somewhat disappointed in his searches, he decided to sit under a (fig) tree and just observe his own mind. In this state, he had what is called an *enlightenment* experience, which is one of self-transcendence and nonduality, where the sense of self, time, and space dissolves into a recognition that reality is *consciousness* and everything else comes and goes within it; nothing has independent existence. It was from this transformative experience of mind and the transcendent nature of consciousness that compassion arose. However, we cannot tap into this "true" transcendent reality because we exist within biological minds that are constantly generating desires, wishes, thoughts, a sense of self, and so forth.

Today, many scientists recognize that the brain does not perceive reality, but rather creates ways of experiencing that allow biological systems to survive and reproduce (Hoffman, 2019; Hood, 2011). Our sensory processing systems are actually processing energy frequencies and translating them into experience. For example, we see a ripe tomato as red, but the tomato is an energy field. Our brains create that experience of red from the light rays falling on the retina. Red does not exist outside the mind (Hoffman, 2019).

This is important because, in the Buddhist tradition, self-compassion is about losing the sense of the individual separate self and having experiences of "being of, all things, that is" consciousness. Indeed, the concept of self-compassion with the focus on "a separate striving self" would not fit this approach because in the domain of pure consciousness, there is no separate self (or selves) to be compassionate to or for (Gilbert et al., 2024). Certainly, the concept of self-love, which has been creeping into Western approaches, is a potentially dangerous distraction. It is through the enactment of *bodhicitta*, the desire to become enlightened to help others experience nondual self-transcendence and thus be free from separate self-illusions, that is key to the compassion motive. This, in turn, directs attention away from the worries of the self, enabling deeper experiences of interconnectedness, or as Siegel (2023) calls it, "intraconnectedness." As Brazier (2013) notes:

> Buddhism was not originally conceived with modern ideas about science, secularism, academic sensibilities, or popular self-development in mind. Nor was the Buddha much interested in stress reduction. One of his most used words was "Strive." Buddhism is or was fundamentally about waking up to a radically changed perspective on life as a whole rather than the application of limited techniques to the treatment of particular

> ailments or tension reduction. Mindfulness, in origin, was not a treatment, and it was one dimension of such awakening. It was concerned with fundamentals rather than symptoms. . . . The Buddha advocated mindfulness as a means to learning, not as a treatment. If it had any effect on stress, it was supposed to increase it, leading the practitioner to a direct experience of impermanence such as would impart a sense of urgency or even crisis life and thereby, in the best case, provoke a breakthrough to a more authentic life. (p. 118)

A Comparison of Contemplative and Evolution Approaches

The Buddhist approach to compassion views the motives for compassion as arising from experiences of insight into the interconnectedness of all things; a form of a radical shift in conscious awareness of nonduality and self-transcendence (Gilbert & Van Gordon, 2023).

This approach should not be confused with an evolutionary and biopsychosocial approach to compassion, *which is rooted* in understanding the evolved mechanisms for self-awareness, the problem of inheriting multiple motivational systems that can be helpful or harmful, including compassion, and the facilitators and inhibitors of their biopsychosocial processes (Gilbert et al., 2024). Nonetheless, many Buddhist practices have been developed and adapted to strengthen the sense of self, not loosen it, precisely to help us cope with the ups and downs of life and the importance of developing a compassionate and moral focus (Ricard, 2015). That focus is not simply because it creates social harmony but because *bodhicitta* motivation also loosens the sense of self and increases the potential for interconnected (or intraconnected) awareness, self-transcendence, and enlightened experiences (Anālayo, 2015; Siegel, 2023).

Concerns have arisen when the practices (e.g., mindfulness) *are used only* for self-regulation and do not point to the moral and ethical basis of (self-) compassion training or the potential for enlightened experience (Condon & Makransky, 2020). In a more complex analysis, the two approaches can and do support each other in complex ways (Gilbert & Choden 2013; Gilbert & Van Gordon, 2023; Gilbert et al., 2024). Whereas the Buddha focused on what he regarded as an ultimate reality of consciousness (Anālayo, 2015; Brazier, 2013), CFT focuses on the "worldly" reality, that whatever is the basis of consciousness, it is biological minds that texture it and create (helpful or harmful) actions in the world. It starts with the fact that all living things are rooted in biological systems created from DNA (Dawkins, 2016; Hoffman, 2019). Indeed, we even share much of our DNA with plant life.

Genes orient all life-forms to struggle to survive, reproduce, and thus replicate. Genes build bodies to carry them around; individual bodies are very short, whereas the information carried by genes exists over millennia. Having said that, around 99% of all living things that have ever existed on this planet are now extinct (Dawkins, 1996). Indeed, for most of planet Earth's history, it has been very hostile to life, with a number of mass extinction of life-forms (Bond & Grasby, 2017). Without them, we, as a species, would not be here. Crucially then, no living entity chose to be what it is. We did not choose the genes that predispose us to both talents and vulnerabilities, including health and illness; we did not choose a brain that has evolved multiple motives and emotions geared toward survival and reproduction and can therefore create a sense of self that wants to defend itself and to struggle and grasp and fulfill desires. Our desires are rooted in motivations that serve our genes in their pursuit of reproduction; we chose none of that. We did not choose our ethnicity, our gender, and the environments we were born into. Yet these environments have profound impacts on the kinds of brains and epigenetic profiles, values, sense of self, and empathic and emotional regulation competencies we come to mature. These are crucial insights when we come to conceptualizing work with concepts of having a self and compassion for our "tricky" brain.

In CFT, this is the beginning of a deeper understanding of self-compassion; the wisdom to recognize that our brains, and the way they texture our consciousness have been created for us, not by us. Sapolsky (2023) goes even further and argues that, because every moment from the beginning of the universe creates the conditions for the next moment, we do not have any free will, but it is all an unfolding of patterns that are co-arising. What we take to be a sense of self is the operating of basic brain algorithms designed for survival and reproduction (Hoffman, 2019; Hood, 2011). Our brain is not set up to give us accurate pictures of reality, including of time and space, but to function for our genes to survive and reproduce. This means that we have a distorted and limited view of any reality (Hoffman, 2019). As such, the motive and emotion algorithms of our brains can orient us to be not only helpful but also harmful. In CFT, we call this *evolutionary wisdom*. It creates a platform of insights to depersonalize and de-shame and create an observer mindfulness-focused orientation to our mind and experience (see Practice C, "Compassion Practice Sequences to Aid Cultivating Compassion Brain, Body, and Mind States," in the Appendix for a sample of CFT practices). With practice, we become aware that various biologically designed and socially textured systems respond to threats or desires that are triggered within us, filling and texturing consciousness with experiences that we can find pleasant, neutral, or unpleasant; desired or undesired; helpful or harmful.

All these will be highly modified by experience, context, and subsequent cognitive processes, but for the moment we can see that part of mindfulness is to become aware of these basic, triggered brain state patterns within us. In other words, we practice mindfulness not to control our thoughts or triggered body states but so that our thoughts and triggered body states do not control us, especially as we confront the challenges of biological living. If we are to take self-compassion *as sensitivity to suffering within ourselves with the desire to alleviate and prevent it*, then we have to begin by understanding the roots and causes of that suffering as lying partly in the way we have been designed by nature. Whereas Buddhism sees the problem of suffering as arising from the illusions of a sense of a separate self and ignorance of our true nature as being part of consciousness, CFT places the source of suffering in evolved motives and emotions that texture consciousness. The CFT approach to self-compassion is rooted in these important insights into how evolved design has sent us difficult challenges, for which compassion is a major source of help.

Neff (2011) highlights the importance not of separating ourselves from *common humanity* but seeing ourselves as all vulnerable to the same challenges and ultimate realties (decay and death) of life. We can become more observant and mindful of what arises in the playing out of these evolved brain systems without blaming or shaming, given that we never chose or built them. CFT argues that evolutionary insights enable us to take responsibility for working with brain systems that can be problematic but that are not of our design or fault. It is when we blame and shame ourselves or believe that what arises in us is our fault that we can get lost in self-criticism and hopelessness. We can help to counteract this personalization of the states of our mind by recognizing just how much of what goes on in our minds was not built or chosen by us, and hence not our fault. This is essential for self-compassion, and indeed all forms of compassion.

Not only is it not our fault that we are shaped the way we are but, in fact, becoming consciously aware of our intentions and emotions is quite late in the information processing chain (Bargh, 2017). The various algorithms of our brain may well have decided how to process information before it turns up in consciousness and we may end up justifying our emotions or behaviors rather than being in control of them. Indeed, the brain may already have decided on an emotion or action before we become conscious of it. Again, this brings us to a crucial element of self-compassion that is based on wisdom and discernment. In the case of CFT, this is knowledge about brains (evolving over hundreds of years for survival and reproduction) and their biological infrastructures. Mindfulness is the ability to detect the arising of problematic emotions, desires, or thoughts without *then* acting them out in harmful ways and not being absorbed into them.

So, for example, one may become aware that, to a certain disappointment, one tends to launch an aggressive attack on oneself (Gilbert, 2022c). If one can notice and stand back from that, note its origins, and not be pulled into it, that can be helpful. In addition, learning to be compassionate to our self-criticism itself and to see it as linked to underlying fears of (say) rejection or abandonment enables us to work with the brain that so easily generates self-attacking thoughts and feelings (Gilbert, 2022c).

Some Biopsychosocial Dimensions of Compassion

Taking a biopsychosocial approach to compassion allows us to begin to identify specific trainings for each of these dimensions. Hence, self-caring compassion and the prevention of suffering have multiple biopsychosocial domains linked to the physical self, the psychological self, and the social self. As noted at the beginning of the chapter, we can see the caring as both (secure base) validating and encouraging to engage with difficulties, functions, and also soothing and grounding functions.

The Physical

To begin with the physical self, like all living things we must take in nutrients to sustain ourselves appropriately. Although this would seem obvious, in our modern world, the way we sustain ourselves can be harmful, and we now suffer from an epidemic of obesity, diabetes, and cardiovascular disease related to poor regulation of diet and exercise. We have allowed the food industry to saturate our foods with salt, fat, and sugar. Because these were hard to come by in our ancestral environments, we find them highly rewarding. These, along with excessively processed carbohydrates, are inflammatory, and inflammatory diets have been linked to poor mental health (Beurel et al., 2020). There are some mental health difficulties, such as anorexia, where individuals struggle to sustain themselves and can become distressed at eating sufficiently to maintain appropriate body weight.

Part of self-compassion, therefore, is the ability to use knowledge to *sustain the body appropriately* for physical and mental health and well-being. In some cases, then, self-compassion is rooted in exercising and eating appropriately and, in other cases, it is rooted in resisting desires (e.g., French fries, chocolate cake, alcohol). We live in a world that constantly promotes overconsumption. In other words, we have created cultures that are out of tune with our evolved biological systems; this is called "mismatch" (Li et al., 2018). Insight into this can take some of the pressures off our tendency to be self-blaming and shaming.

There are many areas where the struggles of ill health require self-compassion. For example, how do we confront a new diagnosis of cancer or dementia or come to terms with chronic pain conditions? One of the first applications of mindfulness in medical settings was for people with chronic pain (Kabat-Zinn et al., 1985). Learning how to work with our emotions of fear, rage, and grief at pain and the life changes these conditions force upon us, can be a very important self-compassion process. Self-compassion therefore can have a clear physical focus.

The Physiology of Caring

Our psychophysiological processes are highly influenced by our relationships, particularly those that are caring versus neglectful or hostile. Indeed, the evolution of caring, particularly in the child–parent attachment context, but also in friendships, evolved supporting genetic and psychophysiological systems. Research has identified various neurophysiological circuits that underpin compassion (Kim et al., 2020; Vrtička et al., 2017) and that specific compassion trainings can stimulate them (Weng et al., 2018). Expressing and receiving compassion are linked to hormones such as oxytocin and endorphins (Kucerova et al., 2023), key processes within the autonomic nervous system, especially the myelinated vagus nerve (Di Bello et al., 2020), and a range of "body processes" (Mascaro & Raison, 2017; Petrocchi et al., 2022). Di Bello and colleagues (2021) have shown that there are different psychophysiological underpinnings to our ability to engage and be sensitive to suffering, in contrast to those that are triggered when we are working out what to do and taking action. Self-compassion, therefore, needs to identify these two different processes.

The Psychological

What is unique about humans is that we have a range of complex cognitive competencies that hone our sense of a separate, self-aware self with needs, desires, and fears. The ways in which we reason, interpret, anticipate, plan, expect, and project are the focus of cognitive-behavioral therapies. They highlight that we can become attentionally overfocused, ruminate, and become oriented to negative aspects (negativity bias).

We can constantly monitor our inner life (of desires, emotions, and fantasies linked with memories and behaviors) against desired ones and feel ashamed of what we find within. We can react negatively when our efforts fail or our ideals are not met. When we experience frustration at not being able to achieve what we want to achieve, and if that is linked to worry, we can feel less lovable and harshly self-critical (Gilbert, 2022c). This is not just having negative thoughts about the self; it is also having hostile internal *emotional textures* to the self (Gilbert, 2020c).

Self-compassion therefore requires us to be mindful of our responses to others and ourselves when we are faced with the challenge of life's setbacks, disappointments, misfortunes, and mistakes. If we launch hostile attacks on ourselves, then we are stimulating the threat systems in our brains and bodies, which are not conducive to well-being (Kim et al., 2020; Long et al., 2010). Hence, in many therapies that focus on self-compassion, addressing harmful self-criticism is often a key focus (Gilbert 2009, 2022c; Neff, 2011).

In addition to addressing self-criticism, there are ways of supporting self-reassurance and encouragement and learning self-regulation skills, such as self-validation and empathic support for planned action (secure base functions; Gilbert et al., 2004, 2017; see Figure 2.1 on page 35).

Competencies of Self-Compassion

Keeping in mind that compassion has two basic components to it means that we can (1) detect, notice, engage, understand, and tolerate suffering and (2) work out how to be helpful and then take the necessary action (Di Bello et al., 2020; Gilbert, 2009). Both require courage and wisdom. Courage without wisdom can be reckless—we might rush in to be helpful but misunderstand the nature of suffering and end up making things worse. Wisdom without courage can be ineffective because we are frightened to act on what we know could be helpful (e.g., standing up against injustice or being more assertive in our positions).

In the first process of noticing and moving toward suffering and engaging with it, we can identify six nonexclusive competencies that include (1) being motivated to pay attention; (2) being sensitive to certain signals of distress, suffering, or need; (3) having personal sympathetic reactions to these observations; (4) being able to tolerate the stress and distress of engaging with suffering without closing down on it; (5) being able to be insightful and empathic and make sense of suffering and its causes; and (6) being nonjudgmental, condemning, or hostile to it.

Although engaging with being empathic and validating suffering can be helpful, if we feel ignorant of how to be helpful, even in small measure, or too fearful, we can feel powerless, overwhelmed, and stuck and switch off (Klimecki & Singer, 2012). It is well-known that when we see major catastrophes on television and feel that the problems are too big or insurmountable, we tend to turn away (Cameron & Payne, 2011). It can be the same with depression. If people feel that their problems are too complex, chronic, insurmountable, and overwhelming, the depression deepens because they disengage from trying to help themselves because they can see no way to do so. There is also clear evidence that people can be frightened of or angrily resist compassion (Kirby et al., 2019). Cameron and colleagues (e.g., Scheffer et al., 2022) have shown that all kinds of costs to being compassionate can lead people to turn off empathy and compassionate engagement. This can be true for self-compassion also, when we think the cost/effort of getting fit and losing weight or facing trauma or depression too high. Therefore, the next aspect of compassion requires us to switch attention from the distress of suffering into generating ideas about what could be helpful and how to do it, even in small ways. And here too there can be fears, blocks, and resistances.

For the "taking action" aspect, CFT identifies six nonexclusive competencies for helpfulness: (1) switching attention from the nature of suffering onto what might be helpful, (2) imagining and running scenarios in one's mind of what might be helpful, (3) using one's capacity for empathic reasoning and problem solving, (4) engaging in specific behaviors to address suffering, (5) attending to the body and grounding the body to enable distress tolerance (e.g., mindfulness and use of vagal breathing when taking action), and (6) having the courage and wisdom to work with the feelings that arise when we take compassionate action. These are depicted in the competency circle in Figure 2.2.

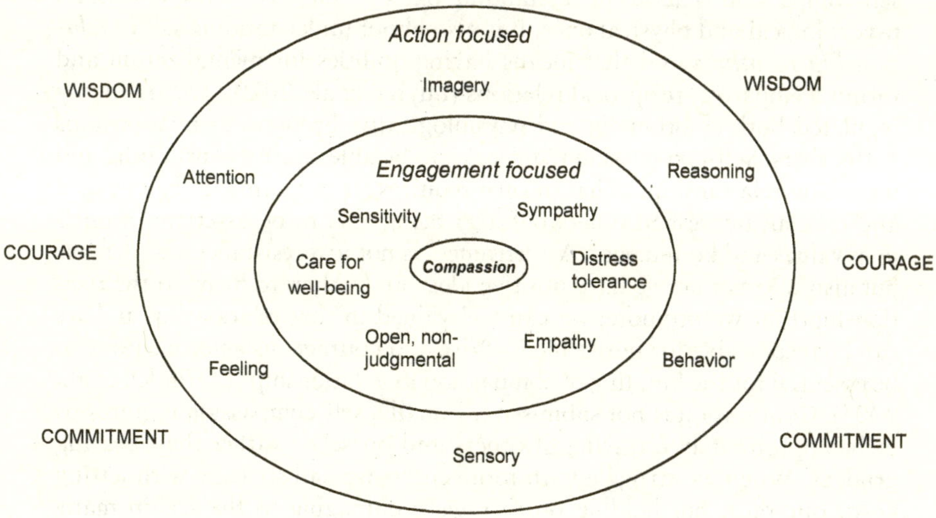

FIGURE 2.2. Twelve competencies of compassion. Adapted from Gilbert (2009), *The Compassionate Mind*, with permission from Little, Brown.

These 12 competencies are exclusive and are used as guides of the value of seeing the two different dimensions to the compassion algorithm: engagement and action. Each of them can be trained, cultivated, and developed, and each of them will contribute to compassion and self-compassion. However, even if we are motivated to be helpful to ourselves or others and know what to do, we don't always translate that into actual actions (Poulin, 2017; Scheffer et al., 2022). For example, as noted, losing weight and getting fit may well be a self-compassion intention, but we may not engage in the necessary behaviors. That requires wisdom, courage, commitment, and the preparedness to make sacrifices to change harmful lifestyles. Self-compassion extends to concerns with the external world, such as the climate. For example, we need to do things that will secure our future and that of our children. Such considerations indicate that self-compassion can be self-focused but also with insightful and wider implications beyond the self.

Social Dynamics

Although we may assume that self-compassion is about being compassionate to the self, that doesn't mean that CFT sees the self as a self-contained island that can provide for all of its emotional and physical needs irrespective of the social environment in which one exists. CFT highlights the importance of the flows of compassion and the evidence that part of self-compassion is about understanding one's *social* needs as well as one's psychological and physical ones. It is also about understanding self *in relationship to others* and that means having abilities for mentalization and forming empathic, reciprocal relations (Luyten et al., 2020). We are highly regulated both emotionally and physiologically through our relationships with others. Self-compassion requires us to be able to create sustaining and nurturing relationships. That in turn requires learning how to be engaged and take an interest in others but also being able to be assertive of one's own values and boundaries. Assertiveness is not just resistance and defense but also means that we have positive ideas and values to bring to the relationship that we promote; we can feel valued in that relationship and we can be responsible for nurturing it. Wise and courageous assertiveness can be essential for the building of compassionate relationships (Arrindell et al., 2005). Compassion is not submissive. Equally, self-compassion requires us to be appropriately forgiving of others and ourselves rather than bearing grudges. When we struggle with forgiveness, we can struggle with letting go of our rage, but holding on to rage is damaging to the self in many ways (Enright & Song, 2020). It is also important for us to be able to apologize in the event we have unintentionally caused distress to others. Hence, assertiveness, forgiveness, and apology are three important parts of self-compassion because these help us to become moral agents, cultivate caring relationships, and more likely flourish and find happiness.

Hence, sustaining relationships requires both caring and sharing with others, taking an interest in them and being responsive to others taking a caring interest in us without being ashamed of being a mutually dependent individual. Shame and narcissistic self-focus can interfere with the creation of sustainable relationships—therefore, self-compassion moderates both of them. Self-compassion requires us to recognize that we are not islands and there are many areas of our lives where we need the help of others to trust appropriately and to show gratitude appropriately. Self-compassion, therefore, also involves a personal humility to recognize that we are interdependent beings who are part of an intraconnected universe (Siegel, 2023). These considerations are important because self-compassion and training in self-compassion have also been shown to have a significant impact on a range of prosocial behaviors (Ferrari et al., 2019). This indicates that compassion needs to be understood as a flow rather than as a unitary process and that the benefits we get from being prosocial are helpful to us (Gilbert, 2020).

Conclusion

Self-compassion is a phenomenon that arises because we have a particular kind of self-aware and monitoring mind that is different from those of other animals: the experience of being self-aware. We have capacities for different forms of reasoning, empathy, self-awareness, and mindfulness. Life confronts us with many challenges, including those that stimulated Siddhartha's search, such as how to cope with disease, decay, and death, along with the threats, losses, and disappointments of life. One source of self-compassion is to pursue enlightenment and, in that way, recognize the illusions of the self. However, this is not an easily obtained state, although studies on psychedelics are exploring approximations of these states and the implications for self-experience.

Whereas in the contemplative sciences compassion arises out of a loosening or even a loss of a sense of a separate self into nonduality experience, in CFT the attention is on the evolved and biopsychosocial mechanisms underpinning compassion. As such, understanding these processes is also the guide for how we train our minds to become more motivated for, and competent in, compassion. Because compassion is like other motives, it can have a range of fears, blocks, and resistances (Kirby et al., 2019; Scheffer et al., 2022). These may arise from life traumas, problems of shame or anger, and other reasons. We may find it difficult to find compassion for parts of ourselves that we dislike or want to dissociate from.

In summary, CFT seeks to stimulate and cultivate compassion as a basic motivation that is linked to ways of thinking about the self and others in the world. As such, it brings on a whole range of psychophysiological processes that are conducive to stress coping, flourishing, and well-being that, in the case of depression, will counteract problems of low motivation, loss of confidence, hopelessness about the future, and self-isolation (see Chapter 13 for more on compassion and depression). For an example of CFT practices, see Practice C, "Compassion Practice Sequences to Aid Cultivating Compassion Brain, Body, and Mind States," in the Appendix.

REFERENCES

Anālayo, B. (2015). *Compassion and emptiness in early Buddhist meditation.* Windhorse.

Arrindell, W. A., Akkerman, A., van der Ende, J., Schreurs, P. J., Brugman, A., Stewart, R. E., et al. (2005). Normative studies with the Scale for Interpersonal Behaviour (SIB): III. Psychiatric inpatients. *Personality and Individual differences, 38*(4), 941–952.

Bargh, J. (2017). *Before you know it: The unconscious reasons we do what we do.* Simon & Schuster.

Beurel, E., Toups, M., & Nemeroff, C. B. (2020). The bidirectional relationship of depression and inflammation: Double trouble. *Neuron, 107*(2), 234–256.

Brazier, D. (2013). Mindfulness reconsidered. *European Journal of Psychotherapy and Counselling, 15*(2), 116–126.

Bond, D. P., & Grasby, S. E. (2017). On the causes of mass extinctions. *Palaeogeography, Palaeoclimatology, and Palaeoecology, 478*, 3–29.

Cameron, C. D., & Payne, B. K. (2011). Escaping affect: How motivated emotion regulation creates insensitivity to mass suffering. *Journal of Personality and Social Psychology, 100*(1), 1–15.

Camilleri, T., Rockey, S., & Dunbar, R. (2023). *The social brain. The psychology of successful groups.* Cornerstone Press.

Cassidy, J., & Shaver, P. R. (Eds.). (2016). *Handbook of attachment: Theory, research, and clinical applications* (3rd ed.). Guilford Press.

Condon, P., & Makransky, J. (2020). Sustainable compassion training: Integrating meditation theory with psychological science. *Frontiers in Psychology, 11*, 2249.

Dalai Lama. (1995). *The power of compassion.* HarperCollins.

Dawkins, R. (2016). *The selfish gene.* Oxford University Press.

Di Bello, M., Carnevali, L., Petrocchi, N., Thayer, J. F., Gilbert, P., & Ottaviani, C. (2020). The compassionate vagus: A meta-analysis on the connection between compassion and heart rate variability. *Neuroscience and Biobehavioral Reviews, 116*, 21–30.

Di Bello, M., Ottaviani, C., & Petrocchi, N. (2021). Compassion is not a benzo: Distinctive associations of heart rate variability with its empathic and action components. *Frontiers in Neuroscience, 15*, 617443.

Enright, R. D., & Song, J. Y. (2020). The development of forgiveness. In L. A. Jensen (Ed.), *The Oxford handbook of moral development: An interdisciplinary perspective* (pp. 402–418). Oxford University Press.

Feldman, C., & Kuyken, W. (2011). Compassion in the landscape of suffering. *Contemporary Buddhism, 12,* 143–155.

Ferrari, M., Hunt, C., Harrysunker, A., Abbott, M. J., Beath, A. P., & Einstein, D. A. (2019). Self-compassion interventions and psychosocial outcomes: A meta-analysis of RCTs. *Mindfulness, 10,* 1455–1473.

Gilbert, P. (1984). *Depression: From psychology to brain state.* Erlbaum.

Gilbert, P. (2000). Social mentalities: Internal "social" conflicts and the role of inner warmth and compassion in cognitive therapy. In P. Gilbert & K. G. Bailey (Eds.), *Genes on the couch: Explorations in evolutionary psychotherapy* (pp. 118–150). Psychology Press.

Gilbert, P. (2009). *The compassionate mind.* Robinson.

Gilbert, P. (2014). The origins and nature of compassion focused therapy. *British Journal of Clinical Psychology, 53,* 6–41.

Gilbert, P. (2016). *Human nature and suffering.* Routledge. (Original work published 1989)

Gilbert, P. (2019). *Living like crazy* (2nd ed.). Annwyn House.

Gilbert, P. (2020). Compassion: From its evolution to psychotherapy. *Frontiers in Psychology, 11,* 586161.

Gilbert, P. (2021). Creating a compassionate world: Addressing the conflicts between sharing and caring versus controlling and holding evolved strategies. *Frontiers in Psychology, 11,* 582090.

Gilbert, P. (2022a). Compassion-focused therapy as an evolution-informed, biopsychosocial science of the mind: History and challenge. In P. Gilbert & G. Simos (Eds.), *Compassion focused therapy: Clinical practice and applications* (pp. 24–89). Routledge.

Gilbert, P. (2022b). The evolved functions of caring connections as a basis for compassion. In P. Gilbert & G. Simos (Eds.), *Compassion focused therapy: Clinical practice and applications* (pp. 90–121). Routledge

Gilbert, P. (2022c). Internal shame and self-disconnection: From hostile self-criticism to compassionate self-correction and guidance. In P. Gilbert & G. Simos (Eds.), *Compassion focused therapy: Clinical practice and applications* (pp. 164–206). Routledge.

Gilbert, P., Catarino, F., Duarte, C., Matos, M., Kolts, R., Stubbs, J., et al. (2017). The development of compassionate engagement and action scales for self and others. *Journal of Compassionate Health Care, 4*(1), 1–24.

Gilbert, P., & Choden. (2013). *Mindful compassion.* Constable Robinson.

Gilbert, P., Clarke, M., Kempel, S., Miles, J. N. V., & Irons, C. (2004). Criticizing and reassuring oneself: An exploration of forms style and reasons in female students. *British Journal of Clinical Psychology 43,* 31–50.

Gilbert, P., Huxter, M., & Choden. (2024). Exploration of evolution-informed compassion-focused therapy and Buddhist approaches to insight meditation: A three-way exploration. *Mindfulness, 15*(5), 1014–1037.

Gilbert, P., & Simos, S. (Eds.). (2022). *Compassion focused therapy: Clinical practice and applications.* Routledge.

Gilbert, P., & Van Gordon, W. (2023). Compassion as a skill: A comparison of contemplative and evolution-based approaches. *Mindfulness, 14*(10), 2395–2416.

Hoffman, D. (2019). *The case against reality: Why evolution hid the truth from our eyes.* Norton.

Hood, B. (2011). *The self-illusion: Why there is no "you" inside your head.* Constable.

Kabat-Zinn, J., Lipworth, L., & Burney, R. (1985). The clinical use of mindfulness meditation for the self-regulation of chronic pain. *Journal of Behavioral Medicine, 8*, 163–190.

Kim, J. J., Cunnington, R., & Kirby, J. N. (2020). The neurophysiological basis of compassion: An fMRI meta-analysis of compassion and its related neural processes. *Neuroscience and Biobehavioral Reviews, 108*, 112–123.

Kirby, J. N., Day, J., & Sagar, V. (2019). The "flow" of compassion: A meta-analysis of the fears of compassion scales and psychological functioning. *Clinical Psychology Review, 70*, 26–39.

Klimecki, O., & Singer, T. (2012). Empathic distress fatigue rather than compassion fatigue?: Integrating findings from empathy research in psychology and social neuroscience. *Pathological Altruism, 5*, 368–383.

Kucerova, B., Levit-Binnun, N., Gordon, I., & Golland, Y. (2023). From oxytocin to compassion: The saliency of distress. *Biology, 12*(2), 183.

LeDoux, J. E. (2020). Thoughtful feelings. *Current Biology, 30*(11), R619–R623.

Li, N. P., van Vugt, M., & Colarelli, S. M. (2018). The evolutionary mismatch hypothesis: Implications for psychological science. *Current Directions in Psychological Science, 27*(1), 38–44.

Longe, O., Maratos, F. A., Gilbert, P., Evans, G., Volker, F., Rockliffe, H., & Rippon, G. (2010). Having a word with yourself: Neural correlates of self-criticism and self-reassurance. *NeuroImage, 49*, 1849–1856.

Luyten, P., Campbell, C., Allison, E., & Fonagy, P. (2020). The mentalizing approach to psychopathology: State of the art and future directions. *Annual Review of Clinical Psychology, 16*, 297–325.

Mascaro, J., & Raison, C. L. (2017). The body of compassion. In P. Gilbert (Ed.), *Compassion: Concepts, research, and applications* (pp. 89–104). Routledge.

Neff, K. (2011). *Self-compassion: The proven power of being kind to yourself.* Hachette UK.

Petrocchi, N., Di Bello, M., Cheli, S., & Ottavianni, C. (2022). Compassion-focused therapy and the body: How physiological underpinnings of prosociality informed clinical practice. In P. Gilbert & G. Simos (Eds.), *Compassion focused therapy: Clinical practice and applications* (pp. 345–359). Routledge.

Petrocchi, N., Ottaviani, C., Cheli, S., Matos, M., Baldi, B., Basran, J. K., & Gilbert, P. (2024). The impact of compassion-focused therapy on positive and negative mental health outcomes: Results of a series of meta-analyses. *Clinical Psychology: Science and Practice, 31*(2), 230–247.

Poulin, M. J. (2017). To help or not to help: Goal commitment and the goodness of compassion. In E. M. Seppälä, E. Simon-Thomas, S. L. Brown, M. C. Worline, L. Cameron, & J. R. Doty (Eds.), *The Oxford handbook of compassion science* (pp. 355–367). Oxford University Press.

Ricard, M. (2015). *Altruism: The power of compassion to change yourself and the world.* Atlantic Books.

Roland, D. (2020). *The power of suffering.* Simon & Schuster.

Sapolsky, R. M. (2023). *Determined: Life without free will.* Random House.

Scheffer, J. A., Cameron, C. D., & Inzlicht, M. (2022). Caring is costly: People avoid the cognitive work of compassion. *Journal of Experimental Psychology: General, 151*(1), 172.

Siegel, D. J. (2023). *Intraconnected: Mwe (Me+We) is the integration of self, identity, and belonging.* Norton.

Spikins, P. (2015). *How compassion made us human: The evolutionary origins of tenderness, trust, and morality.* Spear and Sword Books.

Teasdale, J. D., & Chaskalson, M. (2013). How does mindfulness transform suffering?: I. The nature and origins of dukkha. *Contemporary Buddhism, 12*(1), 89–102.

Vrtička, P., Favre, P., & Singer, T. (2017). Compassion and the brain. In P. Gilbert (Ed.), *Compassion: Concepts, research, and applications* (pp. 135–151). Routledge.

Weng, H. Y., Lapate, R. C., Stodola, D. E., Rogers, G. M., & Davidson, R. J. (2018). Visual attention to suffering after compassion training is associated with decreased amygdala responses. *Frontiers in Psychology, 9*, 771.

Yaden, D. B., Haidt, J., Hood, R. W., Jr., Vago, D. R., & Newberg, A. B. (2017). The varieties of self-transcendent experience. *Review of General Psychology, 21*(2), 143–160

3

Expanding the Contemporary Meaning of "Self"

An Interpersonal Neurobiology Perspective on Inner-Compassion and Intraconnection

Elli Weisbaum
Shelby L. Alsup
Daniel J. Siegel

In this chapter, we propose that the fields of neuroscience, attachment, and mindfulness support an expanded conceptualization of the "self" that goes beyond our individual physical bodies. This orientation toward viewing the self as not wholly separate from other living beings and the wider cosmos can help to dismantle some of the systemic/cultural/social/psychological barriers that often exist in relation to "self-compassion." We apply the transdisciplinary lens of interpersonal neurobiology to explore the concept and experience of the "self."

In interpersonal neurobiology, the focus is on uncovering consilience among a wide range of knowledge streams by weaving together perspectives that thoughtfully integrate science and subjective experience. The central aim is to understand the mind, define and promote mental health, and bring more compassion and kindness into the world (Siegel, 2012). Consilience can be defined as "the convergence of evidence from independent sources and methods of measurement to support one coherent conclusion; connecting concepts, models, and principles from different disciplines to promote the formation of a unified and comprehensive theory" (Mascaro et al., 2020, p. 3). It is through this orientation toward knowledge production that we examine and integrate wisdom from the fields of (1) neuroscience (e.g., looking at neural circuits related to compassion/empathy), (2) attachment (e.g., how "relational integration" can promote secure attachment and therapeutic alliance), and (3) mindfulness (e.g., drawing upon the central

Buddhist psychology concept of non-self/emptiness) to explore and expand the concept of the "self." We also wish to recognize that there are many knowledge streams and perspectives from across scientific, contemplative, and indigenous wisdom traditions that contribute deep insights into the nature of existence that are beyond the scope of what we can fit into this chapter. Therefore, we invite you to consider what is explored here not as wholly comprehensive but as a contribution to a wider dialogue.

Our exploration begins with the proposal that the term *self* may refer to something that does not need to be limited to a separate or singular body. As we explore this proposal, it may be useful to consider that our experience of "self" can be seen to be rooted in our "subjective sensations of being alive, the perspective we have on the world, and the agency we assert in shaping our behavior and interactions" (Siegel, 2023, p. 1). Understanding that our notion of self is often rooted in our sensations, perspectives, and agency can help us see that the idea of a "solo self" (wholly separate from the world around us) is potentially a top-down construction, informed by our subjective lived experience of having a physical body. If we are not aware of this construction, it can become an unconscious reinforcement of a solo self, which can lead to a sense of separation/isolation. This narrative of separation can be an impediment to both inner and outer compassion. In this chapter, we suggest that expanding our conceptualization of the self to go beyond the physical body may be a useful way to help articulate the pragmatic application of compassion—its experience and its cultivation—by using a three-part framework (see Figure 3.1):

1. Inner-compassion (relating to our relationship with our inner landscape/states/mental activities/physical body)
2. Intercompassion (relating to our interpersonal relationships and our interconnectedness with all of nature)
3. Intracompassion (relating to our integrated relationship that differentiates the inner and the inter- and combines these into an integrated whole: me [inner] plus we [inter-] as MWe (Me + We)—our intraconnected identity).

Our aim in this chapter is to provide those interested in promoting self-compassion—to clinicians and beyond—with language and scientific evidence that is accessible and supportive to these efforts. Therefore, we invite you, the reader, to not take our word for any of this. Rather, you are invited to proceed into this chapter with a critical investigative mind to consider how the discussion put forth reflects your own direct experience and understanding of "self" in relation to your inner-, inter-, and intralived experiences.

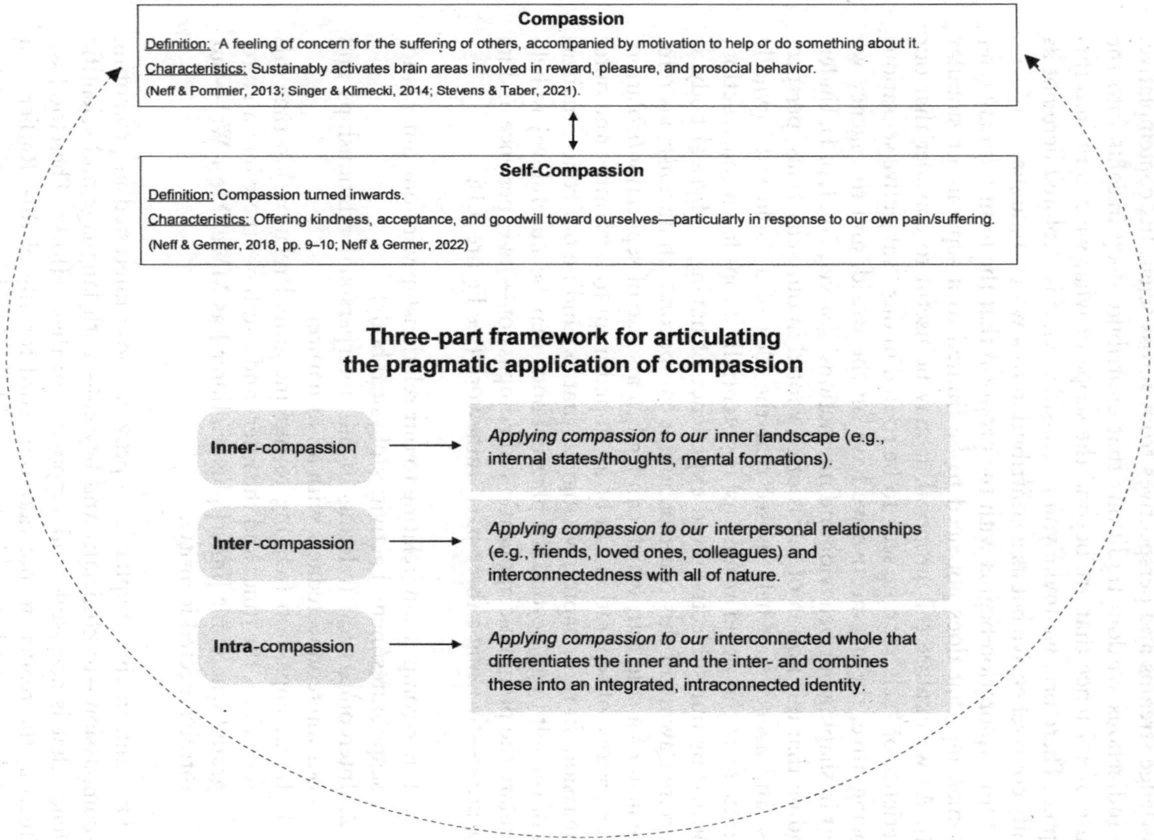

FIGURE 3.1. Three-part framework: pragmatic applications of compassion.

Integrating and Exploring Three Knowledge Streams' Perspectives on the Experience, Concept, and Notion of "Self": Neuroscience, Attachment, and Mindfulness

Neuroscientific Perspectives on "Self"

Similarly to consciousness, the self has become a burgeoning topic in neuroscience. For example, there is an entire area of study around the homunculus and how it creates a full representative map of the physical body (Huang & Sereno, 2018; Muret et al., 2022). There is also a fascinating body of research looking at "visuotactile integration and self-attribution," which explores how the mental maps of our bodies inform our proprioception and sense of *personal space* or *ownership* over the space that we sense we physically "occupy." For example, a well-known study called "The Rubber Hand Illusion" showed that "watching a rubber hand being stroked synchronously with one's own unseen hand causes the rubber hand to be attributed to one's own body" to a degree that participants perceived the position of their own hand as changing (Tsakiris & Haggard, 2005, p. 80). This study, and subsequent replication studies, reveal the interplay among vision, touch, and proprioception to show that visual and tactile stimuli can influence the perceived position of one's own body parts. Studies looking at our perceptions (or misperceptions) of our physical self have also shown that our sense of the space we occupy can readily fluctuate beyond what we might typically consider our "physical" body. For example, if we are holding a tool or driving a car, our sense of the space we occupy grows to encompass the space the tool or car takes up—this is referred to as *peripersonal space* (PPS; Galigani et al., 2020; Ho & Spence, 2009). PPS impacts and informs how we move through space, interact with others, and protect ourselves from external threats (Rabellino et al., 2020). From these examples, we can start to see that there may be cause to problematize the notion that the self is limited only to our physical bodies as a separate entity from the world around us.

Default Mode Network

Understanding our brain's structures and functions can help bring awareness to our inner narratives and how we are constructing and making meaning of our lives. For example, the default mode network, which is linked to mind wandering, ruminating on the future/past, and self-referential processing (Raffone et al., 2019; Zeidan et al., 2019) has been indicated to be involved in our autobiographical sense of self (Philippi et al., 2015; Spreng & Grady, 2010). Ruminating or reflecting on past experiences and using this to inform how we anticipate and plan for future experiences are useful mechanisms for our survival. It is also an interesting example of how our inner narratives of our lived experience can then shape our interpersonal actions. Our autobiographical memory contributes to our sense of the construction of our "unique personal narrative and identity" (Philippi et al., 2015, p. 318). Our inner narrative of "personal identity" is constructed and informed based, in part, on our recollection of lived experiences—which happen in the inter–intra space.

The fundamental etymological question becomes, "Is the personal body, one's individual somatic skin-encased corpus, a synonym for the term *self*?" If the answer is yes, then the body's boundaries are indeed the defining limits of what self is and what it is not. "Who you are"—what your self is—is *only* your body. Is this true—or is there perhaps a difference between the physical body and the self? Being open to such changes in how we have a direct "sense of self" may allow our conceptualizations of what self is to expand.

The Circuitry of Empathy and Compassion

Research on the circuitry of empathy and compassion clearly demonstrates our interconnection to the living beings around us, and that the lines of separation between ourselves and others are inherently blurry. Empirical research on compassion has steadily grown over the past few decades (Mascaro et al., 2020). This has been driven in part by promising findings related to the potential for compassion to address systemic societal issues, such as burnout and anxiety, including for patient populations and those in caregiving professions (Neff, 2023; Singer & Klimecki, 2014; Stevens & Taber, 2021). Neuroimaging tools, such as functional magnetic resonance imaging, have identified the medial orbitofrontal cortex (mOFC), subgenual anterior cingulate cortex (sgACC), and the ventral striatum/nucleus accumbens (VS/NAcc) as some of the central neural systems activated in relation to compassion. These areas of the brain are associated with reward and pleasure and are indicated to inform prosocial behavior. Research has indicated that compassion training can increase prosocial behaviors, fostering feelings of goodwill and friendliness toward other individuals (Singer & Klimecki, 2014). Within the academic literature, compassion is often defined along the lines of "feeling concern for the suffering of others, accompanied by motivation to help or do something about it." This broader definition of compassion can be seen as reflective of the aims embedded in self-compassion. Self-compassion has been characterized by Neff and Germer (2018) as offering kindness, acceptance, emotional awareness, and goodwill toward "ourselves"—particularly in response to our own pain/suffering/challenges—just like we might toward a good friend or someone we love (pp. 9–10). It has been proposed that from a certain viewpoint, "self-compassion is simply compassion directed inward" (Neff & Pommier, 2013, p. 160).

If self-compassion is the inward direction of compassion, then we might consider that outcomes often associated with compassion externally—such as the increase of prosocial behavior—might then also be seen internally. Neff and Pommier (2013) conducted a study with college undergraduates, community adults, and practicing meditators that showed that an increase in self-compassion not only enhances an individual's own psychological health but can benefit others that the individual interacts with. One of the study's central conclusions was that self-compassion goes "hand in hand" with "other-focused concern" or the capacity to have compassion for others. These findings concretely suggest that there is no clear boundary between "self" compassion and compassion for other living beings. Therefore, in this chapter, we are proposing the nomenclature of *inner compassion* for what is commonly called *self-compassion* and *intercompassion* for what is typically called "compassion." This language can be useful for expanding the limiting notion of self. Removing the label of "self" can also help assuage the common concern that self-compassion is "selfish."

In relation to the circuitry of compassion, it can be useful to compare and contrast the circuitry of empathy. Research has shown that empathy activates a distinctly different set of neural systems than compassion. Some of the primary neural systems activated in relation to empathy are the anterior insula and anterior/midcingulate cortex (Singer & Klimecki, 2014; Stevens & Taber, 2021). Research on this circuitry has demonstrated that empathy and compassion represent two unique sets of processes and experiences, both of which play a significant role in one's motivation to help or care for others. This distinction is important, as empathy, particularly in clinical settings, can sometimes be mislabeled as "bad" due to the existence of "empathy fatigue"—which can happen if one remains in empathetic resonance with another (e.g., a patient) over a longer period of time. Compassion is often mislabeled or conflated with the concept of empathetic distress or fatigue—however, research has shown that compassion can be seen as a different neuro "lane" from empathy, one that is prosocial and sustainable over time, rather than fatiguing. Some of the neural systems activated in relation to compassion are the VS/NAcc, sgACC, and mOFC (Singer & Klimecki, 2014; Stevens & Taber, 2021).

Empathy is an integral part of our innate capacity to care for others and is shown to lead toward and inform compassion (Stevens & Taber, 2021). Understanding that our natural ability to empathetically resonate with the experience of others involves the activation of brain regions that would also light up if we ourselves had a similar experience, further suggests that at the neural level, the distinction of "self" and "other" is not as obvious as one might initially think. Recognizing that we are not wholly separate from the people around us and that empathetic resonance over longer periods of time can lead toward behaviors such as withdrawal and burnout, is of particular relevance to clinicians, whose jobs often involve witnessing and holding space for their patients' distress. Encouragingly, research has shown that it is possible to train skill sets that can enhance empathy to promote healthy perspective taking as a motivation to care, while also developing the skill set to switch to the lane of compassion in order to provide care in a way that can be sustainable over the long term (see Practices D.1, "Forgiveness," and D.2, "Connecting to the Collective MWe," in the Appendix).

Reflection: Neuroscience Perspectives on the "Self"

The evidence explored in this section has illustrated that the physiological circuitry of our brains is fundamentally impacted by the physical and emotional experiences of those around us. This supports our proposal of an expanded understanding of the self beyond the physical body. This is reflective of what interpersonal neurobiology has proposed in relation to conceptualizing the mind as part of a complex system—a framework rooted in the field of mathematics—which describes a system that is open to influence outside of itself (Siegel, 2016, pp. 34–35).

We invite you to take a moment now to reflect on this from your own lived experience. Have you ever noticed that your inner world (physically and emotionally) is impacted by the distress or joy of the people around you? Do you find it easy to keep your "self" separate from the emotions those around you are expressing? At an *inter*personal level, when someone else has shown kindness or understanding toward you, how has this impacted the understanding or kindness you are able or willing to show back to them? At an *intra*personal level, when you feel a sense of gratitude or appreciation for a beautiful tree or nature spot, how might this impact the care or kindness you are motivated to offer to the planet?

Secure Attachment Perspectives on "Self"

Attachment: Neural and Relational Integration

We begin forming our earliest attachments in utero, where early communication forms through fetal signaling to the pregnant individual and similarly from the pregnant individual to the fetus (Condon, 1993; DiPietro et al., 2021). Once we are born, the relationship between the infant and the caregiver—the attachment relationship—shapes our experience of self (Bowlby, 1988; Sroufe, 1979). These early experiences lay the foundation for our attachments across the lifespan. Attachment is defined as a relationship between a child and caregiver that activates a psychobiological system that helps facilitate a connection to another person. We think about attachment quality as involving behaviors as well as attachment representations falling on a continuum and oscillating between positive or negative views of inner experience and the seeking or avoidance of connection with others (Ainsworth, 1978). Attachment has long been known as a strong predictor of various health outcomes, including psychological and physical health and well-being (Duschinsky, 2020). Our attachments form through our interconnection within experiences of communication; our neural networks allow us to feel another's experience and shape our own. Early attachments shape neurobiological development and organization and help us to understand how to navigate the challenges and joys of our world. Our deeply interconnected nature is embedded early on before we have developed conceptual understanding and language for what these relationships are to look like. Attachment unfolds through the form of communication where a healthy attachment system includes synchronization, concurrent "dyadic regulation," and communication (Alsup et al., 2020).

Our first attachment experiences, often with our parent or caregiver, form through internalized interactions of an infant or child with their attachment figure. These internalizations are thought to shape our internal representation of both inner and interpersonal experiences that are formed in the mind. Collaborative and integrated communication arises from a space of connection, relation, and resonance operating together in bidirectional harmony (Siegel, 2020). Interconnection flourishes when balanced between *differentiation* and *linkage*. Differentiation occurs in a healthy connection through the established and evident understanding of the inner within the interrelationship. Linkage unfolds in the strong connection that is formed interpersonally. The harmonious intersection of differentiation and linkage is known as integration. In healthy relationships, integration emerges as open awareness, attunement, resonance, and love—it is how we honor differences and promote compassionate linkages. Healthy relational integration can be seen when we are able to link or connect with others while maintaining differentiation. This is reflective of what was explored earlier in relation to the circuitry of empathy and compassion. The concepts of attachment and the linkage and differentiation of integration can be useful for setting healthy boundaries, particularly for those in caregiving professions.

Therapeutic Alliance

As providers, focusing on the core concepts of connection, relating, and resonating must come into play when providing care and establishing an alliance with a patient (Siegel, 2010, 2020). When we explore our interpersonal relationships, we must first reflect on and explore our attachment origins. When thinking about our earliest attachments, secure attachment is understood as the parental embodiment of flexibility and safety wherein the parent acts as an external source of what we can call "inner regulation" for the child (Sroufe, 1979). In other words, dyadic interaction leads to an inner state of soothing internal states of distress. A child who experiences secure attachment feels safe to explore the world around them from a "secure base" knowing that when distress arises, their parents are there to console them and provide comfort as a "safe haven." Ultimately, a secure attachment presents itself in relational integration where there is a recognizable balance of differentiation and linkage and the relationship promotes emotional well-being, safety, and a felt sense of belonging (Siegel, 2020).

These same secure attachments can form across the lifespan, well into adulthood. Attachment often serves as a lens through which we see the world and develop as an individual, communally, and with nature. We can think of attachment as the way we navigate the social landscape, bringing with us our past attachments into those new attachments, with the inherent malleability to reorganize our understanding of "healthy" attachments and relationships (Cozolino, 2014). Having both an inner secure base and an intersafe haven is what is meant by someone having security of attachment.

Reflection: Attachment Perspectives on the "Self"

The research investigated in this section demonstrates how attachment is sought out beginning in early childhood and even prior to this in utero. Knowing the long-standing nature of the human need to connect, we can begin to understand the fundamental elements of our inner survival in part determined by our inter- and intrarelations. Once again, we invite you to reflect on how the evidence discussed in this section resonates (or not) with your own lived experience. At the *inter*personal level, how have your own attachment experiences informed your *inner* capacity for empathy and compassion (perhaps with colleagues, friends, or family)? Or how have your experiences of attachment impacted your sense of belonging or love?

Mindfulness Perspectives on "Self"

Context: Buddhist Psychology and the Work of Thich Nhat Hanh

We have chosen to explore evidence from the field of mindfulness in this chapter as it plays a key role in the scientific literature on how to train and cultivate self-compassion. Neff and Germer have proposed that self-compassion contains three elements: self-kindness, common humanity, and mindfulness (Neff, 2003; Neff & Germer, 2018, pp. 10–11). While mindfulness can be seen to have roots in many wisdom traditions from around the world, for the purposes of our discussion in this chapter, we draw upon concepts related to mindfulness that are rooted in the knowledge stream of Buddhist psychology. The exploration that follows draws primarily upon the work of scholar, peace activist, Nobel Peace Prize nominee, and Zen master Thich Nhat Hanh, who is credited in the literature as coining the phrase *engaged mindfulness* and is considered one of the most influential and prolific contemporary Zen masters and translators of Buddhist practice into contemporary settings (Kyte, 2019).

The concept of compassion is prevalent across the majority of Buddhist discourses. One of the key conceptual frameworks that includes compassion is called the "Four Immeasurable Minds" or the "Minds of True Love" (Nhat Hanh, 1999, pp. 169–175). This framework is referred to as "immeasurable" because the qualities included in the framework, including compassion, are considered to be "limitless"—that is, Buddhist teachings propose that they are longitudinally maintainable and sustainable. This proposal reflects the evidence from neuroscientific studies discussed earlier in this chapter, which indicate that compassion is a replenishing and sustainable state.

Situating the Concept of Emptiness or Non-Self within Buddhist Psychology

In Buddhist psychology, perceiving the "self" as a wholly separate entity is considered one of the two "obstacles" because this perception discounts our inherent interconnectedness or relationality to the beings and world around us (Nhat Hanh, 2011, pp. 87–88). The misperception of a separate self is seen to obstruct or limit our capacity to understand and love our inner selves, or what Buddhist psychology refers to as the five *aggregates* or *territories* that are a reflection of what comprises a human being (Nhat Hanh, 1988, pp. 7–10). The five aggregates (referred to as the five *skandhas*) include body, feelings, perceptions, mental formations, and consciousness (Nhat Hanh, 2001, pp. 27–28). Misconceptualizing the self as separate extends beyond just an inner obstacle and is seen to also impact our capacity for cultivating understanding/love in the context of our interpersonal relationships (e.g., friends, family, colleagues), along with our relationship to the wider cosmos (e.g., animals, plants, minerals, the planet).

Unpacking the Concept of Emptiness or Non-Self

Emptiness or non-self is sometimes misleading or confusing for contemporary scholars, who may at first glance interpret it as a form of nihilism. This interpretation is categorically incorrect. Nhat Hanh states that "emptiness does not mean nothingness or nonexistence; it only means there is no such thing as a separate 'self' entity" (Nhat Hanh, 1988, pp. 7–10; Nhat

Hanh, 2011, pp. 87–88). He states that we should be careful of our assumptions about what is meant by the term *empty* and that we can check our assumptions by asking the clarifying question "What are we empty of?" (Nhat Hanh, 1988, pp. 7–10). The answer, in the context of Buddhist psychology, is that we are empty of a separate self, but full of the cosmos (Nhat Hanh, 2001, pp. 47–48). At first, it may seem contradictory to say that being empty actually means we are full. However, this seemingly paradoxical proposal can be pragmatically understood by examining what elements are necessary for a flower to exist. For example, if the sunshine, the rain, and the Earth did not exist, the flower would also not exist. Therefore, the flower does not exist as a separate self-entity—it must "inter-be" with non-flower elements in order to exist. We can apply this same reasoning to human beings. We know that if oxygen, sunshine, or our parents did not exist, we would also not exist. Therefore, we can think of ourselves as made up of non-self elements. Therefore, we are empty of just one thing: a separate self.

Reflection: Mindfulness Perspectives on the "Self"

The Buddhist proposal that both our physical and mental existence is inherently interconnected with the world around us is reflective of what we explored earlier in this chapter in the sections above on neuroscience and attachment. Similarly to neuroscientific and attachment perspectives, Buddhist psychology recognizes the delusion of separation, while also recognizing the usefulness of conceptualizing/validating our personal inner experiences in relation to our outer experiences. Therefore, Buddhist psychology is not proposing that our inner experiences are not valid but that the existence of inner experiences does not define us as a separate self. This may seem somewhat paradoxical. However, the perspective that reality is made up of multiple truths is found across many disciplines interested in behavior and consciousness. For an example of this, we can look to the different branches of physics, which show reality to have a potential range of probabilities. Classical or Newtonian physics explores absolute certainties (e.g., reality is made up of large separate objects or noun-like entities), whereas studies in quantum physics look at processes related to entanglement or interconnection (e.g., all things are deeply interconnected even if we cannot currently see all their connections and they function more as verb-like, deeply connected events; Siegel, 2016, p. 48; Siegel, 2023).

Once again, we invite you to hold these proposals up to your own lived experience. Can you think of the non-self elements that you would not exist without (e.g., the sun, trees/oxygen, or your DNA)? What implications might the insight of non-self or interconnection have on your relationship to your family/friends or to the planet?

Conclusion

Evidence and concepts from across the fields of neuroscience, attachment, and mindfulness all point toward the physical boundaries of the "self" as being blurry. Work from across these fields illustrates a consilient perspective that the human mind and enskulled brain are informed and changed by both our internal and external lived experiences across our lifespan. How we understand our shared experiences (i.e., inter-) is inextricably linked to our inner and our intra-experiences, not only through our conscious awareness and present-moment mindedness but also through our neural circuitry. The discussion put forth in this chapter demonstrates that the construct we typically label as "self" includes our within and between experiences from early childhood, current relationships, educational/societal systems, occupational spaces, the air we breathe, and even the conversations we have. At the same time, all three fields also acknowledge and point toward the existence of a physiological body/individual human being who has unique and valid inner experiences. These two coexisting realities—that the "self" goes beyond our construction of a solo self *and* that there is an individual with unique inner experiences—may seem somewhat contradictory. Therefore, from the lens of interpersonal neurobiology, the following question arises: "What can we do to find consilience amidst this paradox of the 'self'?" We propose that the terminology of inner, inter-, and intra- can be a useful way to navigate this paradox, particularly in relation to the pragmatic conceptualization and application of compassion (see Figure 3.1).

We have endeavored to triangulate perspectives from the fields of neuroscience, attachment, and mindfulness to form an integrative whole. The central aim is to consider how compassion can be integrated and useful to our inner world in order to inform our interpersonal relationships and support the development of healthy intrarelationships (Figure 3.1), without getting overly caught in the language of "self" versus "other." These distinct—yet not wholly separate—domains are useful as they give us a map for thinking about where and how compassion can be applied (Figure 3.1). This in turn can assist in dismantling the idea that self-compassion is "selfish" or separated from the care we provide to ourselves, others, and our planet.

Buddhist psychology proposes that we do not get caught in any one conceptualization of reality, but rather that we utilize concepts and terms so long as they are useful. Therefore, we propose the language of inner-/inter-/intracompassion not as a comprehensive description of reality but as a pragmatic tool to be taken up for when it is useful. With this in mind, we once again invite you, the reader, to hold up what has been presented in this chapter to your own lived experience. The aim of this is to encourage you to take a *settings approach* (Poland et al., 2009) to the application of what you have just read. We hope this helps you to utilize what has been explored in this chapter in a way that is socially and culturally responsive to the spaces and contexts that you serve, inclusive of your inner/inter-/intraworlds.

REFERENCES

Ainsworth, M. D. S. (1978). The Bowlby–Ainsworth attachment theory. *Behavioral and Brain Sciences, 1*(3), 436–438.

Alsup, S. L., Weisbaum, E., Vogel, T., & Siegel, D. J. (2020). Family relations, friendships, and love. In W. IsHak (Ed.), *The handbook of wellness medicine* (pp. 553–564). Cambridge University Press.

Bowlby, J. (1988). Developmental psychiatry comes of age. *American Journal of Psychiatry, 145*(1), 1–10.

Condon, J. T. (1993). The assessment of antenatal emotional attachment: Development of a questionnaire instrument. *British Journal of Medical Psychology, 66*(2), 167–183.

Cozolino, L. (2014). *The neuroscience of human relationships: Attachment and the developing social brain*. Norton.

DiPietro, J. A., Kivlighan, K. T., Voegtline, K. M., Costigan, K. A., & Moore, G. A. (2021). It takes two: An antenatal to postnatal RDoC framework for investigating the origins of maternal attachment and mother–infant social communication. *Development and Psychopathology, 33*(5), 1539–1553.

Duschinsky, R. (2020). *Cornerstones of attachment research*. Oxford University Press.

Galigani, M., Castellani, N., Donno, B., Franza, M., Zuber, C., Allet, L., et al. (2020). Effect of tool-use observation on metric body representation and peripersonal space. *Neuropsychologia, 148*, 107622.

Ho, C., & Spence, C. (2009). Using peripersonal warning signals to orient a driver's gaze. *Human Factors, 51*(4), 539–556.

Huang, R. S., & Sereno, M. I. (2018). Multisensory and sensorimotor maps. In P. J. Vinken, G. W. Bruyn, & H. L. Klawans (Eds.), *Handbook of clinical neurology* (pp. 141–161). Wiley.

Kyte, L. (2019, October 19). The life of Thich Nhat Hanh. In *Lion's roar: Buddhist wisdom for our time*. www.lionsroar.com/the-life-of-thich-nhat-hanh.

Mascaro, J. S., Florian, M. P., Ash, M. J., Palmer, P. K., Frazier, T., Condon, P., & Raison, C. (2020). Ways of knowing compassion: How do we come to know, understand, and measure compassion when we see it? *Frontiers in Psychology, 11*, 547241.

Muret, D., Root, V., Kieliba, P., Clode, D., & Makin, T. R. (2022). Beyond body maps: Information content of specific body parts is distributed across the somatosensory homunculus. *Cell Reports, 38*(11), 110523.

Neff, K. (2003). Self-compassion: An alternative conceptualization of a healthy attitude toward oneself. *Self and Identity, 2*(2), 85–101.

Neff, K. (2023). Self-compassion: Theory, method, research, and intervention. *Annual Review of Psychology, 74*, 193–218.

Neff, K., & Germer, C. K. (2018). *The mindful self-compassion workbook: A proven way to accept yourself, build inner strength, and thrive.* Guilford Press.

Neff, K., & Pommier, E. (2013). The relationship between self-compassion and other-focused concern among college undergraduates, community adults, and practicing meditators. *Self and Identity, 12*(2), 160–176.

Nhat Hanh, T. (1988). *The heart of understanding: Commentaries on the Prajnaparamita heart sutra.* Parallax Press.

Nhat Hanh, T. (1999). *The heart of the Buddha's teaching: Transforming suffering into peace, joy & liberation.* Harmony Books.

Nhat Hanh, T. (2001). *Peace begins here: Palestinians and Israelis listening to each other.* Parallax Press.

Nhat Hanh, T. (2011). *Peace is every breath: A practice for our busy lives.* Random House.

Philippi, C. L., Tranel, D., Duff, M., & Rudrauf, D. (2015). Damage to the default mode network disrupts autobiographical memory retrieval. *Social Cognitive and Affective Neuroscience, 10*(3), 318–326.

Poland, B., Krupa, G., & McCall, D. (2009). Settings for health promotion: An analytic framework to guide intervention design and implementation. *Health Promotion Practice, 10*(4), 505–516.

Rabellino, D., Frewen, P. A., McKinnon, M. C., & Lanius, R. A. (2020). Peripersonal space and bodily self-consciousness: Implications for psychological trauma-related disorders. *Frontiers in Neuroscience, 14*, 586605.

Raffone, A., Marzetti, L., Del Gratta, C., Perrucci, M. G., Romani, G. L., & Pizzella, V. (2019). Toward a brain theory of meditation. *Progress in Brain Research, 244*, 207–232.

Siegel, D. J. (2010). *The mindful therapist: A clinician's guide to mindsight and neural integration.* Norton.

Siegel, D. J. (2012). *Pocket guide to interpersonal neurobiology: An integrative handbook of the mind.* Norton.

Siegel, D. J. (2016). *Mind: A journey to the heart of being human.* Norton.

Siegel, D. J. (2020). *The developing mind: How relationships and the brain interact to shape who we are.* Guilford Press.

Siegel, D. J. (2023). *Intraconnected.* Norton.

Singer, T., & Klimecki, O. M. (2014). Empathy and compassion. *Current Biology, 24*(18), R875–R878.

Spreng, R. N., & Grady, C. L. (2010). Patterns of brain activity supporting autobiographical memory, prospection, and theory of mind, and their relationship to the default mode network. *Journal of Cognitive Neuroscience, 22*(6), 1112–1123.

Sroufe, L. A. (1979). The coherence of individual development: Early care, attachment, and subsequent developmental issues. *American Psychologist, 34*, 834–841.

Stevens, F., & Taber, K. (2021). The neuroscience of empathy and compassion in pro-social behavior. *Neuropsychologia, 159*, 107925.

Teicholz, T. (2017, October 11). Soul surfer: Rabbi's genius quest for a soulful life ("Einstein and The Rabbi" by Naomi Levy [Flatiron Books]). *Huffington*

Post. www.huffpost.com/entry/soul-surfer-rabbis-genius-quest-for-a-soulful-life_b_59de86f3e4b069e5b833b20c.

Tsakiris, M., & Haggard, P. (2005). The rubber hand illusion revisited: Visuotactile integration and self-attribution. *Journal of Experimental Psychology: Human Perception and Performance, 31*(1), 80–91.

Zeidan, F., Baumgartner, J. N., & Coghill, R. C. (2019). The neural mechanisms of mindfulness-based pain relief: A functional magnetic resonance imaging-based review and primer. *Pain Reports, 4*(4), e759.

4

Working with Challenges of Cross-Cultural Psychotherapy with Self-Compassion

Sydney S. Spears
Tracy Ochester

As more and more therapists integrate the practices and concepts of self-compassion into their work with clients, we are encouraged by their potential to help the therapy dyad navigate the complexities of multiculturalism, especially where clients and therapists hold different cultural identities. Sociocultural self-awareness is a foundational aspect of cultural competency and responsiveness (Sue et al., 2016). It supports the expansion of cross-cultural insight and the necessity to integrate the associated competencies of sociocultural knowledge and skillfulness. The process of cultivating this type of self-awareness requires therapists to authentically acknowledge and understand the meaning of their own regional sociocultural conditioning and identities. Developing this type of self-awareness also engages therapists to explore and address their own cross-cultural knowledge gaps and skill-based limitations, including their biases, values, and assumptions (Sue et al., 2016).

For most therapists, embracing this important work is generally not a quick fix or a learning journey of complete ease. Typically, this process is laden with a degree of discomfort and resistance. When certain difficult emotions are experienced, such as fear, guilt, grief, anger, rage, and shame, the fight–flight–freeze response tends to activate the "unholy trinity of self-criticism, self-isolation, and self-absorption" (Germer & Neff, 2015, p. 43). Some therapists can become derailed by these reactions, which often generate avoidance or minimization of sociocultural influences within cross-cultural relationships and encounters (Hardy, 2023; Stampley & Slaght, 2004).

Since cultivating sociocultural self-awareness can be an emotionally challenging venture, there is a critical need for a supportive resource when engaging in this work. We propose that the practice of self-compassion may be one such resource. In fact, Germer and Neff (2015) conceptualize self-compassion as "the emotional attitude of mindfulness—especially in the context of psychotherapy, in which suffering is the focus of attention" (Germer & Neff, 2015, p. 47). In light of this and in conjunction with our own observations and professional experiences, we speculate that practicing self-compassion may help address some of the challenges of cross-cultural responsiveness.

Research indicates that self-compassion is correlated with an increased capacity for being with difficult emotional experiences (Neff, 2011). This expanded capacity not only supports personal well-being and resilience but it can also be a resource for the advancement of cross-cultural training, competencies, and culturally responsive therapeutic processes. Self-compassion provides a sense of personal grounding and self-kindness that can help clients and therapists persist when uncertainties and challenges inevitably arise. In addition, the practices can be titrated when experiencing strong resistance or intense emotions in relation to cross-cultural work.

In this chapter, we (1) discuss the importance of multicultural responsiveness to the therapeutic alliance, (2) suggest ways that therapists can self-compassionately develop cross-cultural competencies critical for effective responsiveness, (3) explore common cross-cultural challenges, and (4) provide examples of ways self-compassion can support and empower therapists and clients within the therapeutic relationship.

The Importance of Multicultural Responsiveness to the Therapeutic Alliance

Decades of research exploring factors impacting therapy outcomes indicate that the therapeutic alliance, commonly called the therapy relationship, as perceived by the client, accounts for about 30% of the variance (Lambert, 1992). A more recent meta-analysis of 295 independent studies suggested a predictive relationship between alliance and outcomes, with the alliance accounting for about 8% of the variability in treatment outcomes (Flückiger et al., 2018). The therapeutic alliance includes an affective bond as well as an agreement on the goals, objectives, and tasks of therapy, supported through empathy, positive regard, cultural congruence, repair of relationship ruptures, avoidance of countertransference, and matching with the individual client (Tschacher et al., 2015).

According to Lambert (1992), the therapeutic alliance contributes to the largest percentage of change within which the therapist has some influence. The other common factors Lambert observed included extratherapeutic change (40%), expectancy (15%), and techniques (15%). Given this, there is a general consensus that the ability to develop a good therapeutic relationship is crucial to treatment success. This finding presents an important opportunity for therapists to be intentional about having a beneficial impact.

Globally, the heterogeneous expressions of culture and the increase of diverse cultural identities are ubiquitous (Lee et al., 2021). Yet, the overall meaning of culture is not simple, one-dimensional, or static. Cross-cultural psychotherapy involves the unique processes that are involved for therapists and clients when their sociocultural identities and cultural experiences are different from one another, such as race, nationality, foreign identity, socioeconomic class, gender, age, ethnicity, sexual orientation, and religion (Lee et al., 2021).

Within the literature, culture has been conceptualized by various scholars in both its similarities and differences. For instance, Draguns (2004) proposes that cultures tend to differ in their artifact, including their implicit and explicit languages, production systems, and philosophies of life. According to Tseng and Strelzer (2001), cultural identity issues are significant aspects of the self, which highly influence the psychotherapeutic cross-cultural relationship and processes. Draguns posits that psychotherapy always involves a sociocultural context with related client–therapist assumptions, meanings, and shared learning. In consideration of these perspectives, therapists must recognize and understand how different experiences, norms, and worldviews of cultural identity influence and shape the clinical process.

Multiculturalism in clinical practice emphasizes addressing the unique realities and sociopolitical challenges of diverse clients (Sue et al., 2016). This approach supports the significance of cross-cultural sensitivity, awareness, knowledge, and skillfulness necessary to provide effective service, especially when therapists work with unknown client identities.

Within the therapy room, practicing self-compassion can be a useful resource for both clients and therapists when responding to cross-cultural differences and related difficulties that can arise within the therapeutic relationship. At its essence, self-compassion can be an internalized container of kindness, warmth, and empowerment when experiencing cross-cultural misunderstandings, lack of connection, microaggressions, and ruptures. Both therapists and clients can deepen their cross-cultural relationship by learning to respond to their own discomfort and suffering with self-compassion and to each other's relational pain with compassion.

Another important aspect of multicultural practice is therapists' ability to cultivate greater awareness concerning the specific cultural and sociopolitical oppressive experiences of clients. Some of the dominant societal systems of oppression with which many culturally diverse clients interface include patriarchy, sexism, racism, classism, casteism, colonialism, homophobia, transphobia, xenophobia, ableism, ageism, heterosexism, anti-Semitism, religious oppression, body oppression, and beyond. These socially constructed systems sustain a culturally disempowered hierarchical structure for those deemed to have nondominant status (Sue, 2016). Specifically, "diverse clients' experiences, social relationships, and problems in living are influenced and shaped by social, economic, and political systems, as well as by dominant ideologies that shape the theoretical and conceptual contours of these systems" (Sue, 2016, p. 18).

Developing an understanding of these harmful societal dynamics is necessary to prevent the therapy room from becoming a microcosm of these oppressive forces. The resource of self-compassion is a developmental practice that can support therapists in building authentic interest in and curiosity about these forces. The practices can increase their capacity for expanding their sociocultural self-awareness, knowledge, and skillful approaches. For example, when confronted with feelings of guilt or shame for oppressing certain marginalized communities through conditioned biases, self-compassion supports giving ourselves the care, motivation, or empowerment we may need so that we can remain engaged in the work (Neff, 2011).

Developing Cross-Cultural Competencies Critical for Effective Responsiveness

Cultural responsiveness is the practice of responding respectfully and effectively to people with a broad intersection of diversity variables and dimensions. It requires a number of competencies, including attitudes, skills, and practices that can strengthen the therapeutic alliance (Owen et al., 2016) and help prevent and repair ruptures (Miles et al., 2021).

It is widely understood now that cultural responsiveness is a necessary skill for mental health professionals. Many professional associations have attempted to codify standards of cultural competence for the professionals they govern. For example, the National Association of Social Workers (2015) publishes *Standards and Indicators for Cultural Competence in Social Work Practice*, including guidelines for self-awareness, cross-cultural knowledge and skills, empowerment, advocacy, and more. The American Psychological Association (2017) publishes *Multicultural Guidelines: An Ecological Approach to Context, Identity, and Intersectionality*, which includes understanding the role of the social and physical environment, power, privilege, and oppression, the use of culturally adaptive interventions, and taking a strength-based approach.

Several studies have demonstrated that cultural congruence between therapist and client, often through active engagement by therapists in cross-cultural conversations during therapy, enhances the therapeutic alliance (Lee, 2011). In addition, a 2011 meta-analysis demonstrated that when evidence-based treatments were adapted to be congruent with a client's cultural group's beliefs there was a modest effect size over unadapted evidence-based treatments (Benish et al., 2011). From these findings, we might conclude that therapist willingness and capacity for multicultural responsiveness has a significant impact on the therapeutic alliance and, consequently, the efficacy of their services. Yet, there are many challenges that can arise in cross-cultural therapy relationships. How therapists and clients meet these challenges can make all the difference.

Since there is a significant positive relationship between self-compassion and cultural competence (Gottlieb & Shibusawa, 2020), and research indicates cultural responsiveness is essential to a strong therapeutic alliance, it follows that therapist self-compassion may improve treatment outcomes. Viewed in this way, this dynamic set of attitudes, skills, and behaviors becomes an ethical imperative and a matter of justice. Yet, reflections upon and discussions of these issues can be very activating and stressful for many.

Common Challenges in Cross-Cultural Psychotherapy

A recent study by Eichstaedt and colleagues (2021) found that the brutal killing of George Floyd, an American Black man, by a White police officer had a profound negative effect on many Black people. Following this traumatic murder, the researchers indicated there was a stark increase in Black people's psychological and physical health struggles. These reactions were also significantly greater for Black people in comparison to the postreactions of White people. This study's findings support the significance of Hardy's (2023) clinical perspective that many clients of color may harbor invisible wounds in psychotherapy. Being a witness and target of relentless dehumanization, assault, brutality, and personal oppression is often a manifestation of racial trauma. "Cultural trauma occurs when members of a collectivity feel they have been subjected to a horrendous event that leaves indelible marks upon their group consciousness," according to Alexander and colleagues (2004, p. 1). Hardy also noted that when people of color enter psychotherapy, the experiences of race and racial trauma tend to be ignored or misidentified as a sign of stress or other secondary symptoms. This illustrates how differing cultural identities between clients and therapists are often situated in a context of divergent multicultural realities about self, others, and the world.

Cross-cultural psychotherapy involves client–therapist dyads in which each person identifies differently across sociocultural experiences, values, languages, and worldviews. Cross-cultural dyads that can be particularly challenging are those in which the therapist holds identities that are dominant within the cultural context while the client holds identities that are marginalized—for example, a White therapist working with an Asian client or a therapist who identifies as heterosexual working with a client who identifies as a lesbian. "It is imperative for clinicians to understand that culture is always a silent participant in every counseling situation" (Stampley & Slaght, 2004, p. 344). Otherwise, the challenges of developing a safe, compassionate, and attuned cross-cultural alliance may give rise to client–therapist relational ruptures and disconnection.

A therapeutic rupture is a deterioration in the therapeutic alliance that can happen for any number of reasons. Ruptures are inevitable in therapy relationships, but they can be more common and complicated to repair when the therapist and client differ in identity, privilege, and culture. This is because there are so many different cultures, they can intersect, they are ever-changing, and one's expression of and attachment to culture can vary from person to person. Perhaps what matters more than the rupture itself is how the therapist responds to it. The resolution of ruptures is moderately associated with positive patient outcomes (Eubanks et al., 2018).

A key challenge when providing responsive cross-cultural competence in psychotherapy that can lead to a rupture is the lack of therapists' cultural self-awareness of examining their own sociocultural identities, socialization experiences, biases, stereotypes, values, and beliefs (Hardy, 2023; Lee et al., 2021; Sue et al., 2016; Yan, 2008). Another salient therapist limitation involves the lack of personal and professional awareness of their socially constructed dominant identities and how these identities render certain sociopolitical power and privileges (Sue et al., 2016). Consequently, there is a need for therapists to critically examine these issues in order to truly expand their sense of cultural self-awareness. "Without such awareness, the counselor who works with a culturally different client may be engaging in cultural oppression using unethical and harmful practices" (Sue et al., 1992, p. 480).

According to the cross-cultural psychotherapy literature, another challenge experienced by many therapists is their limited multicultural knowledge and training regarding the sociopolitical realities of the diverse clients that they serve, including the impact of systemic oppression, discrimination, cultural worldviews, barriers to services, and cultural trauma (Hardy, 2023; Sue et al., 2016, 2019). This deficiency tends to create a major barrier against developing cross-cultural responsive relationships, especially considering the plethora of cultural differences and identities encountered within therapeutic dyads (Lee, 2011; Sue et al., 1992, 2016).

Limited multicultural knowledge can also sustain therapists' stereotypes and implicit biases. The lack of engaging in professional training to build cultural knowledge when working cross-culturally raises the risk of inflicting harm on clients "which borders on a violation of human rights" (Sue et al., 1992, p. 480). This implies therapists must have adequate and ongoing cultural knowledge about diverse clients' experiences in the world and pay attention to their own cultural identities and worldviews.

Another key challenge in cross-cultural work is related to the lack of multicultural skillfulness when engaging with diverse clients. Culturally responsive therapists are able to integrate multicultural approaches in alignment with building and maintaining attuned cross-cultural relationships, which support positive outcomes (Lee, 2011; Sue et al., 1992, 2016). However, it can be challenging for some therapists to fully understand how to actually practice certain cultural competencies with diverse clients (Lee, 2011; Stampley & Slaght, 2004). For example, a study conducted by Jaladin (2013) examined Malaysian counselors' self-perceived multicultural competencies abilities. The highest reported area of cultural competence among this group was found to be multicultural knowledge and understanding. However, the critical dimensions of cultural awareness and skillfulness were self-perceived as lower in competency. In response to this issue, Lee proposed focusing on cross-cultural competencies that reflect the significance of the therapeutic relationship. Relationally based cultural competencies refer to "a clinician's capacity to attune to an individual client's culturally embedded lived experience and to create shared moments in interactions with the client from a different cultural context" (Lee, 2011, p. 190).

For some therapists, immersion into cross-cultural relationships can harbor certain tensions, fears, difficulties, value conflicts, and negative reactions, which are sometimes projected onto their diverse clients (Yan, 2008). This therapeutic phenomenon is conceptualized as cultural countertransference. It is "often rooted in the clinician's cultural biases and/or insensitivity to cultural differences. The result may be a lack of empathy with a distorted perception of the client" (Stampley & Slaght, 2004, p. 333). In Stampley and Slaght's (2004) examination of cultural countertransference, they found that some clinicians responded to cross-cultural challenges and discomfort by using avoidance and distancing tactics, such as client referrals, client labeling, assigning homework, and avoidance of certain topics. Negating the cultural worldviews, values, and needs of diverse clients not only replicates dynamics of interpersonal and systemic oppression but also increases the likelihood of client mistrust and dyad ruptures (Sue et al., 1992, 2016). Many studies indicate that effective cross-cultural work is advanced when therapists use culturally responsive "modalities and define goals consistent with the life experiences and cultural values of clients" (Sue et al., 1992, p. 481).

In terms of therapists' challenges related to their skillfulness, navigating potential therapeutic microaggressions tends to be another challenge in cross-cultural dyads. Microaggressions are "verbal or behavioral indignities, whether intentional or unintentional, that communicate hostile, derogatory, or negative racial slights and insults that potentially have a harmful or unpleasant psychological impact on the target person or group" (Sue et al., 2007, p. 72). In some contexts, this conceptualization often includes other marginalized groups beyond people of color. Microaggressions are categorized across three types of expressions: (1) microassaults—communicating disrespect; (2) microinsults—violent communication, discrimination, or avoidant actions; and (3) microinvalidations—exclusion, negating, or disregarding (Sue et al., 2016). All of these perceived experiences of harm can disrupt cross-cultural relationships, processes, and positive outcomes, especially when microaggressions are unaddressed, unexamined, and unrepaired.

Considering all of these cross-cultural therapeutic complexities and common challenges embedded within multicultural engagement, it is quite typical for many therapists to struggle with the processes of cultivating effective cultural responsiveness. The overarching competencies of working to develop multicultural self-awareness, knowledge, and skillfulness often require the inclusion of underlying supportive approaches to help navigate the discomfort that can arise when therapists and clients encounter dyad cultural differences, worldviews, harm, and personal biases. To address this gap the practice of mindful self-compassion can be a useful, supportive resource for both therapists and clients when experiencing difficulties within the therapeutic cross-cultural relationship and beyond.

We have provided an example of a self-compassionate practice that can support cross-cultural engagement, understanding of diverse realities, and relational connection. I (Sydney) created this practice for clients who have suffered from ongoing sociocultural oppression and trauma. Many of these clients may be more receptive to initially practicing self-kindness when physical objects are involved, as well as culturally based explorations (see Practice E.1, "My Inner Container of Self-Kindness Exploration," in the Appendix for the full practice).

Supporting and Empowering the Therapy Dyad with Self-Compassion

Self-compassion includes three components: mindfulness, recognition of common humanity, and responding with self-kindness (Neff et al., 2007). Each component can help therapists expand their window of presence to support the important ongoing work of multicultural responsiveness. The mindfulness component of self-compassion helps us hold difficult experiences in loving awareness rather than overidentifying with them. The element of common humanity allows us to view difficulty as part of our shared human experience. We recognize that everyone suffers, though the details are different, and everyone wishes to be happy. Finally, the self-kindness component helps calm our threat response system and activates the self-soothing system, so we can relate more effectively with others and our environment. Modeling of self-compassion by the therapist demonstrates personal sovereignty through self-reflection, self-trust, and permission giving.

A self-compassion practice that can support therapists in the process of rupture and repair is befriending the harsh inner critic (Germer & Neff, 2023, pp. 172–178). In the mindful self-compassion program, participants are invited to get to know their self-critical experience, which the developers call the *inner critic* (Germer & Neff, 2019). The following is one of my (Tracy) experiences of how befriending the inner critic was helpful in developing multicultural responsiveness in my work with clients:

> "I have found the personification of my inner critic to be very useful in the process of cultivating cultural responsiveness and learning from mistakes. By relating to the harsh inner critic as just another part of myself, a part with beneficent intentions but unhelpful methods, I am able to face my mistakes with less reactivity and a greater capacity for learning. Rather than experiencing my imperfections as a threat to be defended against or ignored, I can see them as part of being human and investigate them with curiosity and openness so that I can take empowered action."

In addition to self-awareness and self-empowerment, therapists must recognize the pervasiveness of oppression, the importance of intersectionality of identities, and be willing to challenge and take action to change oppressive structures and practices to promote equity and justice for all. Neff's (2021) Fierce Self-Compassion practice can be quite helpful for some clients in the process of rupture and repair. Bringing to mind the harm they experienced, they are invited to be mindful of any associated emotions and physical sensations. They may find it helpful to think to themselves something like "I see what's happening here, and it's not okay." Next, the client is invited to recognize that they are not alone in experiencing this kind of harm and that *they too* are worthy of care, respect, justice, or whatever they did not receive. Finally, the client can be invited to motivate themselves with encouragement and kindness, to set a boundary, or to take some other needed action to protect themselves from harm while still holding others in compassion.

Neff's (2021) conceptualization of Fierce Self-Compassion as protecting, providing, and motivating can be helpful to both therapists and clients in the action stage of anti-oppression work. Neff says self-compassion helps us cope by acknowledging suffering and working toward needed change, and the brave, empowered clarity engendered through fierce energies can inspire us to push back sustainably against oppression. Yet a balance of *both* fierce and tender self-compassion helps prevent us from falling into complacency on one end of the behavior spectrum, and hostility on the other. The self-acceptance built through self-compassion practice empowers us to remain resilient in the face of overwhelming societal harm (Neff, 2021).

The following cross-cultural segment of a case vignette and a self-compassion practice with me (Sydney) also illustrates the usefulness of self-compassion as a resource when client–therapist challenges arise:

Cross-Cultural Clinical Vignette: Integrating Self-Compassion toward Increasing Therapist Sensitivity, Empowering the Client, and Strengthening the Therapeutic Alliance

During the first session, I shared my core identities—a Black, multiracial, cisgender/woman—with the client. In some regions, the term *cisgender* means identifying with the sex one was assigned at birth. In this case, there were many cultural differences within the dyad, especially divergent gender identities and racial identities. My practice of self-compassion, compassion for the client, and being present with cultural humility has helped me to be aware and attuned to the differences in cross-cultural dyads that lay the critical groundwork for authentic cultural self-acceptance.

In this case vignette, an adult White, transgender woman–identified client requested therapy to address issues related to family relational conflicts and recent experiences of coming out to her parents as a transgender woman. One parent's reactions to the client's coming out generated the client's sadness, frustration, and a sense of nonacceptance of her gender identity. During this time, the client was experiencing several concurrent identity-based, relational, and role shifts, including gender identity–transitioning processes, a recent divorce, relocating to her parents' home, and starting a new academic program to cultivate a new career.

During recent sessions, the client had been sharing her frustrations about the conflicts with the nonaccepting parent, as well as two different interpersonal microaggressive experiences in which transphobic and oppressive comments were made in the presence of the client. The client reacted to these situations with natural anger and voiced her frustration regarding these harmful experiences of nonacceptance of her trans identity and the trans community. As a result, she struggled with excessively ruminating about these microaggressions, which increased her stress and anxiety load as she was trying to cope with navigating a more expansive life.

The client and I had a very organic cross-cultural conversation about her experiences, feelings, self-observations, microaggressions, and relationships. I mentioned the possible need to practice self-kindness/self-compassion to build a sense of wise, empowered choices toward the external experiences of nonacceptance, harm, and injustice. The client shared that she needed to be kinder to herself. This was an important client self-assessment. Then, I invited the client to reflect upon the self-kind actions that might decrease her struggles with external nonacceptance and support the client's sense of agency and self-acceptance. The client has been practicing self-compassion by noticing negative thoughts and interrupting this by mindfully acknowledging feelings and remembering that it is okay to be self-kind, imperfect, and sometimes not knowing. The client said this is what ultimately matters. This perspective is true when practicing developing the vital inner empowerment of self-acceptance. It is important for clients who experience oppression to construct an authentic self that is scripted by the client—not by the oppressors of the outer world.

I (Sydney) developed a self-compassion-based meditation script that therapists and culturally diverse clients can share as a possible dyad experience (see Practice E.2, "Self-Compassion for My Social and Cultural Identities," in the Appendix).

Conclusion

This chapter provided an exploration of the utility of integrating self-compassion practices in multicultural psychotherapy to address the complexities of common cross-cultural challenges. As Stampley and Slaght (2004) concluded, it is imperative for therapists to understand that "it is virtually impossible to avoid the influence of culture on clinical behavior" (p. 345). Considering the challenges involved in providing cross-cultural psychotherapy, practicing self-compassion rather than overidentification of shame, self-judgment, and self-isolation can advance the essential awareness, knowledge, and skillfulness required for cultivating greater cultural responsiveness. Additionally, self-compassion can serve as a therapeutic cross-cultural anchor and inner resource when emotional pain and difficulties arise. Emotionally supportive and insightful practices, such as mindful self-compassion, are crucial resources for both therapists and clients in navigating the challenging yet fruitful terrain of cross-cultural psychotherapy, ultimately leading to more resonance and positive outcomes.

REFERENCES

Alexander, J. C., Eyerman, R., Giesen, B., Smelser, N. J., & Sztompka, P. (2004). *Cultural trauma and collective identity*. University of California Press.

American Psychological Association. (2017). *Multicultural guidelines: An ecological approach to context, identity, and intersectionality*. www.apa.org/about/policy/multicultural-guidelines.pdf.

Benish, S. G., Quintana, S., & Wampold, B. E. (2011). Culturally adapted psychotherapy and the legitimacy of myth: A direct-comparison meta-analysis. *Journal of Counseling Psychology, 58*, 279–289.

Draguns, J. G. (2004). Resocialization into culture: The complexities of taking a worldwide view of psychotherapy. In R. W. Brislin, S. Bochner, & W. J. Longer (Eds.), *Cross-cultural perspectives of learning* (pp. 273–289). Halsted Press.

Eichstaedt, J. C., Sherman, G. T., Giorgi, S., Roberts, S. O., Reynolds, M. E., Ungar, L. H., & Guntuku, S. C. (2021). The emotional and mental health impact of the murder of George Floyd on the US population. *Proceedings of the National Academy of Sciences of the United States of America, 118*(39), e2109139118.

Eubanks, C. F., Muran, J. C., & Safran, J. D. (2018). Alliance rupture repair: A meta-analysis. *Psychotherapy, 55*(4), 508–519.

Flückiger, C., Del Re, A. C., Wampold, B. E., & Horvath, A. O. (2018). The alliance in adult psychotherapy: A meta-analytic synthesis. *Psychotherapy, 55*(4), 316–340.

Germer, C., & Neff, K. (2019). *Teaching the mindful self-compassion program: A guide for professionals*. Guilford Press.

Germer, C., & Neff, K. (2023). *Mindful self-compassion teacher guide*. Center for Mindful Self-Compassion.

Germer, C. K., & Neff, K. D. (2015). Cultivating self-compassion in trauma survivors. In V. M. Follette, J. Briere, D. Rozelle, J. W. Hopper, & D. I. Rome (Eds.), *Mindfulness-oriented interventions for trauma: Integrating contemplative practices* (pp. 43–58). Guilford Press.

Gottlieb, M., & Shibusawa, T. (2020). The impact of self-compassion on cultural competence: Results from a quantitative study of MSW students. *Journal of Social Work Education, 56*(1), 30–40.

Hardy, K. (2023). *Racial trauma: Clinical strategies and techniques for healing invisible wounds*. Norton.

Jaladin, R. A. M. (2017). Perceived multicultural counseling competence of Malaysian counselors: An exploratory study. *Journal of Multicultural Counseling and Development, 45*(2), 127–148.

Lambert, M. J. (1992). Psychotherapy outcome research: Implications for integrative and eclectic therapists. In J. C. Norcross & M. R. Goldfried (Eds.), *Handbook of psychotherapy integration* (pp. 94–129). Basic Books.

Lee, E. (2011). Clinical significance of cross-cultural competencies (CCC) in social work practice. *Journal of Social Work Practice, 25*(2), 185–203.

Lee, E., Greenblatt, A., & Hu, R. (2021). A knowledge synthesis of cross-cultural psychotherapy research: A critical review. *Journal of Cross-Cultural Psychology, 52*(6), 511–532.

Miles, J. R., Anders, C., Kivlighan, D. M., III, & Belcher Platt, A. A. (2021). Cultural ruptures: Addressing microaggressions in group therapy. *Group Dynamics: Theory, Research, and Practice, 25*(1), 74–88.

National Association of Social Workers. (2015). *Standards and indicators for cultural competence in social work practice.* NASW Press. www.socialworkers.org/Practice/NASW-Practice-Standards-Guidelines/Standards-and-Indicators-for-Cultural-Competence-in-Social-Work-Practice.

Neff, K. (2011). *Self-compassion: Stop beating yourself up and leave security behind.* Morrow.

Neff, K. (2021). *Fierce self-compassion: How women can harness kindness to speak up, claim their power, and thrive.* Harper.

Neff, K. D., Kirkpatrick, K. L., & Rude, S. S. (2007). Self-compassion and adaptive psychological functioning. *Journal of Research in Personality, 41*(1), 139–154.

Owen, J., Tao, K. W., Drinane, J. M., Hook, J., Davis, D. E., & Kune, N. F. (2016). Client perceptions of therapists' multicultural orientation: Cultural (missed) opportunities and cultural humility. *Professional Psychology: Research and Practice, 47*(1), 30–37.

Stampley, C., & Slaght, E. (2004). Cultural countertransference as a clinical obstacle. *Smith College Studies in Social Work, 74*(2), 333–347.

Sue, D. W., Arredondo, P., & McDavis, R. J. (1992). Multicultural counseling competencies and standards: A call to the profession. *Journal of Counseling and Development, 70*(4), 477–486.

Sue, D. W., Bucceri, J., Lin, A. I., Nadal, K. L., & Torino, G. C. (2007). Racial microaggressions and the Asian American experience. *Cultural Diversity and Ethnic Minority Psychology, 13,* 71–78.

Sue, D. W., Rasheed, M. N., & Rasheed, J. M. (2016). *Multicultural social work practice.* Wiley.

Sue, D. W., Sue, D., Neville, H. A., & Smith, L. (2019). *Counseling the culturally diverse: Theory and practice* (8th ed.). Wiley.

Tschacher, W., Haken, H., & Kyselo, M. (2015). Alliance: A common factor of psychotherapy modeled by structural theory. *Frontiers in Psychology, 6*, 421.

Tseng, W. S., & Strelzer, J. (Eds.). (2001). *Culture in psychotherapy: A guide to clinical practice.* American Psychiatric Publishing.

Yan, M. C. (2008). Exploring cultural tensions in cross-cultural social work practice. *Social Work, 53*(4), 317–328.

5

Why Does Self-Compassion Work?

Implications for Psychotherapy Practice

José Ramón Yela Bernabé
Antonio Crego Díaz

Research has proposed self-compassion as one of the mechanisms of therapeutic change, explaining why mindfulness-based interventions may work (Duarte & Pinto-Gouveia, 2017; Evans et al., 2018; Sevel et al., 2020; van der Meulen et al., 2021). Moreover, interventions focused on self-compassion are effective in enhancing well-being and produce significant improvements in a variety of psychological problems, such as eating behavior, rumination, lack of self-compassion, stress, depression, overidentification with aversive experiences, self-criticism, psychological distress, and anxiety, among others (Ferrari et al., 2019; Kirby, 2017; Wilson et al., 2019). Research has also highlighted the benefits of self-compassion on the therapists' own well-being and mental health, and on the improvement of their professional skills as care providers (Crego et al., 2022).

However, as Germer and Neff (2019) have noted, it is important to deepen our knowledge of the mechanisms of the action of self-compassion interventions and how beneficial effects are produced. This chapter explores why self-compassion works, aiming to connect self-compassion with other psychological processes proposed as factors involved in change in psychotherapy. Based on the identification of such mechanisms of change, in this chapter we present orientations that may help therapists strategically introduce the cultivation of self-compassion into their interventions.

Self-Compassion as a Mechanism of Therapeutic Change

Self-compassion has been proposed to explain the beneficial effects of various interventions. For example, self-compassion has been regarded as one of the processes through which the mindfulness-based stress reduction program would produce its effects (Evans et al., 2018; Sevel et al., 2020). Self-compassion has also been reported as a key process in research analyzing the effects of mindfulness-based cognitive therapy (Kuyken et al., 2010), attachment-based compassion therapy (Montero-Marin et al., 2020), and other mindfulness-based interventions (Duarte & Pinto-Gouveia, 2017; van der Meulen et al., 2021). Moreover, self-compassion has been found to account for the effects of acceptance and commitment therapy (ACT) interventions on problems such as clinical perfectionism (Ong et al., 2019), fear of cancer recurrence (Fishbein et al., 2022), and chronic pain (Carvalho et al., 2021).

In addition, self-compassion has been suggested as a factor that may have an influence on other mechanisms of change (i.e., assuming a *moderating role*). For example, in people with chronic pain, Carvalho and colleagues (2019) have found that the relationship between cognitive fusion and depression is buffered when individuals can respond to perceived personal flaws and shortcomings with self-kindness and warmth. Similarly, the possible protective role of self-compassion has been found in a study by Farr and colleagues (2021) where the levels of self-compassion attenuated the effects of experiential avoidance on depression. As the authors remark, this finding yields an important conclusion for clinicians: Self-compassion-based interventions that target experiential avoidance may be highly beneficial in reducing depressive symptoms.

Identifying How Self-Compassion Interventions Are Connected with Beneficial Effects

Research on self-compassion interventions, and especially on the mindful self-compassion (MSC) program (Germer & Neff, 2013, 2019; Neff & Germer, 2018), have highlighted the role of psychological flexibility-related variables, such as experiential avoidance, acceptance, and presence of meaning in life. For example, Yela and colleagues (2021) found that the connection between changes in self-compassion and the beneficial effects of the MSC program was explained by reductions in experiential avoidance that also emerged as an MSC training effect. Zaw and colleagues (2022) conducted a randomized controlled trial, with the experimental group receiving the MSC training and a wait-list control group. The explanatory mechanism analyzed in this research was "acceptance," referring to a mental attitude of openness, receptivity, nonjudgment, and equanimity toward internal and external experiences, instead of experiential avoidance, where attempts are made to suppress, alter, or avoid disturbing thoughts and emotions. The results revealed that participants in the MSC group had a higher level of acceptance and a lower level of perceived stress than the control group. Furthermore, acceptance fully explained the effect of the experimental condition on perceived stress.

Other research has also provided evidence suggesting the link between self-compassion and increases in psychological flexibility that may occur during the interventions. For example, Yela and colleagues (2020) found that meditators presented higher levels of self-compassion and better levels of mental health compared to a group of nonmeditators. Furthermore, those who meditated regularly had better mental health than occasional meditators, and occasional meditators reported higher levels of self-compassion and mental health than nonmeditators. In all cases, the association between self-compassion and mental health was explained by meaningfulness and experiential avoidance. Higher levels of self-compassion were associated with a greater presence of meaning in life and lower experiential avoidance.

Viskovich and Pakenham (2020) randomly assigned participants to a web-based ACT program or a wait-list control. Participants in the treatment group significantly enhanced their levels of self-compassion, among other mental health-related variables, in comparison to the control group. Interestingly, the improvements in self-compassion were explained by psychological processes, such as reduced experiential avoidance and cognitive fusion, and enhanced values-based living and present-moment awareness (mindfulness).

Misurya and colleagues (2022) analyzed data from people exposed to traumatic events. The researchers found that, in this sample, levels of self-compassion were positively connected with experienced posttraumatic growth through psychological flexibility.

Research has also suggested other mechanisms by which self-compassion effects are produced. For instance, the association between self-compassion and various psychopathology and well-being outcomes can be explained based on decreased cognitive rumination, positive coping, greater resilience, and a balanced time perspective.

How Emotion Regulation Contributes to Explaining Self-Compassion's Positive Effects

The research has also identified a remarkable link between self-compassion and emotion regulation. Low levels of self-compassion may impact depression through deficits in emotional regulation and, in particular, through experiential avoidance. A review by Inwood and Ferrari (2018) identified three studies where emotional regulation was proposed as a variable explaining the connection between self-compassion and symptoms of posttraumatic stress disorder in people who suffered trauma, stress in clinical psychologists in training, and unipolar depression in a clinical sample. The results suggest that habitual use of self-compassion influences mental health by facilitating emotional regulation and enabling negative emotions to be processed. Specifically, self-compassion may be associated with improvements in depressive symptoms by enhancing tolerance to negative emotions. The increased ability to tolerate negative feelings may improve the integration and processing of emotions and contribute to reducing the use of maladaptive emotion regulation strategies, such as avoidance (Inwood & Ferrari, 2018; Neff & Germer, 2013).

Self-Compassion and the Regulation of Shame

The regulation of the emotion of shame, in particular, has received great attention among self-compassion authors (Germer, 2023). The alleviation of shame is a mechanism that has been suggested to explain how self-compassion generates changes in psychotherapy (Callow et al., 2021). Shame is a "self-conscious" emotion characterized by negative self-evaluations and can be associated with the real or imagined rupture of social bonds. In this regard, shame is connected with the need for relatedness (Ryan & Deci, 2000) and the core yearning for belongingness (Hayes, 2019). Similarly, Germer and Neff (2019) consider that shame is an "innocent" emotion because we all naturally experience the need to belong to a community. The failures concerning the need to feel accepted, valued, and loved by other people, and experiences of indifference, abandonment, and rejection may be associated with shame. Concerning cognition, shame is characterized by negative nuclear core beliefs, again connected with failures to satisfy basic needs for competence and relatedness: "I am deficient, imperfect"; "I am not worthy of being loved"; "I am alone"; "I am helpless"; "I am inadequate"; and "I am a failure." These negative core beliefs may elicit conditional beliefs (e.g., "If I show myself to others as I am, then they will reject me") or dysfunctional attitudes, such as dependency (e.g., "I need the approval of others to be happy") and perfectionism (e.g., "I must be perfect if I want to be accepted").

The feelings of shame may arise at any stage of life, when security in relationships is compromised, or social position is at risk (i.e., the satisfaction of the need for belongingness is threatened). However, according to self-compassion literature, childhood is a critical period. The feelings of shame may be prompted by early experiences of childhood emotional neglect and abuse, exposure to harsh criticism, feelings of isolation and invisibility due to exclusion and stigmatization of social minorities, and intergenerational transmission of trauma and shame.

Research has found that childhood abuse is associated with emotional dysregulation through low levels of self-compassion (Barlow et al., 2017).

As Inwood and Ferrari (2018) noted, the symptomatology of childhood trauma and abuse may reduce a person's ability to be self-compassionate through multiple pathways and have an impact on self-compassion's components: negative evaluations of trauma, such as self-blame, shame, and elevated self-criticism, are likely to impede kindness toward oneself while disconnection from others is likely to challenge a sense of common humanity and chronic hyperarousal can make mindfulness difficult.

The use of experiential avoidance to cope with emotions is a typical maladaptive strategy in trauma-related mental health problems; it is a response incompatible with self-compassion. In this regard, providing self-compassion skills may facilitate an adaptive emotional regulation in people suffering trauma, allowing them to down-regulate hyperarousal, and enabling them to compassionately (self-kindness vs. self-criticism) experience (mindfulness vs. overidentification/rumination) and process (common humanity vs. shame/isolation) negative emotions and manage suffering. Interestingly, the MSC program considers that shame is perpetuated by silence. The idea of silence—muted or suppressed shame-related feelings, thoughts, and memories—is consistent with the suggested role of experiential avoidance as a mechanism involved in problem maintenance: A first task is to admit to ourselves that we have these beliefs, then we should offer compassion for the suffering we experience, and when we feel confident enough we can share our emotions with others (Germer, 2023; Germer & Neff, 2019).

Implications for Clinical Practice and Recommended Practices

Drawing from the findings on the mechanisms of action of self-compassion interventions, some suggestions can be made for applied clinical psychologists and other practitioners:

1. Experiential avoidance can be proposed as a core target of self-compassion interventions. Suffering depends to a large extent on the resistance we put up to pain, placing value on the ability to accept pain, as opposed to experiential avoidance. Reducing avoidant behaviors (and cultivating acceptance), in their multiple varieties, can significantly contribute to the efficacy of self-compassion interventions and training. To a greater extent, self-compassion practices contribute to exposing the person to unwanted experiences by increasing awareness of an inner life where aversive feelings, memories, and thoughts are present. For example, through formal and informal practices where mindfulness is cultivated, participants come into contact with potentially aversive inner experiences, with a

nonreactive and open attitude, as opposed to escaping or avoidance. Here, the habitually used "escape or avoidance" mechanism is broken, as we can see in recommended Practice F.1, "Labeling Emotions," in the Appendix (Germer & Neff, 2019).

2. In addition, self-compassion techniques contribute to changing the relationship between the person and those potentially unwanted inner experiences. Self-compassion interventions emphasize that thoughts, memories, emotions, and sensations, however painful they may be, are part of our shared human nature, and the individual is encouraged to maintain a benevolent and compassionate attitude toward oneself while engaging in contemplative practices. As we can see in recommended Practice F.2, by adding a self-kind, warm, nonjudgmental perspective while fostering common humanity interpretations, the meaning of aversive stimuli changes (see Practice F.2, "Pause for Self-Compassion," in the Appendix).

Progressively, the awareness of pain, distressing thoughts, hard feelings, negative emotions, and problematic memories enables responses of self-care and nurture, gentleness, and a feeling of belonging, which may be intrinsically reinforcing behaviors. Again, as taught in the MSC program, self-compassion is not a means to stop suffering but rather we give ourselves compassion because we suffer (Germer & Neff, 2019). In this vein, Wilson and Murrell (2004) state that "exposure in the context of values gives both the client and the therapist something meaningful to dignify the suffering that treatment produces" (p. 140).

3. As can be seen in recommended Practice F.3, using self-compassion practices with clients suffering from anxiety and depressive symptoms could facilitate an adaptive emotion regulation process. Participants in self-compassion training learn to increase tolerance to their negative emotions, which is a crucial competence for the maintenance and recovery of mental health. In addition, exposure versus avoidance may facilitate the compassionate processing of difficult emotions and contribute to managing suffering (Inwood & Ferrari, 2018; see Practice F.3, "Soften–Soothe–Allow," in the Appendix).

4. The cultivation of self-compassion also entails a reminder of what matters to that person (i.e., personal values; Germer & Neff, 2019). Recommended Practice F.4 emphasizes that values are in the service of finding meaning in life. In this regard, formulating and living by a vow may contribute to clarifying and expressing values, which at the same time represents a self-compassionate behavior in itself. Expressing loving-kindness can also be practiced as vows if they reflect our core values, such as "May all human beings be happy and free from suffering," or "May I learn to

love all beings" (see Practice F.4, "Discovering Our Core Values," in the Appendix).

Moreover, there is a connection between core values and the satisfaction of basic psychological needs. In self-compassion programs, the answer to the question "What do I need to give myself now to take care of myself?" is essential and refers us back to motivational variables well studied in psychology: basic psychological needs (Ryan & Deci, 2000) and core yearnings (Hayes, 2019), such as competence, belonging, self-determination, and so forth. These motivational variables are at the service of finding the psychological adaptation of the subject.

Here, adding kindness, presence, and connectedness to self- and other-directed actions is both an expression of core values and a psychologically flexible form of satisfying basic human needs. Self-compassion practices are related to the satisfaction of needs and yearnings in multiple ways. For instance, working on a sense of common humanity may be viewed in connection with the human yearning for belonging, the cultivation of mindfulness may contribute to satisfying the yearning for being fully present in the here and now, and self-kindness may fulfill the yearning for a values-based living, among other possible links. Moreover, self-uncompassionate behavior may also be considered in the light of human yearnings, as inflexible or maladaptive attempts to satisfy needs. For example, isolation may paradoxically be a means to keep others away from discovering one's failures or vulnerabilities in an attempt to remain part of the group (i.e., belonging), overidentification may be seen as maladaptive behavior that seeks to find extreme coherence or find orientation by focusing on the past or the future, and self-critical behavior may be an exemplar of dysfunctional attempts to be "perfect" to feel competent. These ideas are consistent with Ryan and Deci's (2000) view that excessive control, nonoptimal challenges, and lack of connectedness may disrupt the actualizing of inherent human tendencies (i.e., relatedness, competence, and autonomy) and result in detrimental outcomes, such as lack of initiative, apathy, alienation, distress, and psychopathology.

5. In particular, knowing the connections between shame, experiential avoidance, and the yearning for belonging can help therapists understand the mechanisms of maintaining suffering. Feeling shame is an aversive emotion that prompts social avoidance behaviors aimed at self-protection from being rejected by the group (i.e., the yearning for belonging is under perceived threat), as the person uncompassionately self-evaluates as inappropriate, unworthy, or objectionable. Similarly, the study of the connections between self-compassion and attachment-related problems may benefit from considering mechanisms of experiential avoidance in the context of satisfaction of social needs.

Conclusion

When we suffer, the definition of self-compassion itself entails a calling to be warm and kind to ourselves (values clarification), to be open to experience the emotions that arise (mindfulness), and to understand that suffering is purely human (common humanity), that it is part of life and that there is no reason to isolate or be ashamed of it (acceptance). Working on self-compassion in psychotherapy contexts has benefits for both the client and the therapist. But why does self-compassion work? Several mechanisms have been proposed, highlighting the role of experiential avoidance. Figure 5.1 humorously illustrates how avoiding experiences can lead to stagnation. Cultivating self-compassion is related to reduced experiential avoidance and greater acceptance of potentially disturbing thoughts, emotions, and other internal experiences.

In addition, developing self-compassionate attitudes is associated with adaptive emotional regulation and contributes to meaningful living, especially by helping to satisfy the human need for connection and belonging. These psychological processes can be introduced in therapeutic contexts through practices such as the ones presented aimed at connecting with difficult emotions (see Practice F.1, "Labeling Emotions," in the Appendix),

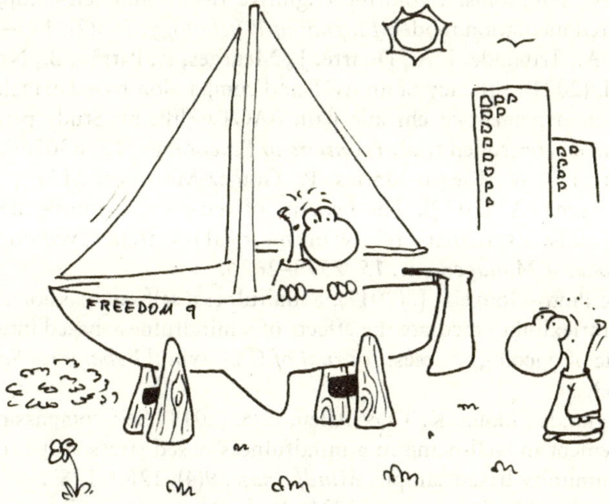

I KNOW, DRY DOCK SAILING IS LESS FUN THAN REAL SAILING, BUT IT IS LESS SCARY

FIGURE 5.1.

identifying moments and ways to give compassion to oneself (see Practice F.2, "Pause for Self-Compassion," and Practice F.3, "Soften–Soothe–Allow," in the Appendix), and contributing to a life based on implementing personal values (see Practice F.4, "Discovering Our Core Values," in the Appendix).

ACKNOWLEDGMENTS

Preparation of this chapter was funded by a research grant from the Spanish Ministry of Science and Innovation, the Spanish State Research Agency, and the European Regional Development Fund (Project PID2021-125918OB-I00, funded by MCIN/AEI/10.13039/501100011033/FEDER, EU).

REFERENCES

Barlow, R., Goldsmith Turow, R., & Gerhart, J. (2017). Trauma appraisals, emotion regulation difficulties, and self-compassion predict posttraumatic stress symptoms following childhood abuse. *Child Abuse and Neglect, 65,* 37–47.

Callow, T. J., Moffitt, R. L., & Neumann, D. L. (2021). External shame and its association with depression and anxiety: The moderating role of self-compassion. *Australian Psychologist, 56,* 70–80.

Carvalho, S. A., Pinto-Gouveia, J., Gillanders, D., & Castilho, P. (2019). Pain and depressive symptoms: Exploring cognitive fusion and self-compassion in a moderated mediation model. *Journal of Psychology, 153*(2), 173–186.

Carvalho, S. A., Trindade, I. A., Duarte, J., Menezes, P., Patrão, B., Nogueira, M. R., et al. (2021). Efficacy of an ACT and compassion-based eHealth program for self-management of chronic pain (iACTwithPain): Study protocol for a randomized controlled trial. *Frontiers in Psychology, 12,* 630766.

Crego, A., Yela, J. R., Riesco-Matías, P., Gómez-Martínez, M. Á., & Vicente-Arruebarrena, A. (2022). The benefits of self-compassion in mental health professionals: A systematic review of empirical research. *Psychology Research and Behavior Management, 15,* 2599–2620.

Duarte, J., & Pinto-Gouveia, J. (2017). Mindfulness, self-compassion and psychological inflexibility mediate the effects of a mindfulness-based intervention in a sample of oncology nurses. *Journal of Contextual Behavioral Science, 6*(2), 125–133.

Evans, S., Wyka, K., Blaha, K. T., & Allen, E. S. (2018). Self-compassion mediates improvement in well-being in a mindfulness-based stress reduction program in a community-based sample. *Mindfulness, 9*(4), 1280–1287.

Farr, J., Ononaiye, M., & Irons, C. (2021). Early shaming experiences and psychological distress: The role of experiential avoidance and self-compassion. *Psychology and Psychotherapy: Theory, Research, and Practice, 94*(4), 952–972.

Ferrari, M., Hunt, C., Harrysunker, A., Abbott, M. J., Beath, A. P., & Einstein, D.

A. (2019). Self-compassion interventions and psychosocial outcomes: A meta-analysis of RCTs. *Mindfulness, 10*(8), 1455–1473.

Fishbein, J., Judd, C. M., Genung, S., Stanton, A. L., & Arch, J. J. (2022). Intervention and mediation effects of target processes in a community oncology clinic-based randomized controlled trial of acceptance and commitment therapy. *Behaviour Research and Therapy, 153,* 104103.

Germer, C. (2023). Self-compassion in psychotherapy: Clinical integration, evidence base, and mechanisms of change. In A. Finlay-Jones, K. Bluth, & K. Neff (Eds.), *Handbook of self-compassion: Mindfulness in behavioral health* (pp. 379–415). Springer.

Germer, C. K., & Neff, K. (2013). Self-compassion in clinical practice. *Journal of Clinical Psychology, 69*(8), 856–867.

Germer, C. K., & Neff, K. D. (2019). *Teaching the mindful self-compassion program: A guide for professionals.* Guilford Press.

Hayes, S. (2019). *A liberated mind: The essential guide to ACT.* Random House.

Inwood, E., & Ferrari, M. (2018). Mechanisms of change in the relationship between self-compassion, emotion regulation, and mental health: A systematic review. *Applied Psychology: Health and Well-Being, 10*(2), 215–235.

Kirby, J. N. (2017). Compassion interventions: The programs, the evidence, and implications for research and practice. *Psychology and Psychotherapy: Theory, Research and Practice, 90*(3), 432–455.

Kuyken, W., Watkins, E., Holden, E., White, K., Taylor, R. S., Byford, S., et al. (2010). How does mindfulness-based cognitive therapy work? *Behaviour Research and Therapy, 48*(11), 1105–1112.

Misurya, P., Shukla, V., & Anand, P. V. (2022). Self-compassion and post traumatic growth: The mediating role of psychological flexibility. *Psychreg Journal of Psychology, 6*(2), 113–124.

Montero-Marin, J., Van Gordon, W., Shonin, E., Navarro-Gil, M., Gasión, V., López-del-Hoyo, Y., et al. (2020). Attachment-based compassion therapy for ameliorating fibromyalgia: Mediating role of mindfulness and self-compassion. *Mindfulness, 11*(3), 816–828.

Neff, K. D., & Germer, C. K. (2013). A pilot study and randomized controlled trial of the Mindful Self-Compassion program. *Journal of Clinical Psychology, 69*(1), 28–44.

Neff, K. D., & Germer, C. (2018). *The mindful self-compassion workbook: A proven way to accept yourself, build inner strength, and thrive.* Guilford Press.

Ong, C. W., Barney, J. L., Barrett, T. S., Lee, E. B., Levin, M. E., & Twohig, M. P. (2019). The role of psychological inflexibility and self-compassion in acceptance and commitment therapy for clinical perfectionism. *Journal of Contextual Behavioral Science, 13*, 7–16.

Ryan, R. M., & Deci, E. L. (2000). Self-determination theory and the facilitation of intrinsic motivation, social development, and well-being. *American Psychologist, 55*(1), 68–78.

Sevel, L. S., Finn, M. T., Smith, R. M., Ryden, A. M., & McKernan, L. C. (2020). Self-compassion in mindfulness-based stress reduction: An examination of prediction and mediation of intervention effects. *Stress and Health, 36*(1), 88–96.

van der Meulen, R. T., Valentin, S., Bögels, S. M., & de Bruin, E. I. (2021). Mindfulness and self-compassion as mediators of the Mindful2Work Training on perceived stress and chronic fatigue. *Mindfulness, 12*(4), 936–946.

Viskovich, S., & Pakenham, K. I. (2020). Randomized controlled trial of a web-based acceptance and commitment therapy (ACT) program to promote mental health in university students. *Journal of Clinical Psychology, 76*, 929–951.

Wilson, A. C., Mackintosh, K., Power, K., & Chan, S. W. (2019). Effectiveness of self-compassion related therapies: A systematic review and meta-analysis. *Mindfulness, 10*(6), 979–995.

Wilson, K. G., & Murrell, A. R. (2004). Values work in acceptance and commitment therapy: Setting a course for behavioral treatment. In S. C. Hayes, V. M. Follette, & M. M. Linehan (Eds.), *Mindfulness and acceptance: Expanding the cognitive-behavioral tradition* (pp. 120–151). Guilford Press.

Yela, J. R., Crego, A., Buz, J., Sánchez-Zaballos, E., & Gómez-Martínez, M. A. (2021). Reductions in experiential avoidance explain changes in anxiety, depression, and well-being after a mindfulness and self-compassion (MSC) training. *Psychology and Psychotherapy: Theory, Research, and Practice, 95*, 402–422.

Yela, J. R., Crego, A., Gómez-Martínez, M. A., & Jiménez-Goméz, L. (2020). Self-compassion, meaning in life, and experiential avoidance explain the relationship between meditation and positive mental health outcomes. *Journal of Clinical Psychology, 76*, 1631–1652.

Zaw, P. P., Takahashi, Y., & Thein, K. S. (2022). Mindful self-compassion training online and perceived stress: Exploring moderation of awareness and mediation of acceptance. *Journal of Behavioral Science, 17*(1), 113–124.

PART II

A Self-Compassion-Based Clinician

What Shapes and Informs Practice

6

Exploring the Interplay between Therapeutic Presence and Self-Compassion in Psychotherapy

Shari Geller

Bringing ourselves to the present moment with clients is a powerful and compassionate approach to meeting the client and the depth of their suffering. This way of being allows clients to feel seen, heard, and felt, which provides the refuge to explore their suffering and trauma within the safety of the therapeutic relationship. Therapeutic presence provides the landscape by which effective therapy can ensue—both for clients to open and engage in deep therapeutic work, as well as for therapists to feel grounded yet immersed and attuned to what is needed in the present moment.

Compassion is a key component in the embodiment of therapeutic presence (Geller & Greenberg, 2022). It is the fabric underlying the ability to be fully available and engaged with and for the client in service of their healing. Self-compassion is an important first step for therapists to generate compassion with others as it helps to both cultivate presence and work with barriers to presence, such as self-doubt and shame (Geller, 2017). This chapter aims to explore therapeutic presence in the context of psychotherapy and the relationship of compassion and self-compassion to therapeutic presence. An empirically validated model of therapeutic presence and related research is shared, followed by a dialogue on the neurophysiology of presence informed by polyvagal theory. The role of compassion and self-compassion is discussed in relation to both cultivating therapeutic presence and helping overcome the barriers to presence. A final discussion includes how training and professional development in therapeutic presence would benefit from including self-compassion practices to both generate therapeutic presence and to work with the barriers.

Therapeutic Presence: Understanding the Essence

A brief review of the research helps us to understand the essence of therapeutic presence, commencing with an empirically validated model describing its overarching qualities (Geller & Greenberg, 2002, 2022).

Definition and Model of Therapeutic Presence

Therapeutic presence is a way of *being* in the therapeutic encounter that enhances the *doing* of therapy (Geller, 2017; Geller & Greenberg, 2022). It involves therapists offering their whole self physically, emotionally, cognitively, relationally, and spiritually to the client and the therapeutic encounter (Geller, 2017; Geller & Greenberg, 2002, 2022). An empirically validated model of presence developed by Geller and Greenberg (2002, 2022) encompasses (1) *preparation* for presence (a) *in life* and (b) *before and during* sessions; (2) *process* (in session) of presence, which involves (a) being *receptively attuned* to clients' experience moment-to-moment, (b) being *inwardly attuned* to therapists' own experience and resonance with clients, and (c) being in *contact and extending* self to the client from that receptive and inward place of attunement; and finally, (3) *embodied experience*, which includes simultaneously (a) *grounding* within self, (b) *immersion* in the moment with the client, (c) a sense of *expansion* and larger sense of spaciousness, and (d) *compassion* or *being with and for* the client and in service of their healing.

Therapists' self-care is also essential in the model of therapeutic presence as it supports therapists in remaining attuned within themselves, and responsive to their clients' moment-to-moment verbal and nonverbal experiences (Geller, 2017). A core element of self-care is self-compassion by which therapists can learn to bring warmth, kindness, and a sense of common humanity to their emotions and their inner experience. This helps them to show up in the therapy room and meet their clients' moment-to-moment experiences with presence while holding their inner resonance of pain and the challenges that may emerge internally in the process.

Therapeutic Presence Research

Extensive research demonstrates that the therapeutic alliance is the most consistent predictor of therapeutic outcomes and change (Norcross & Lambert, 2019). Yet contributions to the alliance are less understood. A growing body of evidence suggests therapeutic presence is a common factor integral to generating psychological and emotional safety, developing strong therapeutic alliances, and optimizing the effectiveness of therapy transtheoretically (see Geller & Greenberg, 2022, for a literature review).

Foundational research using the Therapeutic Presence Inventory for therapists' and clients' perceptions of their therapist's presence (TPI-T and TPI-C, respectively; Geller et al., 2010) suggests that therapeutic presence is a positive predictor for therapeutic alliance across multiple modalities (Geller et al., 2010; Pos et al., 2011). Importantly, clients' experiences of their therapist's presence is associated with ratings of a positive alliance and a successful session outcome across emotion-focused therapy (EFT), person-centered therapy (PCT), and cognitive-behavioral therapy (CBT) (Geller et al., 2010).

The Neurophysiological Basis of Therapeutic Presence: Insights from Polyvagal Theory

Stephen Porges's (2011) polyvagal theory elucidates how therapeutic presence may lead to therapeutic change. Briefly, polyvagal theory highlights the two (hence the term *poly*) pathways traveling within the vagus nerve located in the parasympathetic branch of the nervous system: a dorsal vagal pathway and a ventral vagal pathway (Porges, 2011). The dorsal vagal pathway reflects when we are shut down. For example, when a person feels overwhelmed or "in danger" in a relationship or in general (a fight-or-flight response of the sympathetic nervous system), their system may subsequently shut down and freeze (dorsal vagal response), as in the case of clients with dissociation from trauma. Alternatively, the ventral vagal pathway, also known as the social engagement system, responds to safety cues and supports regulation in relationships (Geller, 2018; Geller & Porges, 2014; Porges, 2011). When the ventral vagal system is activated through a safe connection in relationships, we calm down and our nervous system regulates. Therapeutic presence, for which compassion is central, can help optimize this ventral vagal pathway by exercising clients' neural muscles to feel safe with others (Geller & Porges, 2014).

Research affirms that clients who experience their therapist as present have a stronger therapeutic alliance and session outcome (Geller et al., 2010; Pos et al., 2011). To enhance clients' perceptions and experiences of their therapist's presence, therapists must communicate and embody this state. Polyvagal theory delineates how this is possible through vocal prosody, open body posture, soft facial expression, and attentive eye gaze. Clients receiving their therapists' presence can experience safety on a neurophysiological level (Geller & Porges, 2014). Over time, repeatedly journeying back to this state of safety allows clients to "feel felt" (Siegel, 2010), met, and understood, thus creating space for vulnerable expressions of emotion and optimal engagement in therapy.

Therapists' presence is known to co-regulate clients' emotions (Geller, 2018). In clinical terms, if therapists express a sense of calm and compassion through their presence, clients will feel safe in resonance, as emotions, bodies, and brains are bidirectionally linked (Geller, 2017; Geller & Porges, 2014). Alternatively, if therapists are not grounded, present, and compassionate, then they can be thrown off their center or dysregulated by their clients' emotional overwhelm.

Compassion and Self-Compassion: Facilitating the Cultivation of Therapeutic Presence

Compassion is core to the embodied experience of therapeutic presence and can be developed through the cultivation of self-compassion (Geller, 2017). Self-compassion means caring for our suffering in the way we would care for someone we truly love. Kristen Neff and Christopher Germer (2018), developers of the Mindful Self-Compassion program, describe three components of self-compassion:

1. *Mindfulness*, which involves noticing one's experience and suffering moment-to-moment without judgment.
2. *Common humanity*, which includes recognizing the shared human element of suffering and that we are not alone.
3. *Self-kindness* toward ourselves and our suffering rather than self-judgment. Overall, mindfulness and self-compassion approaches encourage therapists to integrate personal practices that strengthen qualities of attention, awareness, warmth, compassion, and sensitivity, and in turn optimize attunement with clients and strengthen therapeutic relationships (Geller & Greenberg, 2022; Germer, 2023).

Although presence and compassion are distinct, they often elicit similar effects (i.e., safety) and are seemingly complementary. Across multiple studies, Stellar et al. (2015) found that heightened vagal activity was linked to viewing compassion-evoking stimuli in comparison to controls, and participants who rewatched one of the compassion-evoking videos experienced greater respiratory sinus arrhythmia (a measure of vagal activity), which was once again associated with subjective and objective measures of compassion. In psychotherapy, approaching pain with compassion frees us from resistance and opens us to feeling a profound sense of connection and safety with clients (Germer, 2023).

The Relationship between Mindfulness and Therapeutic Presence

Although there is a relationship between mindfulness and therapeutic presence, the two constructs are distinct. While mindfulness tends to be a technique for practicing present-centered focused awareness in the here and now, presence encapsulates a personal experience of embodiment with the intention of being in a compassionate and healing therapeutic relationship. Mindfulness practices can be taught to therapists to help sharpen their attention, self-regulation, and presence, and they can be taught to clients to help them self-regulate. However, therapeutic presence is a quality that is specific to therapists in their way of being and relating with clients.

Research suggests mindfulness practice helps to cultivate the experience of therapeutic presence by enhancing the focused attention required for the embodied experience of *immersion* (Bourgault & Dionne, 2019; Geller & Greenberg, 2002, 2022; Vinca, 2009). By reducing stress, anxiety, and burnout, and increasing self- and emotional regulation, mindfulness helps therapists sustain a level of psychological well-being and steadiness to approach clients' intense emotions with a sense of equanimity. For example, counselors trained in mindfulness showed a greater ability to be present in sessions with clients and with themselves (Tannen et al., 2019). This allowed them to feel more attuned to clients, more secure in themselves, and be a more effective instrument in their clients' therapeutic process.

While mindfulness supports the cultivation of therapeutic presence, a study by Bourgault and Dionne (2019) suggests that self-compassion mediates this relationship. Mindfulness was found to enhance therapeutic presence by strengthening self-compassion and reducing psychological distress. The authors proposed that self-compassion contributes to an awareness of oneself, of others, and of the relationship between them, infused with warmth and kindness, which ultimately strengthens the relational bond.

The Relationship between Self-Compassion and Presence

Self-compassion is not only a core element of therapeutic presence, but it also strengthens the embodied experience of presence. To embody compassion and presence fully, therapists require a level of acceptance and self-compassion with their own moment-to-moment experience (Geller & Greenberg, 2022).

Self-compassion is a helpful way of working with therapists' internal barriers to being present (e.g., self-doubt, shame, self-criticism). When uncertain about how to approach or respond to a client who is suffering, self-compassion can soften the critical voice that is activated and distracting from the unfolding of the moment. Self-compassion also helps therapists to work through the deeper experiences that have contributed to their self-doubt, and process some of the original emotions by accessing them with compassion. It encourages therapists to be with their own humanness and vulnerability, which strengthens the human-to-human connection that therapeutic presence can invite. The work of self-compassion is feeling the pain that underlies one's own self-doubt and offering a kinder and softer approach to ourselves.

How Does Self-Compassion Support Therapists in Cultivating and Embodying Therapeutic Presence?

A key aspect of therapeutic presence is self-care and self-compassion. Self-compassion can act as an antidote to the emotional work of therapy. It is offering to the self a way of approaching and resolving difficult emotions with acceptance and kindness.

There are numerous benefits to self-compassion for therapists. Self-compassion reduces burnout and fatigue in health care professionals (Raab, 2014). In a sample of psychologists, Finlay-Jones and colleagues (2015) found that self-compassion also decreases stress by reducing challenges in regulating emotions. Finally, self-compassion can enhance positive emotions, including social connectedness, optimism, curiosity, competence, happiness, and well-being (Neff et al., 2007). The vitality and flow that can be accessed through self-compassion practice can support therapists in staying open to clients and their suffering while remaining calm and energized.

Regular practice can help therapists to access self-compassion when in session. Examples of helpful practices from the mindful self-compassion program include affectionate breathing, breathing in and out compassion, and loving-kindness (see Practice B, "Giving and Receiving Compassion," in the Appendix, and Neff & Germer, 2018, for practice examples). Research has demonstrated that loving-kindness meditation, and compassion practices for health care professionals can increase therapists' presence and related qualities contributing to the effectiveness of the therapeutic process (see Geller & Greenberg, 2022, for sample studies).

Cultivating Therapeutic Presence with Self-Compassion Practices

Based on the evidence that these qualities can be trained and applied across therapeutic approaches, researchers are beginning to envision modules that could be integrated into training programs (see Geller & Greenberg, 2022, for a more extensive discussion). Several self-compassion practices can help support the cultivation of presence, as well as the positive well-being of therapists. See Neff and Germer (2018) and Geller and Greenberg (2022), as well as the Appendix in this book, for detailed descriptions of these practices.

Mindfulness and Self-Compassion Practices from the Mindful Self-Compassion Program

Mindfulness and self-compassion practices help to enhance attention, awareness, warmth, compassion, and sensitivity, which are foundational to the qualities of therapeutic presence, such as attunement, empathy, and the development of positive therapeutic alliances (Geller & Greenberg, 2022; Germer, 2023). The following practices are pulled from and inspired by the Mindful Self-Compassion program (Neff & Germer, 2018).

Soothing touch is the ground of self-compassion practice. This involves resting a hand on a place on your body where you feel your emotional or physical pain. Touch activates the caregiving system and parasympathetic nervous system, just as it calms babies down when they are in distress. A soothing touch is also helpful when experiencing challenging emotions, such as the pain therapists may feel in their bodies as they resonate with their clients. This promotes presence, gestures to clients that you are feeling their pain, and nonverbally invites them to do the same with their pain (see Practice G, "Soothing or Supportive Touch," in the Appendix).

Soften–soothe–allow is a practice that can help to soften underneath difficult emotions, such as shame and sadness. It involves becoming aware of emotions in the body and labeling them without judgment (mindfulness), softening the emotions, soothing them with kindness and touch, and allowing them to be there. This can help therapists to stay present with difficult emotions that arise both in and out of session (see Practice F.4, "Soften–Soothe–Allow," in the Appendix).

Relational self-compassion: Compassionate listening involves two or more people. It focuses on listening in silence to another talk about a poignant experience. "Pings" are little internal taps or moments of salience that the listener feels in their own body as they resonate with the client (Neff & Germer, 2018). Learning to listen to the pings helps therapists use their whole body, a key aspect of therapeutic presence, to listen and resonate with clients as they recount challenges. Eventually, therapists can then use these pings to share with clients what touches them and to validate, empathize, or maintain meaningful contact with their experience.

Cultivating Presence Before and In Session

The first overarching quality in the model of therapeutic presence, preparing for presence, involves therapists intentionally setting aside personal concerns, needs, preconceptions, expectations, beliefs, and theories (Geller, 2017). Research endorses engaging in practice for even 5 minutes before a session leads to a stronger therapeutic alliance and session outcome (Dunn et al., 2013; Geller & Greenberg, 2002). The following practice can be used before the session:

P.R.E.S.E.N.C.E. Practice

The following acronym encompasses all aspects of presence, such as contact with self and others (Geller, 2017).

- Pause.
- Relax into this moment.
- Enhance awareness of your breath.
- Sense your inner body with compassion; bring warm awareness to your physical and emotional body.
- Expand sensory awareness outward (seeing, listening, touching, sensing what is around you).
- Notice with kindness what is true in this moment, both within you and around you. Notice the relationship between the internal and the external.
- Center and ground (in yourself and your body).
- Extend and make compassionate contact (with clients, or others).

Embodied Presence Practice: Core Body Centering

A core presence practice to embody the experience of presence and ground oneself prior to session can be found in Practice H, "Embodied Presence Practice: Core Body Centering," in the Appendix. An audio recording is also available at *www.guilford.com/tyano-ronen-materials*. Therapists can also use this practice in session to recenter when their attention moves away from the moment or emotions become overwhelming.

Overcoming Barriers to Therapeutic Presence with Self-Compassion

Rumi shares in his famous quote that the task is not to find love but rather to remove the barriers to love (paraphrased and taken from Geller, 2017). The same is true for presence. This begins with therapists bringing compassionate awareness to barriers and reactions, which includes being able to discern internal personal barriers, such as countertransference, from useful information such as interpersonal responses (noticing therapists' responses to clients' interpersonal styles) or resonance (noticing the feelings clients experience resonating in the therapist's body, which helps deepen empathic understanding of the other). This starts with a sense of embodied self-awareness, and self-compassion practice can help with developing this as well as working with countertransference responses, such as personal triggers, feeling overwhelmed, or shutting down.

The barriers to engaging intimately and being present in the moment in a psychotherapeutic encounter can arise *internally* from within the therapist (i.e., personal triggers, difficulty with uncertainty, emotional shutdown, self-doubt, shame, burnout) or *externally* from the client (i.e., hopelessness, emotion dysregulation, personality styles, dying or death) or the relationship (i.e., therapeutic ruptures). Self-compassion is ideal for working with and softening these barriers. While the distinction between internal and external is helpful to conceptually understand these challenges, even those that emerge externally (e.g., client's anger) are ultimately internal challenges, as they can serve as a personal trigger evoking therapists' own vulnerability. It is important for therapists to notice their loss of presence, come back to the moment through their compassionate awareness of their bodies, and bring themselves back into present-moment sensory contact with their clients. A fuller discussion of barriers and challenges to presence (as well as tools to work with these) can be found in other publications (see Geller, 2017; Geller & Greenberg, 2022).

The Role of Self-Compassion in Navigating Barriers to Presence

Self-compassion is particularly helpful when working with barriers such as therapists' shame, self-doubt, impostor syndrome, and related burnout. These common challenges can interfere with therapists' ability to be present and attuned with clients. Self-compassion practice (i.e., "self-compassion break" or "soften–soothe–allow") can help generate awareness of the underlying pain (i.e., shame) and the need that is related to that (i.e., need for respect or acceptance), and to offer that to ourselves with kindness and compassion. Similarly, in working with dying and death, self-compassion is imperative as compassionate care involves being fully present with others in their fear, pain, and suffering, without shutting down or feeling overwhelmed (Geller & Greenberg, 2022).

Practices to Implement with Barriers to Presence in Session

Two main practices are highlighted below, specifically designed to work with barriers to presence.

Pause, Notice, and Return

During experiences of overwhelm, helplessness, or disconnection in session, a simple yet profound *pause*, *notice*, and *return* (PNR; Geller, 2017) practice can be helpful. This involves three steps:

1. *Pause* to ask yourself what is coming up for you.
2. *Notice* what led to this feeling, nonjudgmentally and with compassion, and taking a moment to visualize yourself putting it aside for the time being.
3. *Return* awareness to the present moment through intentional breathing, grounding, and direct focus back to the client from this place of inner stability.

It is important to take time outside of the session when personal triggers arise to work with these and not just continuously put them aside in session.

Giving and Receiving Compassion

Giving and receiving compassion (see Practice B, "Giving and Receiving Compassion," in the Appendix) is a powerful practice in dealing with barriers that occur in sessions. Developed by Christopher Germer and adapted from traditional Tonglen practice based on Tibetan Buddhism, this practice is helpful for therapists when feeling overwhelmed with emotion, blocked, or shut down within themselves or with their clients. When therapists notice themselves becoming distant or shut down in connection with clients, they can take a deep in-breath while offering compassion to the distress and an out-breath while offering compassion to their client. They can then continue with this natural rhythm of inhaling for themselves and exhaling for their client until a sense of reconnection is felt and established. Of course, like all presence and self-compassion practices, it is important to engage this as a formal practice outside of session, and then, once familiar, it can be used in session to reconnect with a client in a moment of disconnection.

Applying the Interplay between Therapeutic Presence and Self-Compassion

The following clinical vignette (adapted from Geller & Greenberg, 2022) demonstrates how integrating mindful and self-compassion practices, such as breath awareness, core body centering, and PNR, can help therapists notice when they are not present, work with their distraction, and bring their attention back to the moment:

> A's grief over the loss of their father had become difficult to handle. Their therapist, R, found herself having an aversive response to upcoming appointments, noticing her fatigue and internal voice saying that she needed a break from

clients in general. R realized that something larger was at play inside herself, particularly the lack of competency she felt in not affecting a shift in A's grief and complete loss of motivation.

R's awareness of her nonpresent state arose as she anticipated with dread the upcoming session. She used her presence practice by engaging in a 5-minute presession practice (body centering with a soothing touch) to bring herself into a more open and centered place. R felt more available when she approached the door to welcome A in.

As the session began, A spoke in their usual way about their lack of motivation, deep sadness, and sluggishness. R began to experience that open, compassionate, and centered place start to slip away, and a voice in her head taunted her about her inability to help them. As R invited her attention back into the moment with a kind inner voice, she saw A in a way she had not before. She noticed this 40-year-old lawyer with the vulnerable posture of a little child, wringing their hands as they spoke. R felt a resonance of despair in her body, experienced discomfort in her chest, and placed a hand on her heart. She reflected to A the deep despair she saw in their eyes, with a warmth in her voice and soft eye contact, and queried their feeling of being incapable in response to the death of their father. A's eyes began to well up, and they looked at her in a way she had not seen before, with deep sadness yet relief. They quieted for a moment and then spoke about the loss of not only their dad but also the only person who believed in them. They spoke of the taunting they had experienced by their sisters and even their mother growing up, and how their dad would always quietly support them and tell them how great they were. Their tears flowed as they expressed their fear that they would be incapable of succeeding without the presence of their father.

After the session ended, A commented that they felt "softer" and more understood. They began to express an understanding and compassion for the depth of their pain and loss and were hopeful that they could continue to process their grief of their father and regain a sense of peace.

Reflection

This therapist's practice before the session, as well as in session, of noticing her shutdown and returning to a sense of grounding and centeredness through mindfulness and self-compassion allowed her to bring her attention and focus fully back into the moment. This was possible through prior mindfulness and self-compassion practice so that she could quickly recognize what she was feeling, bring kindness to it, and realign her body and her attention. As the therapist listened to and trusted her internal resonance ("pings"), she could reflect back this awareness while staying present and compassionate with herself and in contact with the client. This allowed her client to express a deeper opening and feel understood. She could stay or return to presence and compassion and hence be with despair without feeling overwhelmed or turning away so that the client could feel understood and express the layers of grief that they were experiencing.

Conclusion

In this chapter, we delved into the intricate and profound interplay between therapeutic presence and self-compassion within the realm of psychotherapy. This chapter also highlights the significance of a therapist's presence for transformative therapeutic relationships and the role of self-compassion in both cultivating therapeutic presence, as well as working with therapists' barriers to presence. This chapter also underscores the reciprocal nature of this relationship, revealing that as therapists practice self-compassion, their presence strengthens. This generates clients' safety in the relationship with their present-centered therapists, allowing them to be better equipped to engage authentically within the therapeutic space. This symbiotic dynamic enriches the therapeutic alliance, leading to more meaningful and enduring therapeutic outcomes. Self-compassion practices have the added benefit of helping therapists work through the barriers to presence, as well as relate to their own and their client's pain and suffering with kindness and warmth, heightening their ability to be present.

As the field of psychotherapy continues to evolve, research in therapeutic presence and self-compassion brings to light a nuanced understanding of how these two experiences coalesce to create a powerful foundation for healing and transformation. Training in psychotherapy would benefit from a foundational module in therapeutic presence, including self-compassion skills to both cultivate presence and work with barriers to presence (see Geller & Greenberg, 2022, for a sample module). Programs incorporating therapeutic presence and self-compassion are already showing positive benefits for psychotherapy trainees (Boellinghaus et al., 2013; Tannen et al., 2019).

This chapter not only advances theoretical perspectives but also offers practical implications for therapists seeking to enhance their therapeutic effectiveness. By recognizing the profound synergy between therapeutic presence and self-compassion, practitioners can refine their approaches, ultimately fostering an environment for clients to explore, heal, and flourish.

REFERENCES

Boellinghaus, I., Jones, F. W., & Hutton, J. (2013). Cultivating self-care and compassion in psychological therapists in training: The experience of practicing loving-kindness meditation. *Training and Education in Professional Psychology, 7*(4), 267–277.

Bourgault, M., & Dionne, F. (2019). Therapeutic presence and mindfulness: Mediating role of self-compassion and psychological distress among psychologists. *Mindfulness, 10*(4), 650–656.

Dunn, R., Callahan, J. L., Swift, J. K., & Ivanovic, M. (2013). Effects of pre-session centering for therapists on session presence and effectiveness. *Psychotherapy Research, 23*, 78–85.

Finlay-Jones, A. L., Rees, C. S., & Kane, R. T. (2015). Self-compassion, emotion regulation and stress among Australian psychologists: Testing an emotion regulation model of self-compassion using structural equation modeling. *PLoS One, 10*(7), e0133481. https://self-compassion.org/wp-content/uploads/2015/08/Finlay_Jones.pdf.

Geller, S. M. (2017). *A guide to cultivating therapeutic presence.* American Psychological Association.

Geller, S. M. (2018). Therapeutic presence and polyvagal theory: Principles and practices for cultivating effective therapeutic relationships. In S. Porges & D. Dana (Eds.), *Clinical applications of the polyvagal theory: The emergence of polyvagal-informed therapies* (pp. 106–126). Norton.

Geller, S. M., & Greenberg, L. S. (2002). Therapeutic presence: Therapists' experience of presence in the psychotherapeutic encounter. *Person-Centered and Experiential Psychotherapies, 1*(1–2), 71–86.

Geller, S. M., & Greenberg, L. S. (2022). *Therapeutic presence: A mindful approach to effective therapeutic relationships* (2nd ed.). American Psychological Association.

Geller, S. M., Greenberg, L. S., & Watson, J. C. (2010). Therapist and client perceptions of therapeutic presence: The development of a measure. *Journal of Psychotherapy Research, 20*(5), 599–610.

Geller, S. M., & Porges, S. W. (2014). Therapeutic presence: Neurophysiological mechanisms mediating feeling safe in therapeutic relationships. *Journal of Psychotherapy Integration, 24*(3), 178–192.

Germer, C. (2023). Self-compassion in psychotherapy: Clinical integration, evidence base and mechanisms of change. In A. Finlay-Jones, K. Bluth, & K. Neff (Eds.), *Handbook of self-compassion* (pp. 379–416). Springer.

Neff, K., & Germer, C. (2018). *The mindful self-compassion workbook: A proven way to accept yourself, build inner strength, and thrive.* Guilford Press.

Neff, K. D., Rude, S. S., & Kirkpatrick, D. (2007). An examination of self-compassion in relation to positive psychological functioning and personality traits. *Journal of Research in Personality, 41*(4), 908–916.

Norcross, J. C., & Lambert, M. J. (Eds.). (2019). *Psychotherapy relationships that work: Vol. 1. Evidence-based therapist contributions.* Oxford University Press.

Porges, S. W. (2011). *The polyvagal theory: Neurophysiological foundations of emotions, attachment, communication, and self-regulation.* Norton.

Pos, A., Geller, S., & Oghene, J. (2011). *Therapist presence, empathy, and the working alliance in experiential treatment for depression.* Paper presented at the 42nd annual meeting of the Society for Psychotherapy Research, Bern, Switzerland.

Raab, K. (2014). Mindfulness, self-compassion, and empathy among health care professionals: A review of the literature. *Journal of Health Care Chaplaincy, 20*(3), 95–108.

Siegel, D. J. (2010). *The mindful therapist: A clinician's guide to mindsight and neural integration*. Norton.

Stellar, J. E., Cohen, A., Oveis, C., & Keltner, D. (2015). Affective and physiological responses to the suffering of others: Compassion and vagal activity. *Journal of Personality and Social Psychology, 108*(4), 572–585.

Tannen, T., Daniels, M., & Koro-Ljungberg, M. (2019). Choosing to be present with clients: An evidence-based model for building trainees' counselling competence. *British Journal of Guidance and Counselling, 47*(4), 405–419.

Vinca, M. (2009). *Mindfulness and psychotherapy: A mixed methods investigation*. Unpublished doctoral dissertation, Penn State University.

7

The Power of a Self-Compassionate Mindset

Shauna Shapiro
Shayda Roohparvar
Jill Lillie

This chapter aims to explore the power of a self-compassionate mindset to strengthen both professional effectiveness and personal well-being for therapists. Though the practice of compassion has been central to the world's perennial wisdom traditions for thousands of years, the empirical study of self-compassion is relatively new to the field of psychology. Since 2003, when the first empirical paper on self-compassion was published (Neff, 2003), research on self-compassion has grown exponentially. Although self-compassion has received a great deal of attention in recent years, with most of the research focusing on self-compassion as an important psychological resource with significant benefits in terms of psychological and physical well-being, significantly less attention has been given to the role of a self-compassionate mindset for therapists. We begin by discussing the important question: What is a self-compassionate mindset and why is it essential for therapists? We then explore how therapists can cultivate a self-compassionate mindset and discuss specific practices and interventions to do so. We conclude with a discussion of how a self-compassionate mindset can support clinicians personally and professionally.

Self-Compassion Simply and as an Alchemy

Self-compassion is most succinctly defined as treating ourselves as we would treat a dear friend who is having a hard time. We learn to bring kindness, affection, and tenderness to our own suffering. We learn to be on our team, instead of berating or rejecting ourselves.

And yet, self-compassion does more than simply soothe and help us feel better. It provides us with the life raft we need to navigate through the tough times. By deepening our self-compassion, we discover untapped reserves of strength, resilience, and wisdom that help us survive the storm, *and* we strengthen our resources to better navigate future storms. This is one of the alchemical powers of self-compassion: It simultaneously soothes the negative and grows the positive.

And yet, self-compassion is not our typical response when the going gets tough. Instead, we tend to fall back on habitual coping mechanisms that are ineffective and can be downright harmful. When faced with adversity, many of us respond by turning on ourselves, our minds filled with self-judgment and shame. We mistakenly believe this will somehow motivate us to change. But if our mind is clouded by shame, we can't see our behavior patterns clearly and we just keep repeating them. Shame robs our brain of the resources it needs to respond effectively to a challenging situation.

When we feel shame, the amygdala—the part of our brain that is central to memory, decision making, and emotional responses—triggers a cascade of norepinephrine and cortisol, chemicals that increase our stress level, narrow our perspective on perceived "threats," and inhibit our cognitive flexibility. Shame puts us in the grip of our fight, flight, or freeze survival response, thereby inhibiting the learning centers of the brain.

If we want to learn from our mistakes and keep from repeating them, we need a compassionate mindset, not shame. This is an essential mindset for therapists. It not only gives them the tools to learn from their mistakes, but it also models for their clients a healthy and adaptive way to respond to challenges.

The willingness to face the darker parts of ourselves and the darker parts of life takes courage. This courage is born of compassion—compassion for ourselves and one another. As we practice self-compassion, we learn not only to confront and grow from our struggles and sorrows but to connect with the sufferings and sorrows of others. This capacity to bring compassion to our own and others' suffering is essential for therapists.

What Is Self-Compassion?

So, what *is* self-compassion? Self-compassion comprises three core elements as articulated by Kristin Neff (2003): mindfulness, kindness, and common humanity.

1. *Mindfulness* helps us see clearly that we are in pain. We need to be aware of pain before we can heal it. And yet, facing pain is not easy, as many distractions exist to lure our consciousness away from what we

fear or dislike. Mindfulness provides the nonjudgmental "witness state" of consciousness that helps us see our pain clearly and *choose* to comfort and soothe it instead of succumbing to ingrained reactions of shame or avoidance.

2. *Kindness* is the process of actively soothing ourselves: offering support and care when we are in pain. Importantly, we're not soothing ourselves to make the pain go away. We're soothing ourselves *because* we are in pain. When things go wrong, we often try to suppress the pain, berate ourselves, or leap into problem-solving mode. But once again, imagine how you might support a friend who is suffering. Would you tell your friend to forget about it? Would you call your friend an "idiot"? Would you start barking out orders and instructions? Or would you offer your friend kindness, let them know you care; that no matter what happened or what will result from it, you love them?

3. *Common humanity* reminds us that we are not alone in our suffering. Our belief that this is "my" personal problem and that we are the "only one" suffering isolates and separates us. Common humanity helps us recognize that other people also get divorced, have sick children, or make mistakes. Self-compassion helps us reframe our situation in light of our shared human experience. When we recognize our common humanity and don't take things so personally, we experience a greater sense of connection, comfort, and calm.

These three elements work together to create a self-compassionate mindset. Through training, we can strengthen and grow all three elements and deepen our ability to bring compassion to each moment of the therapeutic process and beyond. Below we explore how a self-compassionate mindset can benefit therapists, and then we review the literature on practices and interventions to cultivate self-compassion in therapists.

A Self-Compassionate Mindset

Research shows that a self-compassionate mindset is important for therapists, impacting both their personal and professional well-being. One of the main struggles therapists face is the prevalence of burnout and "compassion fatigue," which has been extensively studied across populations of caregivers. Its prevalence rates have been reported to affect between 40 and 80% of caregivers (McCray et al., 2008). Doing intense emotional labor that requires therapists to empathically connect to and potentially be overwhelmed by their client's experiences can negatively impact therapists. This is problematic in that it can be emotionally draining and difficult on the mental health of the caregiver (Eriksson et al., 2018). Equally important, it can reduce the quality of care that the patients receive (Raab, 2014). For both the therapist's own sake and the sake of their patients, they need to find a way to manage and mitigate their feelings of burnout and compassion fatigue.

A self-compassionate mindset has been demonstrated to be an effective means of counteracting and even preventing caregiver burnout. Burnout is caused by empathic distress, where the caregiver can feel the other person's affective state, is aware that the source of their emotional response stems from the other person, and then is negatively impacted by it. It's been found that people respond to this distress by either avoiding the distressing situation or by overly identifying with and inappropriately attempting to help the person they are connected to (pathological altruism). A self-compassionate mindset has tools to help combat this distress. We next discuss how self-compassion helps the therapist regulate their own emotions and see things clearly.

For example, research has shown that when individuals imagined themselves from the patient's perspective, they experienced higher distress compared with people who were able to differentiate between themselves and the patient (Lamm et al., 2007). The ability to not be overwhelmed by their empathic response allowed caregivers to be able to help the other not out of their desire to alleviate their distress but out of their genuine compassion for the other and desire to help.

Not only has a self-compassionate mindset been demonstrated to help the therapist's well-being but it's also been demonstrated to increase their professional skills. Therapists high in self-compassion are more present; suffer less from stress, anxiety, and depression; and can attend and respond to their clients (Dorian & Killebrew, 2014). In addition, therapists high in self-compassion are more self-aware and flexible in their thinking, which enhances the therapist's ability to engage in more effective therapy (Gockel et al., 2013). Increasing the therapist's ability to better utilize their skills results in better outcomes for their client.

Training Self-Compassion

Benefits of Mindfulness-Based Interventions

How does the therapist train for self-compassion? Mindfulness-based interventions (MBIs) are the most widely used therapeutic practices used to train for self-compassion. The literature is growing exponentially with studies demonstrating the efficacy of self-compassion training (Neff, 2023).

Studies show that people with greater self-compassion have less depression (Neff et al., 2020), anxiety (Gockel et al., 2013), shame, and stress (Neff et al., 2020)—and greater happiness and well-being (Neff & Germer, 2012), as well as life satisfaction, optimism, resilience, and performance (Neff et al., 2020).

The Research

In this section, we summarize the literature on MBIs for the health care community, specifically focusing on the ability to increase self-compassion. Research shows that training health care professionals in a self-compassionate mindset is most strongly supported through MBIs (Ferrari, 2019). While other methods are being explored, three key MBI practices emerge, with the most robust evidence supporting the training of a compassionate mindset: (1) mindfulness-based stress reduction (MBSR), (2) mindful self-compassion (MSC), and (3) self-compassion training for health care communities (SCHC).

Mindfulness-Based Stress Reduction

A notable self-compassion intervention for the therapist is MBSR. Although self-compassion is not explicitly taught in the MBSR intervention, research shows that it does indeed increase self-compassion in participants (Shapiro et al., 1998), as well as decrease burnout in health care professionals (Shapiro et al., 2005). Originally developed by Jon Kabat-Zinn in 1979 for patients with chronic pain, MBSR techniques are now widely used by health care professionals to prepare for and protect against the risk of occupational-related psychological problems faced by therapists and other health care professionals (Kabat-Zinn et al., 1985).

MBSR training methods include formal and informal practices. The formal practice of mindfulness is the practice of meditation, while informal mindfulness is being aware and present in the everyday moments of our lives. The formal training for mindfulness practices found in MBSR is delivered in a training class for 2.5 hours each week over 8 weeks, with a 1-day retreat. MBSR intervention for the therapist involves development in the following areas: meditative practices of sitting meditation, body scan, hatha yoga, breathing work, and loving-kindness meditation (Segal et al., 2002). Mindfulness practices also contain informal mindfulness meditation techniques that can be applied in everyday work life.

Research shows interesting MBSR research data. One of the first published mindfulness studies in health care by Shapiro and colleagues (1998) examined the effects of MBSR training on medical students. Results demonstrated that mindfulness training protected empathy and compassion and reduced depression and anxiety in students in the MBSR course compared to a wait-list control group of students. Further support of MBSR as a compassion training for health care workers showed positive outcomes in Shapiro's randomized study of medical professionals from the Veterans Affairs health care system in 2005. After completing the MBSR training program, the study participants reported (1) decreased overall psychological distress, (2) decreased stress, (3) decreased job burnout, (4) increased overall life satisfaction, and (5) increased self-compassion (Shapiro et al., 2005).

MBSR continues to be an effective intervention. The training method benefits the health care community. A 2021 meta-analysis reviewed 30 pieces of literature and found MBSR useful for health care professionals. The study concluded that MBSR is effective in reducing health care professionals' anxiety, depression, and stress, and is beneficial to overall wellness (Hofmann et al., 2010).

Mindful Self-Compassion

MSC is a compassion-based program that combines mindfulness and compassion practices to cultivate a self-compassionate frame of mind (Germer & Neff, 2019). Learning to bring kindness to oneself when suffering occurs is a key component of the MSC training course developed by Kristin Neff and Christopher Germer. Originally designed for nonclinical populations as a resource-building intervention, MSC is now specifically being applied to train caregivers in self-compassion. Mindfulness, kindness, and common humanity are the core components of a compassionate mindset (Germer & Neff, 2019).

MSC training develops the three key elements of self-compassion. Cultivating mindfulness, kindness, and common humanity are the components shown to combat burnout and compassion fatigue (Germer & Neff, 2019). MSC training is an existing 8-week group educational training program. The training is 2.5–3 hours per class session with one 4-hour retreat class. During the 8 weeks, participants are asked to engage in 30 minutes of formal or informal mindfulness practice at home.

The first MSC compassion program took place in 2010. A randomized and controlled trial of the program was completed 3 years later by Neff and Germer in 2013. Study results show that MSC training cultivates the capacity for a more sustainable approach to personal challenges or to the challenges of being a caregiver (Neff & Germer, 2012). Additional studies have confirmed the positive impact of MSC on therapists, showing that MSC training builds resources and grows one's capacity for self-compassion (Germer & Neff, 2019).

Self-Compassion for the Health Care Communities

SCHC uses the principles of MSC. Neff and Germer (2019) derived and developed SCHC training to benefit health care professionals specifically. Applicable to the therapist, SCHC addresses the need for training self-compassion skills with health care professionals. Given that care workers generally have limited extra time outside of work, SCHC is intentionally designed to deliver the full benefits of MSC training in less time during the workday.

SCHC trains in less time. The MSC 8-week training program that met for 2.5 hours weekly was condensed into a 6-week program held in 1-hour sessions during the workday. The abbreviated training was accomplished by focusing on retaining content and delivering practical self-compassion tools that health care professionals can use on the job to help health care communities, including therapists, notice their stress at the moment that it is occurring (Neff et al., 2020). Research studies showed that the efficacy of the SCHC program resulted in significantly increased self-compassion well-being and reduced secondary traumatic stress burnout among health care professionals (Neff et al., 2020).

Studies support the use of informal self-compassion practices during times of struggle. Therapists can learn how to soothe their own pain by activating their parasympathetic nervous system. A therapist can learn to relax this system of nerves through self-compassion exercises, such as breath work or supportive touch, such as putting one's hand on one's heart and speaking kindly to oneself (Germer & Neff, 2019). Another practice carried over from MSC to SCHC is a practice particularly designed for caregivers called "compassion with equanimity," which reminds caregivers that while they can help others, they are not in complete control of the outcome of the health care encounter (see Practice J.2, "Self-Compassion with Equanimity," in the Appendix; Germer & Neff, 2019). An example used in SCHC is learning to focus the "in-breath" on compassion for the self and the "out-breath" on compassion we give to others. To conduct this type of soothing touch practice, see Practice G, "Soothing or Supportive Touch," in the Appendix.

Last, in their 2013 study, Germer and Neff state that a compassionate state of mind is operationalized by three elements of compassion: kindness, a sense of common humanity, and mindfulness. The SCHC training is tailored for the health care worker and thus benefits the health care community, including the therapist. As stated in the 2022 mega-study done by Crego, the practice of training for self-compassion brings numerous professional benefits. The study concluded that training for these skills protects from burnout and compassion fatigue and supports therapeutic efficacy. While recognized as beneficial, self-compassion training is not widespread in the therapeutic community. The opportunity for therapists to train for MSC continues to be accessible, as the mega study showed that online training was as effective as face-to-face coursework (Crego et al., 2022).

Self-Compassion in Practice

The research suggests that a self-compassionate mindset is beneficial for a therapist's personal and professional well-being, and it can be cultivated. Self-compassion does more than just help us feel better. It provides us with the life raft we need to navigate through the tough times. By deepening our self-compassion, we discover untapped reserves of strength, resilience, and wisdom that help us survive the storm, *and* we strengthen our resources to better navigate future storms. This is one of the alchemical powers of self-compassion: it simultaneously soothes the negative and grows the positive. The key is to practice self-compassion using all three elements: mindfulness, kindness, and common humanity. It is through their synergistic co-arising that transformation occurs. For a basic meditation practice adapted from Germer and Neff (2019) to get started, see Practice A, "Self-Compassion Break," in the Appendix.

Another practice that can be helpful is to write a letter to yourself about a current struggle in your life, or an area where you feel inadequate and want to motivate yourself to change. But this letter has a special twist. In this letter to yourself, write *as if you were talking to a dear friend* facing the same concerns as you. How might you respond to your friend? What might you say? How might you support them? Try not to think too much about organizing your words or thoughts. Simply write from your heart.

After writing the letter, put it in an envelope and mail it to yourself. When you receive it, see if you can slowly reread it, letting the words soothe and comfort you. The key to self-compassion is to practice. It is a skill that can be cultivated through training (see Practice I, "Self-Compassion in Practice," in the Appendix).

Why We Sometimes Feel Worse before We Feel Better

When we practice self-compassion, strong and painful emotions may arise at first. This is understandable. Self-compassion takes us into the depths of our hearts where we hold our most painful and tender memories and experiences. As we practice self-compassion, it can unveil these pains, allowing them to rise to the surface of our consciousness.

We have accumulated a great deal of suffering over a lifetime, and often have suppressed it in order to function. As we begin to practice self-compassion, we are inviting this pain to surface and heal. Sometimes this can feel overwhelming (Neff & Germer, 2018). If this happens to you, remember that it's natural to feel these strong and painful emotions. It is important to keep offering yourself compassion, especially for the painful emotions that are arising. You can use your mindfulness to explore with openness and curiosity where you feel the emotions in your body. If the experience becomes too distressing, it is okay to simply pause and say to yourself, "This is really hard. It's time to rest and take a break. I can come back to this when I'm ready."

Self-compassion is not a quick fix, and there is no need to push an overly intense experience. Self-compassion takes strength, courage, and faith. We encourage you to trust the process and allow yourself to slowly let in more self-compassion, and more kindness, a few degrees at a time. Change happens in small increments. We know this from experience: We can't instantly erase an unproductive habit and attain a behavior we want. Yet instead of seeing this as a normal process of change, we tend to punish ourselves each time we "fail."

Personal change is not linear. There are stops, detours, setbacks, serendipities, and surprises. Transformation is longitudinal and it is experiential. Layer upon layer, we literally integrate new ways of thinking, feeling, and behaving as we lay down new pathways in our brains and then let these pathways express themselves in our thoughts, words, and actions.

Conclusion

Research on the benefits of a self-compassionate mindset for therapists is in its infancy—however, the preliminary data are strong, and future research is needed. Teaching self-compassion explicitly provides therapists with tools so that they can learn to be kind to themselves in a more direct way. Self-compassion must be experienced to be known. As the behavior of supporting oneself is practiced, neuronal pathways are established, and being self-compassionate becomes more of a habit. Self-compassion begins with an intention to be kind to oneself. Then it becomes a practice. Then it becomes a habit. Eventually, it is simply who you are.

While the body of self-compassion research is growing, comparatively little research has been devoted to understanding its unique role for therapists. Continued exploration is needed with the goal of determining how we can more effectively integrate self-compassion training and a self-compassionate mindset into therapeutic training. There are many unanswered questions and a substantial amount of work that needs to be done in order to facilitate the growth of a meaningful and illuminative understanding of how to best do this.

Methodologically, there is a need for much greater care in the design of studies. This includes such elements as grounding research, in theory, to guide the development of research expectations, selecting participants in a way that ensures sufficient power and generalizability of findings and/or allows for detailed examination of theoretically relevant mechanisms, processes, and outcomes, utilizing study designs that permit the examination of changes and effects both cross-sectionally and longitudinally, resisting the tendency of overrelying on a single methodology (e.g., self-report measures, translational imaging technologies).

Rigorously designed randomized controlled samples with large sample sizes and diverse populations are needed to elucidate how best to train self-compassion in therapists. Finally, future research needs to determine the impact of the therapist self-compassionate mindset on patient outcomes. It can be hypothesized that increasing therapist self-compassion will produce positive synergistic benefits for their clients, including greater attunement, enhanced therapist compassion for clients, and improved therapeutic relationships. As we cultivate the ability to meet our own pain with compassion, we strengthen our ability to meet others' pain with compassion.

The collaboration of a self-compassionate mindset and therapeutic process is still in its infancy, yet it seems this furthering may prove enriching for both therapist and client, and lead to greater understanding, healing, and enhancement of the human mind and heart.

REFERENCES

Crego, A. (2022). The practice of training for self-compassion brings numerous professional benefits. *Journal of Self-Compassion, 1*(1), 1–15.

Crego, A., Yela, J. R., Riesco-Matías, P., Gómez-Martínez, M. Á., & Vicente-Arruebarrena, A. (2022). The benefits of self-compassion in mental health professionals: A systematic review of empirical research. *Psychology Research and Behavior Management, 15*, 2599–2620.

Dorian, M., & Killebrew, J. E. (2014). A study of mindfulness and self-care: A path to self-compassion for female therapists in training. *Women and Therapy, 37*(1–2), 155–163.

Eriksson, T., Germundsjö, L., Åström, E., & Rönnlund, M. (2018). Mindful self-compassion training reduces stress and burnout symptoms among practicing psychologists: A randomized controlled trial of a brief web-based intervention. *Frontiers in Psychology, 9*, 2340.

Ferrari, M., Hunt, C., Harrysunker, A., Abbott, M. J., Beath, A. P., & Einstein, D. A. (2019). Self-compassion interventions and psychosocial outcomes: A meta-analysis of RCTs. *Mindfulness, 10*(8), 1455–1473.

Germer, C., & Neff, K. (2019). Mindful self-compassion (MSC). In I. Itvzan (Ed.), *Handbook of mindfulness-based programmes: Mindfulness interventions from education to health and therapy* (pp. 357–367). Routledge.

Gockel, A., Cain, T., Malove, S., & James, S. (2013). Mindfulness as clinical training: Student perspectives on the utility of mindfulness training in fostering clinical intervention skills. *Journal of Religion and Spirituality in Social Work: Social Thought, 32*(1), 36–59.

Hofmann, S. G., Sawyer, A. T., Witt, A. A., & Oh, D. (2010). The effect of mindfulness-based therapy on anxiety and depression: A meta-analytic review. *Journal of Consulting and Clinical Psychology, 78*(2), 169–183.

Kabat-Zinn, J., Lipworth, L., & Burney, R. (1985). The clinical use of mindfulness meditation for the self-regulation of chronic pain. *Journal of Behavioral Medicine, 8*(2), 163–190.

Lamm, C., Batson, C. D., & Decety, J. (2007). The neural substrate of human empathy: Effects of perspective-taking and cognitive appraisal. *Journal of Cognitive Neuroscience, 19*(1), 42–58.

McCray, L., Cronholm, P., Bogner, H., Gallo, J., & Neill, R. (2008). Resident physician burnout: Is there hope? *Journal of Family Medicine, 40*(9), 626–632.

Neff, K. D. (2003). Self-compassion: An alternative conceptualization of a healthy attitude toward oneself. *Self and Identity, 2*(2), 85–101.

Neff, K. D. (2023). Self-compassion: Theory, method, research, and intervention. *Annual Review of Psychology, 74,* 193–218.

Neff, K. D., & Germer, C. K. (2013). A pilot study and randomized controlled trial of the mindful self-compassion program. *Journal of Clinical Psychology, 69*(1), 28–44.

Neff, K. D., & Germer, C. K. (2018). *The mindful self-compassion workbook: A proven way to accept yourself, build inner strength, and thrive.* Guilford Press.

Neff, K. D., Knox, M. C., Long, P., & Gregory, K. (2020). Caring for others without losing yourself: An adaptation of the mindful self-compassion program for healthcare communities. *Journal of Clinical Psychology, 76*(9), 1543–1562.

Raab, K. (2014). Mindfulness, self-compassion, and empathy among health care professionals: A review of the literature. *Journal of Health Care Chaplaincy, 20*(3), 95–108.

Segal, Z. V., Teasdale, J. D., Williams, J. M., & Gemar, M. C. (2002). The Mindfulness-Based Cognitive Therapy Adherence Scale: Inter-rater reliability, adherence to protocol and treatment distinctiveness. *Clinical Psychology and Psychotherapy, 9*(2), 131–138.

Shapiro, S. L., Astin, J. A., Bishop, S. R., & Cordova, M. (2005). Mindfulness-based stress reduction for health care professionals: Results from a randomized trial. *International Journal of Stress Management, 12*(2), 164–176.

Shapiro, S. L., Schwartz, G. E., & Bonner, G. (1998). Effects of mindfulness-based stress reduction on medical and premedical students. *Journal of Behavioral Medicine, 21*(6), 581–599.

8

Cultivating the Practice of Self-Compassion

Galia Tyano Ronen

> If you want others to be happy, practice compassion.
> If you want to be happy, practice compassion.
> —HIS HOLINESS THE DALAI LAMA (1998, p. 115)

When I was young, I joined a Zen center. I have a clear-embodied memory of the *zazen*—sitting on the cushion with my back erect, facing the wall for 45 minutes. The sitting was followed by 115 bows. After the dharma talk, the teacher answered some questions. Most of the answers were the same. He would look at the person and hit the floor with his hand saying in a determined voice, "Practice! Just practice!"

What I understood was that I had to try harder so my practice would be perfect and I would be an excellent student and Zen practitioner. I got up every morning at dawn, bowed, and sat. I was determined to make the effort needed to practice and strive for perfection. Over time, I started practicing mindfulness and eventually mindful self-compassion. Bringing a self-compassion approach helped me know that I could stop the striving and have a compassionate attitude toward myself and the practice.

We seek a balanced life, so it demands practice since it is not a natural thing for us as human beings. We want to stay aware and not numb ourselves in the face of suffering, especially when we are therapists. When we are in the presence of suffering, we can give it the space it needs, so we can have a better perspective. Creating a soft inner container by practicing self-compassion will enable us and our clients to befriend difficult emotions, thoughts, and sensations. Otherwise, our suffering will grow or tend to stay. We need to cultivate our self-compassion and act from a mindful stance to contribute to others, have boundaries, and a clear distinction between our inner world and the client's to resource ourselves because we are being called upon to be present to help others.

Mindfulness and self-compassion practices enable us to address suffering that sometimes numbs us. Wisdom and insight can be cultivated through our deeper practices to cultivate resilience on any level. In this chapter, we explore:

- The importance for therapists to practice mindfulness and inner and outer compassion meditation.
- The nature of suffering and the ways to set an intention to alleviate it as based on Buddhist psychology.
- The different qualities that comprise self-compassion and the ways therapists can cultivate them. Guidance is offered to help us sustain a regular practice.

For us to understand the ways we can practice and the ways to alleviate suffering, we first explore the nature of suffering itself according to the Buddhist tradition to provide therapists with a foundation for building a practice.

The Four Noble Truths

Mindfulness is the aware-balanced acceptance of the current experience. We are paying attention to our lives and becoming wiser and free from suffering. The Buddha refers to the Four Noble Truths (Osen, 2021) as a framework of understanding beyond our use of automatic pilot mode. The Buddhist doctrine uses the term *suffering* (*dukkha*) as a broad sense of dissatisfaction (Rahula, 1986).

In the First Noble Truth, the Buddha explained that pain is inevitable and suffering is optional. Pain is inherent because life is unpredictable, difficult, ever-changing, and painful by its nature, not because we are doing it wrong.

The Second Noble Truth states that there is an origin of suffering, which is our attachment to desire. There is a big difference between pain and suffering. Pain is part of life, but suffering is optional. Suffering happens because we struggle with our life experiences and are unable to accept them. Every relationship and experience changes, which causes us to feel the pain of separation and loss. Every moment in life has pleasant and unpleasant parts, and most of them happen at the same time. Craving anything is suffering.

According to the Third Noble Truth, it is possible to end suffering and live happily and cultivate a spacious, awake, compassionate, and involved mind. We can have goals and plans and still be able to let go of them if they don't work out. We can condition the mind for clarity, stability, and freedom so that pains and joys can come and go. This is a freeing, tranquil experience.

The Fourth Noble Truth shows us that there are different ways to end suffering. One of the ways to end suffering is mindfulness and self-compassion practice. As Sylvia Boorstein (1995) says, "Suffering is manageable." We can manage it and not be afraid of it. We can see how we are trapped in our stories and how things change and resolve. We are kinder to ourselves when we see how much pain is conditioned to clinging. Even if things are pleasant, everything is disappointing. After all, nothing lasts.

Suffering and Its Nature

We are kinder to ourselves when we see how much pain is conditioned to clinging. In the following case vignette, we can witness suffering and its nature and how compassion can relieve this. (Identifying details have been disguised to ensure client confidentiality.)

> "I can't take it anymore. I just can't take it anymore," the client says.
>
> Sitting in front of her, I'm feeling the lack of energy in my body, my hips are placed heavily on the armchair, my back is arching, and my head is heavy.
>
> "I just want someone to take all this away from me, for someone else to take care of him. I can't see him like this, so sick. It breaks my heart. It's clear to me that it's mine, that it's on me, it's always all on me. . . ."
>
> She looks at me, full of sadness, exhaustion, and pain. I feel the same feelings inside me as well. My body is shrinking—this inner state . . . that I too experience at certain moments.
>
> The two of us sitting in a room lit by the early morning light, each resonating with fatigue from carrying the load on all levels.
>
> In her case, a woman more or less my age, the progressive illness of her partner. In my case, it was a day full of meetings and many tasks, which started last night.
>
> Our breathing synchronizes, naturally, without any special guidance, slow and deep.
>
> Almost like a big sigh. Together.
>
> We are both seeking a way to continue, how to become a rock in an ocean of stormy waves.
>
> She describes her events, and I place (consciously and naturally for me) the palm of my hand on my heart. This action allows me to bring a supportive and comforting touch, for me. I check with her about what supportive contact is right for her.
>
> She tries different types of touch until she finds the one that suits her. We sit there together, placing a compassionate hand on great pain and fatigue, paving our way to the rest of our meeting.

I, for myself, enable compassionate self-support. And she, for herself, through the option offered to her, and the two of us together.

"How nice it is to rest for a moment like this together," she says with a certain relief on her face, her eyebrows more relaxed now.

I smile at her.

We arrived at an island, at a refuge, and soon we will sail on, continuing our journey.

Can Self-Compassion Relieve Suffering?

The possibility for both the therapist and the client to develop self-compassion forms the basis of therapeutic work that is based on mindfulness and compassion practice. When we encounter suffering compassionately, there is less internal resistance and less immediate reactivity. There is inner space along with experiencing a deep connection to others.

Compassionate consciousness can develop when we, as therapists, practice compassion for ourselves and others. The mind is in a contracted state, perceived suffering, whenever there is any grasping or aversion toward something. The mind unconsciously tries to escape the situation by increasing the grasping or aversion, in a way that only keeps it stuck or even makes things worse. Unfortunately, this further grasping contracts it even more, setting up a vicious circle in which the mind is trapped. The more we develop an awareness of our mind states and untangle it from grasping by creating space, the more relief we feel and accessible it becomes. (See Practice J.1, "Sitting Compassion Meditation Practice," in the Appendix.)

Pema Chodron (2022) explains three traditional categories of suffering according to the Buddha. The *suffering of suffering*, or ordinary suffering, is the term used to describe the outer layer of suffering: neglect, poverty, hunger, homelessness, and violence. There's a deeper layer of suffering, which is the *suffering of impermanence*, which refers to the human desire for things to remain the same. It doesn't recognize the ever-changing experience of life. The most subtle of all is called *all-pervasive suffering*, which refers to wanting our situation to remain stable—not wanting insecurity, uncertainty, or experiencing feelings like anxiety. To be free of all-pervasive suffering means to allow these feelings to be present without struggling against them.

Gardening the Mind and Heart

When we want to cultivate and grow a pragmatic vegetable garden, other unknown plants also start to grow in between. In nature, one could not survive without the other. It's our judgment and mindset that drive us to grow a clean vegetable garden, aspire to productivity, and cultivate a goal-oriented competitive product. In life, we need to accept all of it.

When it comes to cultivating the practice of self-compassion, usually we pursue the same path. As we regard most of our everyday tasks, we tend to push ourselves in a very harsh way to get better at it, to have more, and to succeed in whatever area in life. To cultivate a garden, we need a certain level of acceptance, curiosity, willpower, space, supportive conditions, perseverance, patience, resilience, and grit to handle challenges. As Angela Duckworth (2016) points out in her book *Grit*, for us to succeed we need passion and perseverance, effort, interest, firmness of mind spirit, and courage to continue the path for a long-term goal or state of mind.

When we try to cultivate a garden, we have passion for the idea of it, eating the tasty vegetables we cultivated ourselves, to produce and enjoy. We could feel the passion attached to the thought. When trying to implement these ideas into real life, we find new dimensions that are based on information coming from our experiences. Most of the time there is a gap between the idea and the reality. The part that takes over usually is our habits and patterns that derive from the survival mode in our brain. If our dominant pattern is to flee, we will abandon the whole idea. If we are used to fighting over it, we will persevere and might succeed, but with unbalanced effort that might end in burnout as well. There is immense importance in understanding the different elements underlying the cultivation of the garden of our mind and heart through practice.

It is important to pay attention to not "fall in love" with the idea of practicing meditation and its positive influence on us, or our clients. Instead, we can build an intention inside of us, being less attached to the results, and open with curiosity to the process. When we can be mindful of the different elements that are the qualities that are cultivated through practice, our whole approach and mindset might change and we might be able to practice in a satisfying, self-gratifying way, enjoying the process, the "vegetables," and the "useless plants."

Cultivation of Qualities of the Mind and Heart to Support a Healing Process

What is compassion made of? What "plants" do we grow in our garden? What qualities do we cultivate when practicing mindfulness and compassion? It might be easier for us to track the development of each one of them over time. Our intention is not to achieve a certain level in any of the qualities, but rather to have clues that will point us in the direction of the practice. We usually have a hard time noticing the path that we are walking, so this is a way for us to have signs along the way, indicating to us that change is occurring although almost unnoticeable.

Many beneficial qualities are generated when therapists and clients practice mindfulness, compassion, and self-compassion. I will name just a few, as there are many of them. Across modalities, effective therapy sessions share the quality of a strong alliance supported by these qualities (Raue et al., 1997). The greatest value of meditation practice for the psychotherapist, inside and outside the session, is forming psychotherapy skills, such as compassion, empathy, attention, presence, and a wider perspective on pain and suffering (Chung, 1990; Deikman, 2001; Geller & Greenberg, 2022; Henley, 1994). Through these qualities we can self-monitor to see how they develop over time with practice and how they are helpful as personal well-being and therapist and client work. This is not setting an aim for us, but rather an intention of developing with time one or more qualities with a kind appreciation toward ourselves for the will to practice and be present to the practice's qualities. By the mere action of cultivation, we put effort, energy, and perseverance into our growth and the growth of others. The practice of meditation and psychotherapy was developed to alleviate suffering through introspection and action. Introspection brings a closer observation of thoughts, emotions, and feelings, as well as insights into the patterns and early wounds that influenced their creation.

Qualities Generated through Compassion Practice

General Intention for Growth

As impermanence is at the core of our being and the development of our body, mind, and spirit, we walk the path of life intending to grow and understand the mysteries of life.

Healing

The growing capacity to hold and accept painful experiences enables the transformative healing process and relief from suffering.

Awareness

The practice lets us observe the mind without getting lost in it or identifying with it. We learn to remain centered and see the replication of the neurotic conflicts. We offer this to ourselves and our clients by being with them and assisting them in letting go of their histories. We are invited to come back to awareness again and again, practicing the ability to notice things happening inside and outside of ourselves. Being in touch with our inner processes and expectations enables us to pause and embody a larger, authentic version of ourselves and our clients.

Being in Contact

We cultivate making continual contact with our experience by returning to what's most true at the moment. We simply practice attending to what is without changing it so we are in true contact with the whole realm that the client brings.

The Contingency of Experience

We can be with our client's experience because we know from our practice that everything is impermanent. Nothing remains. This helps us tolerate for the moment what our clients might not.

Self-Love

Self-love holds different facets, such as compassion and empathy, acceptance and gentleness, firmness, and determination. As we evolve in the practice, we discover areas of interest that bring us joy. We can learn new healthier coping skills and accept that we don't need to be perfect to be worthy of love. We set clear boundaries in our relationships, and it enables us to accept ourselves and treat ourselves with kindness and respect, nurturing our growth and well-being.

Acceptance

In the process of learning to tolerate our discomfort and pain, practice gives us the ability to endure the same processes as our clients. The more we accept our own experience, the more we can truly accept our clients' experience. This quality provides the therapist and the client relief from suffering by the mere nonjudgmental awareness of the present and creating a trustworthy environment and relationship.

Tenderness/Gentleness

When we practice self-compassion, we allow ourselves to be gentle with ourselves, which leads us to be gentle with our clients. Not just by deep listening and empathizing but by having a soft gaze and a tender heart, knowing the secret path to the heart.

Courage

Courage is the ability to stand up for values, make decisions, and take decisive action. Courage also entails the willingness to challenge and disrupt deeply ingrained beliefs and is not necessarily a positive capability.

Determination

How do we act in the world? We all have different voices inside of us. Some voices want to achieve a goal and others don't, so they hold us back. We have the power to choose which of the conflicting voices will lead at any given moment. When we practice, it reinforces our determination and self-discipline. We empower the voices we pay attention to.

Self-Discipline

Self-discipline is focusing on what is most meaningful, despite many distractions inside and outside of ourselves. It is spending time and energy on the things that add value to our lives. We practice self-commitment, perseverance, and the ability to sustain an engagement and remain determined and patient, even when efforts take a long time to bear fruit. In the same way that clients come week after week to a session, the practice is following a rhythm and needs a commitment.

Centering

When we practice, we must be in the here and now in a state of open-ended embodied presence. Gradually, we might develop the capacity for an embodied centered presence, free from preoccupation with projecting and defending a particular self-image or a psychological need for upholding a certain worldview that provides a sense of safety. This influences the deep presence of us and our clients.

Inner Peace

Mindfulness and self-compassion meditation are useful for cultivating wisdom and the ability to discriminate, which can bring inner peace. Through the practice of meditation, we recognize the elements of human suffering that are not neurotic and are therefore not susceptible to psychotherapeutic treatment. Our clients want to fix their suffering because they assume they are supposed to be happy, but some pain is inherent to the human condition. The beginning of a meditation practice may reveal unseen possibilities and invite us to step back and reframe the situation.

Gratefulness

The sense of gratefulness encompasses relating to others, the material, and the natural world with a sense of appreciation, gratitude, and joy. A basic appreciative attitude helps build a connection and trust and is thus conducive to creative and collaborative action. This can be helpful in the therapeutic process, as there is less concern with defending an ego conception and being absorbed with predefined ideas and an easier way to appreciate helpful qualities in various situations one finds oneself in.

Deep Listening

During practice, we cultivate our ability to listen inwardly. This contributes to our ability to listen to others, foster genuine dialogue, advocate our views skillfully, and manage conflicts constructively. When we learn to listen to our clients with the same degree of wholeheartedness and undistractedness, the relationship, trust, and profound process with our clients are likely to happen.

Curiosity

For us to feel safe, we embrace the known and predictable and tend to walk less in the land of uncertainty. To be curious asks us to leave the path we know already and walk the unknown with fresh eyes and an open heart. Becoming aware of our reactions, emotions, and identifications, we develop curiosity and a willingness to be vulnerable, change, and grow. We develop flexibility and curiosity about alternative ways of perceiving and interpreting various issues. This is very valuable for the psychotherapy process, as there is a possibility to experiment with various ways of thinking, feeling, and working with issues.

Humility

We learn to trust and listen deeply to our experience, the client's, and the relationship. Meditation helps therapists remain mindful of both the client's and their own limits, capacities, self, and other connections, which teaches humility. The understanding and experience of interconnectedness and intraconnectedness (Siegel, 2022) brings a sense of being part of a larger whole—this is a humble feeling. Intraconnectedness reveals how our culture may give us a message of separation as an individual, isolated self, but a wider perspective unveils that who we are may be something broader than the brain, bigger even than the body, and fundamental to social systems and the natural world. Our body-based self, the origin of a *Me*, is not only connected to others but connected within our relational worlds themselves—a *We*, forming the essence of how we belong and our identity.

Not Knowing: Looking at Things with Fresh Eyes

When we let go of our expectations of each moment through meditation practice, creative possibility and real growth arise. As therapists, we go through many training sessions, learn, and follow many theories. When we practice, we let go of our models and sometimes even our confidence in diagnostic labels. We can look at the world with fresh eyes. Psychoanalyst Wilfred Bion (1967/1988) said, "The purest form of listening is to listen without memory or desire" (p. 18). Bion issued his edict that all analysts should free themselves from willful behavior, just refraining from memory and desire. Bion encouraged leaving "psychological comfort" for the more exciting prospect of venturing "forth into the unknown" to risk the terror. He understood that if clients remained "untouched by analysis," then he needed to suspend all previous psychoanalytic thinking, such as Freud's and Klein's, to allow for a clean start and a new model to be born.

The Motivation to Alleviate Suffering: Compassion

According to Buddhist thought, the awakened mind has three qualities. The first, compassion, is an expression of the greatest strength and a gesture of bravery. We welcome and allow the sorrows of other people to touch us. We can connect, heart-to-heart. At the same time, it is extremely, heartbreakingly ordinary. Our self-compassion meditation practice teaches us how to open our hearts and how to stabilize within the open state so that every time we are touched, we are not also knocked down. Instead, we are stronger in our vulnerability, and the ability to remain soft and open under all circumstances to our clients.

Loving Heart: Cultivation of Empathy

Empathy is the capacity to accurately understand and feel what other people feel, whereas compassion adds the quality of wanting to relate to other people with benevolence. Practicing allows us a way to be with the suffering of our clients and let empathy and compassion arise.

Equanimity

Meditation practice helps us to cultivate respect for the integrity of another person's experience and recognize that they are the owners of their own experiences. It leads to equanimity or mental calmness. While we give everything we have to offer, within the framework of the therapy relationship, we also recognize the limits of our ability to change anybody (see Practice J.2, "Self-Compassion with Equanimity," in the Appendix).

Perspective Skills

Our view of the world is based on a limited and selective set of data and complemented by assumptions and judgments not necessarily backed up by proven facts. It leads us to try to understand perspectives that are very different from one's own. We learn to see the client's worldview, attitudes, and beliefs in contrast to our own beliefs. We learn about our feelings, body sensations, and emotions and begin to see how our own needs can interfere with the treatment. By practicing, we simply see things for what they are.

Joy

It is possible, even in the midst of tremendous pain, to enjoy life. We can feel joy, not because everything is fine but even though it's not. We are capable of recognizing and being in contact with it, which could be a model for us and then pass it on to our clients.

Intimacy

Practicing involves the creation of an intimate relationship with our inner world—our body, mind, and spirit. It involves a gentle, close connection and an opportunity to learn about ourselves from the inside. We learn to trust what we find with genuine contact. With time, this intimacy will enable close relations with the world. This is a very gentle act that will influence the relationship with our clients and enhance a gentle view of themselves.

Creativity

Creative work involves weaving something wonderful and new out of ingredients that already exist in the world. Our mind produces something unique made from our own experiences, memories, and histories. When we practice, we tap into the ability to generate and develop original ideas and innovate, and imagine how things could be if done differently. This virtue is essential for us to enable the view of the client's stories in a new way.

Trust

Trust often is understood as an outcome, rather than a skill or a basic attitude. We might learn to trust the practice itself as a space of intimate meeting with ourselves and our body sensations. We can develop trust by offering ourselves compassion and skillfully reparenting ourselves with kindness toward our experience, especially by practicing self-compassion. Then trust in the process, in the client's ability to thrive, and in ourselves, rises.

Maintaining a Steady Mindfulness and Compassion Practice

Most people who try to maintain a steady practice fail at it over time. This is why we need to find ways to support us in planning and building a sustainable intimate practice. It is possible to practice in many different ways, paving our path to the heart. Imagine that every day we walk the same path toward ourselves. We admire the view and get to know every plant and creature on the path. It's the way to create a neurological pathway. We practice formally, sitting, lying down, standing, or walking, and in a nonformal way, doing everyday activities in a mindful, compassionate way (Germer et al., 2005; see Practice J.3, "Meditation in Action," in the Appendix, for a practice to help us be with suffering).

Planning a Regular Practice

We naturally judge everything, including the practice of mindful awareness, which at first, we may feel we won't be able to do. For us to establish a meditation practice, we need to have the intention of doing so. Perhaps we want to maintain physical health or create stability in our minds and open our hearts. We can plan our practice as we start slowly and make it doable. Decide to meditate, for example, 10 minutes a day. When we have decided on the frequency of the practice for 1 month, then we can decide if we want to do it more. We can practice at the same time every day or experiment with different times of day. Choose a place for your practice that is comfortable and where you enjoy being. Keeping it tidy and inspirational helps us as well. It is better to be consistent than to practice for a long time (10 minutes per day, 4 days a week rather than 40 minutes, 1 day a week). As you sit down to practice, declare your intention: "Now is my time to practice. Everything else will wait." When we miss a practice, we are compassionate with ourselves. As none of us is perfect, we will miss some practices. It would support us to read some text or listen to a dharma talk, as these will deepen our practice.

Cultivation of Self-Compassion

The perception of practice is different when we cultivate self-compassion because every small gesture that is done for ourselves, anything we do during our day-to-day life, or in a formal sitting meditation if done with loving awareness and intention to alleviate suffering, contributes to a practice of healing and growing compassion. The compassion is directed to us, as therapists, and to our clients as well (see Practice G, "Soothing or Supportive Touch," in the Appendix, for a practice to help us warm our practice).

Sustaining a Practice over Time

The practice of meditation and psychotherapy offers "containers" to support us. Just like the structure of the therapy, the integrity of the therapist, the respect for the boundaries of the relationship, and the confidentiality support the process. In meditation, there are several supportive ways to stay close to difficult experiences. Sitting in a group and listening to the teachings gives instruction that can help us understand and guide our practice. Teachers can provide support to tolerate things that we might not otherwise put up with.

Creating the Habit of Practice

We all have habits that we do unconsciously because we do them so often. New neural pathways are formed when we repeat a behavior. The more a brain circuit fires, the easier it becomes for our brain to do whatever that circuit controls without conscious thought. In the beginning, we have to think about each action consciously. Eventually, after we practice enough, we no longer have to. One area involved in habitual behavior is the striatum, which releases chemicals that inhibit the complex thinking part of our brain for that task (Hanson & Mendius, 2009). Our brain is efficient, and then it's free to think about other things.

Habits have three key ingredients: a cue, a behavior, and a reward. A cue is something that triggers a behavior, and this is followed by the reward. Rewarding a behavior can create a craving, and this is what makes habits so strong. Neurons in the brain can fire and give us chemical rewards. Once a habit and a reward are tied together, those reward neurons fire before we do the behavior. The chemistry of our brain is constantly changing in response to everything from learning to moving to hunger. These chemical releases are short-lived, but over time, if the same behaviors are repeated, the physical structure of the brain is changed (Lazar, 2005). When it comes to making a habit, whether it's learning guitar or meditation, there's simply no substitute for repetition.

Reward System

The rewards derived from this practice are not seen as a ripe tomato that grew in our garden or through a deep feeling of inner peace, but rather by the development of the qualities mentioned in the prior section or by an act of compassion to ourselves that is rewarding by itself. At the beginning of a garden creation, nothing is growing, and like the meditation practice, it consists of continuous, repetitive, constant intention, attention, and action. Watering and giving fertilizers to the plants hidden in the soil, is gratifying in the same way we give ourselves the kindness we need and practice. The focus is on the organic process, the circle of growth, when cultivating the soil of practicing self-compassion. We make the practice its reward, without relying on external ones. To support us, we need to cultivate mindful self-discipline.

Mindful Self-Discipline

Self-discipline allows us to bring rhythm, focus, and empowerment into our lives and be the best version of ourselves. It helps us discern wisely and purposefully what is beneficial for us and what isn't. We learn to say no to things that are attractive now but are not beneficial in the long term, so we can say yes to something more meaningful. As Abraham Lincoln (1861) said, "Discipline is choosing between what you want now and what you want most" (Dienstmann, 2021, p. 113). This process requires bravery, strength, awareness, and perseverance so we can live with greater fulfillment and well-being. Mindful self-discipline is based on meditation and awareness rather than forcefulness. We can practice it, as it invites us to harmonize all parts of ourselves in pursuit of a meaningful goal, rather than beat ourselves up. The first step would be to *choose what matters to us*—our values—that is where our goals and aspirations come from. The second step would be to *direct and follow our thoughts, emotions, fears, and triggers* pointing in the direction of our values. Then we are proactive in creating, manifesting, and shaping our life and future. The next step would be to *sacrifice the lower joy to the higher joy*, done gently and kindly toward ourselves. It invites us to harmonize all parts of ourselves in pursuit of a meaningful goal, like practicing meditation, rather than beat ourselves up. Mindful self-discipline helps us keep the practice by asking, "How will you live your aspirations today?" Then pay attention every day to the ways we are *choosing ourselves* and respecting that choice—aspirations over desires (Dienstmann, 2021).

Challenges to Practice

What happens when we hit the wall? And the practice stops? What forces do we have there? At that moment we need *sisu* (Lahti, 2023). *Sisu* is a Finnish word that describes a universal psychological embodied capacity. It is a life force—an extraordinary determination and courage in the face of extreme adversity. It is the point where we feel that we have come to the edge of our preconceived capacities but we don't give up; we enter the zone of *sisu*. It's beyond grit—it is a long-term effort for a goal that you've set your mind and heart to—it takes commitment and perseverance to practice every day. In a *sisu* moment, we unearth something that we weren't previously aware of and we keep on going. Grit, resilience, and perseverance are all cognitive qualities that indicate the use of our thinking. *Sisu* is a visceral energy. Willpower is not only a matter of how we use our minds and how much of this mental toughness we have but also how we increase our strength through our bodies. Practicing meditation is an embodied practice that can maintain *sisu* and also draw forces from it. Those people who are high on *sisu* can see beyond the limitations of this moment. They know *sisu* inside out because they practiced. If we have been leading our lives so that our go-to is always toughness, eventually it will come at the cost of our self-care. It's going to come at the cost of harshness toward ourselves and toward others as well. We need to have both of those—a gentle power. Some might need to be able to toughen up in a certain moment and have more *sisu* and determination. For some, it might mean that they need to start to open to a little bit of gentleness and softness so that they don't get blinded by their self-reliance mode. We have *sisu*, and it's a universal capacity.

Exercise: Building Sisu

As an exercise, we can take a moment to note the moments in our lives where we have overcome something that we thought we could not overcome and endure. So by doing that exercise, we start to see those moments. What were they? Then the second layer is to write down what the key thing was that allowed you to overcome. What was something that you did? What changed the narrative at that moment? Was it some kind of an activity or an action, or was it another human?

The purpose of this exercise is to bring awareness to this capacity within us. Moreover, it is important to practice some gentleness toward ourselves. It also means that we forgive ourselves for those times when we weren't so gracious and graceful and we didn't do so well because what is in the past is in the past. To look into the future with this action mindset is also part of *sisu*. So, that's a chance to be gentle with ourselves.

Disillusion

Acceptance of not having the ideal vegetable garden and having some purposeless plants indicates self-forgiveness. The nonperfect garden—yet with a strong will to continue and give space to the practice that is by itself gratifying as an act of love and acceptance—deepens the cultivation of all the values that represent and are part of self-compassion. We often want our practice to be continuous and fulfilling; our clients might feel the same. Bringing a self-compassionate attitude enables us and our clients to continue, to support each other, and to sustain the mindfulness and compassion practice.

Creating a Ritual for the Therapist and the Clients

Our mind exists the way it does because we have repeated the same reactions countless times since we were born. We build up conditioning that is limiting for us and doesn't give us a lot of freedom. To strike a new path and build a new life, we have to repeat good habits over and over again. It takes time and brings lots of healing. We can build with our clients a ritual at the beginning and ending of a session to turn the attention to the present moment inviting a compassionate attitude, connecting to our bodies with awareness and kindness, letting whatever arises to be present as it is.

Community (*Sangha*) as a Support System

Having a support system is crucial for our personal and global success. Therapists need to practice themselves to bring practice to the clients. We are built to need community. We can find a support system by reaching out to a group around us and practicing with them. The group helps support the action itself and offers the caring of others toward us and of us toward others.

Therapist and Client: Mini-*Sangha*

In the same way that the therapist needs support from a group, the client needs support from the therapist (Germer, 2009). It is helpful for clients to practice with the therapist and receive recorded practices tailor-made especially for them. This is a vulnerable place for the therapist—the simple act of deep listening and being together—to stop and be aware of the patterns automatically used by the client. The alliance between the therapist and the clients enables support and creates a different setting that respects boundaries and yet enables a deeper embodied way of relatedness. Cultivation of practice with the client enables holding the memory of a time when the feeling was better, although we know that it will not always be so.

Conclusion

During the therapeutic process, the therapist and the client build a stronger connection to their inner goodness, nature, and resources. It enables them to support the motivation to practice, even without seeing immediate results. It offers the possibility to build resilience, embrace the not-knowing, trust, and cultivate intimacy with ourselves and our inner and outer lives with others. The therapist's practice creates a safe harbor to come back to for the therapist and the client as well. We are experimenting to find ways to practice. We come to the practice with deep listening to our own needs, to the signals (Rothschild, 2000), and doing our best to attend to these needs. As a therapist, it gives satisfaction to get closer to one's own needs, reparenting ourselves with self-compassion as a creative process (Neff, 2003).

Making the practice simple and enjoyable for us are key elements that help us sustain the practice. In this intimate process, we trust the inner container without judgment and the outer support systems. We need to create our practice routine, do what we love, what we find interesting and useful for us, practice our favorite practices and what we find easy. We do it for ourselves as a creative experiment, being playful, based on deep listening.

The invitation to us, as therapists, to turn toward ourselves and help ourselves with self-compassion requires practice: both daily mindfulness and self-compassion practice. We set an intention and must remember to act with compassion toward the attempt to practice and be compassionate. There is a tremendous benefit of meditation practice to the therapist in cultivating qualities of mind that support a healing therapeutic relationship and well-being. Meditating helps us connect with the beautiful and joyful parts of our life and to accept the long journey of our life. We just need to decide if we want to walk the path this way.

As Carlos Casteñeda (1974) writes in the book *The Teachings of Don Juan*:

> Does this path have a heart? If it does, the path is good; if it doesn't, it is of no use. Both paths lead nowhere; but one has a heart, the other doesn't. One makes for a joyful journey; as long as you follow it, you are one with it. The other will make you curse your life. One makes you strong; the other weakens you. (p. 82)

REFERENCES

Bion, W. (1988). Notes on memory and desire. In E. B. Spillius (Ed.), *Melanie Klein today: Developments in theory and practice: Vol. 2. Mainly practice* (pp. 17–21). Taylor & Frances/Routledge. (These notes were first published in 1967 in *The Psychoanalytic Forum, 2*, 272–273, 279–280.)

Boorstein, S. (1995). *It's easier than you think: The Buddhist way to happiness.* HarperOne.

Casteñeda, C. (1974). *The teachings of Don Juan: A Yaqui way of knowledge.* Pocket Books.

Chodron, P. (2022). *Embracing the unknown.* www.soundstrue.com

Chung, C. Y. (1990). Psychotherapist and expansion of awareness. *Psychotherapy and Psychosomatics, 53*(1–4), 28–32.

Dalai Lama, H. H., & Cutler, H. (1998). *The art of happiness.* Eastin Press.

Deikman, A. (2001). *Spirituality expands a therapist's horizons.* www.buddhanet.net/psyspir3.htm.

Dienstmann, G. (2021). *Mindful self-discipline: Living with purpose and achieving your goals in a world of distractions.* Live and Dare.

Duckworth, A. (2016). *Grit: The power of passion and perseverance.* Scribner/Simon & Schuster.

Geller, S. M., & Greenberg, L. S. (2022). *Therapeutic presence: A mindful approach to effective therapeutic relationships* (2nd ed.). American Psychological Association.

Germer, C. K. (2009). *The mindful path to self-compassion: Freeing yourself from destructive thoughts and emotions.* Guilford Press.

Germer, C. K., Siegel, R. D., & Fulton, P. R. (Eds.). (2005). *Mindfulness and psychotherapy.* Guilford Press.

Hanson, R., & Mendius, R. (2009). *Buddha's brain: The practical neuroscience of happiness, love & wisdom.* New Harbinger.

Henley, A. (1994). When the iron bird flies: A commentary on Sydney Walter's "Does a systemic therapist have Buddha nature?" *Journal of Systemic Therapies, 13*(3), 50–51.

Lahti, E. E. (2023). *Gentle power: A revolution in how we think, lead, and succeed using the Finnish art of sisu.* Sounds True.

Lazar, S. W. (2005). Mindfulness research. In C. K. Germer, R. D. Siegel, & P. R. Fulton (Eds.), *Mindfulness and psychotherapy* (pp. 220–238). Guilford Press.

Neff, K. D. (2003). Self-compassion: An alternative conceptualization of a healthy attitude toward oneself. *Self and Identity, 2*, 85–102.

Osen, A. (2021). *The Four Noble Truths and eightfold path of Buddhism—the mindfulness bell: A guide to everyday life.* Independently published.

Rahula, W. (1986). *What the Buddha taught.* Grove Press.

Raue, P., Golfried, M., & Barkham, M. (1997). The therapeutic alliance in psychodynamic-interpersonal and cognitive-behavioral therapy. *Journal of Consulting and Clinical Psychology, 65*(4), 582–587.

Rothschild, B. (2000). *The body remembers: The psychophysiology of trauma and trauma treatment.* Norton.

Siegel, D. J. (2022). *Intraconnected: MWe (Me + We) as the integration of self, identity, and belonging.* Norton.

9

Self-Compassion

A Powerful Addition to Trauma Therapy

Susan M. Pollak

As a clinical psychologist, I have been treating traumatized individuals of all ages and genders since 1990, guided by the pioneering work of psychiatrist Judith Herman. Her ground-breaking book *Trauma and Recovery* (Herman, 1992) changed our understanding and treatment of trauma. The field has grown tremendously over the past few decades, and our understanding of the prevalence of trauma across the life cycle and across cultures has increased dramatically. This recognition has led to the development of new modalities of treating trauma in clinical settings, most notably seen in internal family systems (IFS), eye movement desensitization and reprocessing (EMDR), sensorimotor psychotherapy, and somatic experiencing.

The focus of this chapter is on the application of self-compassion, which has evolved from the theory and practice of mindfulness. When combined with new developments in trauma therapy, the skills of self-compassion can be profoundly healing. My intention here is to bring together current theories, research, and clinical illustrations that inform how self-compassion can be used effectively in trauma therapy.

What Is Trauma?

What do we mean by *trauma*? Trauma specialist Pat Ogden (2015) writes that "any experience that is stressful enough to leave us feeling helpless, frightened, overwhelmed, or profoundly unsafe is considered a trauma" (p. 66). It is not only the story of something that happened a long time ago, it's also the residue of the pain, horror, and fear that continue to live inside us. It is crucial to include social history, as trauma is frequently rooted in systems of oppression.

The Trauma of War

An understanding of the trauma of war is a good place to begin our inquiry as it offers a useful historical template for understanding the impact of trauma on the mind and body. In his integrative, scholarly, and comprehensive book *The Body Keeps the Score*, Bessel van der Kolk (2014) writes, "Being traumatized means continuing to organize your life as if the trauma were still going on—unchanged and immutable—as every new encounter or event is contaminated by the past" (p. 53). People often report that it feels like their physiology, posttrauma, has changed. For many survivors, van der Kolk maintains, conventional talk therapy is "virtually useless" (p. 72), and he offers an integrative approach. He argues that trauma is one of the greatest public health issues we face. Psychiatrist Mark Epstein (2013) also takes a broad historical perspective and asserts that trauma is the bedrock of psychology.

Current theory underscores that for trauma treatment to be effective, we must engage the body, mind, and brain. Given that so many survivors are replaying and reliving the past, learning to shift into the present moment can itself be healing. This is a basic foundation of mindfulness. An excellent working definition of mindfulness, adapted from psychologist Christopher Germer (2013), is that mindfulness is the awareness of present experience with acceptance (p. 7).

How to Introduce Mindfulness and Compassion into Trauma Therapy

Mindfulness and compassion practices are not for everyone, and some patients may feel uncomfortable exploring their experience of fear and discomfort. Helping survivors get curious about emotional pain and suffering is an important first step to utilizing mindfulness in trauma treatment.

It isn't necessary to provide a synopsis of Buddhist philosophy, which might make some patients recoil. We don't need to use the words *mindfulness* or *compassion* at all, as for some people it has religious or New Age connotations. It is simpler to call it "attention training" or "skills training." The clinician can simply state that there is good research on this approach, and it might help manage the symptoms. Then offer to try it together as "an experiment." It is also important for clinicians to keep it very short, no more than a few minutes. Doing the practices with the therapist provides support and comfort and helps if fears and anxieties arise. If the patient decides that mindfulness and compassion are not for them, there should be no pressure about that choice.

When working with trauma survivors, I keep the following points in mind, which I have gathered from decades of experience and study:

Establish Safety and Stability

This is a process that can take time, often months, if not years. One of the most useful tools I know of is Daniel Siegel's (1999) "window of tolerance" (see Figure 9.1). This is something I often teach my patients so we can work together to recognize dysregulation and arousal. It is a tool that can help an individual learn to function in daily life. I like to think of it as a barometer of how one is managing daily life. With trauma, even seemingly minor stressors can cause someone to feel anxious, angry, or dissociated, leading to either hyperarousal or hypoarousal. One way to conceptualize this model is when you are inside the window of tolerance, you can manage whatever is happening in your life. While you may feel stress or discomfort, you feel you can deal with it. If you are feeling outside the window of tolerance, hyperaroused, you may be feeling angry, anxious, out of control, or overwhelmed. On the other hand, if you are hypoaroused, you may feel spacey, numb, or frozen. Some report feeling shut down. The important clinical question is how do you get back within the window of tolerance?

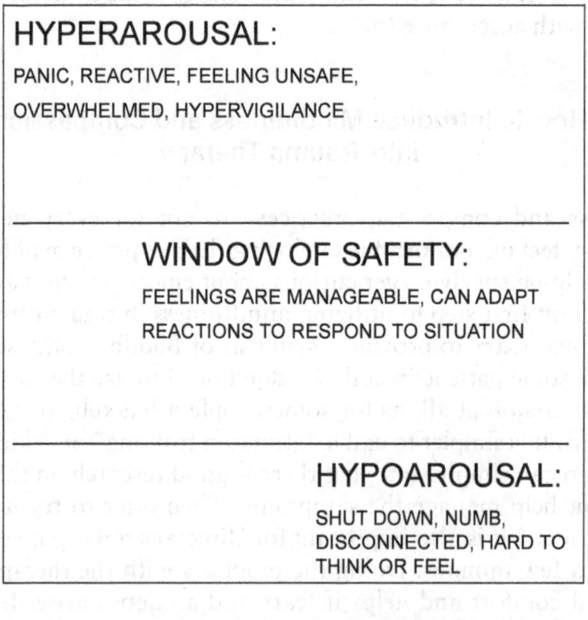

FIGURE 9.1. The window of tolerance.

Simple mindfulness techniques can help. These are my favorite exercises to bring a person back to the window of tolerance:

1. Ask your client to describe three things in your office (or on the Zoom screen). This is a useful anchor as it brings them back to the present moment and helps them connect to the relationship.
2. Orienting in the present moment with your voice is helpful as well. The therapist can simply say, "You are with me. This is [say current date and time]. You are safe."
3. Supportive touch is another self-compassion intervention that can help bring survivors into the window. Try putting a hand on the heart or a hand on the heart and belly. Take a breath or two, feeling the warmth of your touch. (For an extensive practice, see Practice G, "Soothing or Supportive Touch," in the Appendix.)

While many survivors mistakenly believe that complete emotional catharsis is the way to heal, this often increases symptom arousal. Catharsis is not an indication of emotional integration. It is also important to realize that different people have different windows of tolerance. Survivors need to understand their own unique window to help self-regulate.

Keep Eyes Open

While many meditation centers teach mindfulness by starting with eyes closed, this can often be a trigger for trauma survivors. It is important to be able to see what is happening in one's surroundings to increase a sense of agency and control, as can be illustrated in this case vignette (identifying details in all case vignettes have been disguised to ensure client confidentiality):

> One patient, Margaret, who was severely traumatized, could not settle into our sessions until she looked under the sofa and chairs in my office. When I inquired about this, she responded that she needed to know that "no one was hiding under the sofa." When I let her know I understood that she wanted to make sure that things were safe, her trust in me and our work increased. I also assured her I would do everything I could to keep her safe. When I started to teach her basic mindfulness and compassion skills, we started with open eyes so she was aware of all that was happening around her.

It's Fine to Slow Things Down

It is not necessary to bring in mindfulness and compassion in every session, as is shown in this case vignette. After an intense session, my client Roberto let me know the following week that he just needed to talk as he was integrating the racial trauma he experienced as a child growing up. It is important to find a pace that feels comfortable and that people do not feel rushed to "get over" their trauma.

> For example, Roberto found it grounding and soothing to look out the window in my office, focusing on a large tree with deep roots. Connecting with the external world helped expand his perspective and gave him hope that he could create a different life. I have found that anchoring in the larger world has been useful for survivors, as it helps them move out of their individual concerns to connect with the life around them.

Another modification that is useful to offer is short mindfulness breaks rather than extended formal meditation. There is growing interest and research in the power of informal practices that are just 1–3 minutes long. Zindel Segal et al.'s (2012) accessible and practical work on mindfulness-based cognitive therapy can increase motivation to practice as well as agency and confidence. Daniel Siegel (2010) has argued that teaching patients about the brain mechanisms during trauma and after can offer a useful model for what happens in emotional distress.

Clinically, and this can be challenging, the goal is to co-design a practice that is accessible (and even pleasant) for our patients. Framing it as a *mini-vacation* or *a time just for you* can help inspire patients to practice and help create a refuge during the storms and aftershocks of trauma.

Don't Start with the Breath

As skilled therapists will offer modifications to make the practice accessible and keep the client from harm, it is important to offer variations to fit the needs of different patients and keep them safe. For patients who are generally well integrated, concentrating on the breath is an excellent and often-taught practice. Those who can be dissociative, struggle with moderate anxiety, or have a history of respiratory illness, asthma, and trauma often do not feel comfortable with the practice of following the breath. Unfortunately, this is the first practice taught in many meditation classes. Many meditation teachers, such as Sharon Salzberg, and trauma pioneers such as Judith Herman, find it better to work with practices of listening to sounds, noticing sensations on the periphery of the body, or walking. It is easier to start by listening to sounds in the present moment. Finding the right fit, or right combination of practices can enhance the potential for a positive outcome.

For patients with trauma, beginning with the simple practice of "awareness of sound" is generally a gentle introduction (see Practice K.1, "Awareness of Sounds," in the Appendix). It is best to keep it short, just 3–5 minutes. Many patients find it easier to keep their eyes open.

> One of my clients, Maria, had a history of sexual abuse and posttraumatic stress disorder (PTSD). She was interested in the benefit of mindfulness, but

she became anxious and panicked when she tried to feel her breath. "Awareness of sounds" was a technique that worked for her and helped her come into the present moment. When she became agitated or found herself stuck in a disturbing memory of the past, listening to the sounds of the street traffic in the city helped her anchor in her new life, which was so different from the rural home where she had been abused. As Maria practiced, she found pleasure in the sounds of her current life, and her flashbacks and PTSD began to lessen. We added a phrase that supported the changes she made in her life and helped her stay in the present: "That was then, this is now."

Researchers have found that even a moment of mindfulness can make a difference. As Williams and his colleagues (2007) stress, it doesn't have to be complicated; "it may simply involve a shift in the way we pay attention" (p. 71). By anchoring in the present moment, with warmth and compassion, we can disrupt the ruminative thoughts that can perpetuate PTSD, anxiety, and depression. These practices can be done informally as well. Maria incorporated this practice into her daily life and listened while on a bus or subway or washing dishes. Zen teachers encourage us to practice by incorporating "small moments, many times." When a disturbing memory or thought would arise, Maria would think of it as "just noise" and allow it to arise and then fall away, not getting pulled into the story. Often walking into her apartment or giving herself a hug were useful techniques.

Research on Self-Compassion and Responses to Trauma

Many patients in my practice blame themselves for trauma, feeling that they were somehow at fault or deserved abuse—van der Kolk (2014) calls this a dominant emotion, "shame becomes the dominant emotion and hiding the truth the central preoccupation" (p. 67). These reactions of shame and blame are discussed in Herman's (2023) groundbreaking new book *Truth and Repair.* Over the past decade, Herman and her colleagues have been studying the impact of self-compassion on traumatized patients (Scoglia et al., 2018). In summary, they have found that self-compassion is related to an increase in resilience. It can decrease the severity of PTSD. It can mitigate the shame and self-blame that are so common in survivors. It also reduces the emotional numbing that many patients experience in their bodies. It can help patients find the inner strength to turn toward painful emotions and not be overwhelmed by the impact of what they have experienced (see Practice K.2, "Self-Compassion Lifesaver," in the Appendix, for a practice to introduce self-compassion into trauma therapy).

Molly was a college freshman who had little dating experience. She tried very hard to fit in with her new and more sophisticated classmates. A group of friends invited her to a party that was off campus. She was excited but nervous. A charming, attractive man approached her and seemed interested in her. She was taken by his charisma and was flattered. She had limited experience with alcohol or dating. He kept bringing her drinks and chatting with her. She became very drunk very quickly.

When her classmates couldn't find her at the end of the evening, they went searching for her. They found her alone and sobbing—she had been raped.

They brought her to the emergency room at the local hospital, where she was treated. She was a virgin and the sex had been rough. Rape crisis counseling was suggested. Molly started therapy at her college health service. She was filled with shame and enormous self-blame and couldn't believe that she had let this happen. Molly couldn't sleep, stopped eating, and was unable to go to her classes. She was diagnosed with acute PTSD. It turned out that she had been drugged as well.

"What a brilliant start to freshman year," Molly said sarcastically, shaking her head and crying. Her parents were religious, and she didn't feel she could tell them. She was too ashamed to talk to her roommates. She kept replaying the incident over and over in her head and berating herself for her "stupidity." Her body felt numb. The therapist at the counseling center had seen all of this before. She gave Molly skills to help her calm and soothe her hijacked nervous system, trying the "Self-Compassion Lifesaver" (see Practice K.2 in the Appendix). At first, Molly was in denial, and it took some work for her to acknowledge what had happened to her. "But why me?" she kept asking. Realizing that many women have these experiences was helpful and decreased the blame. Molly's therapist reassured her that she had done nothing wrong. "I thought I was the only one who was so foolish," she said. They stayed with this practice for a number of weeks, which Molly called a "lifesaver."

The step of offering herself kindness was the most difficult but ultimately the most helpful. "I'm from a family where you don't show any weakness or any emotion. It's like a foreign language for me. I learned the language of high achievement growing up, and how to drive myself relentlessly. Where I grew up it wasn't okay to be vulnerable. This was not the education I expected to get my freshman year."

As part of her healing, Molly volunteered to work on the school's sexual abuse hotline, helping other women who had been victimized. With time, therapy, and learning to support others, Molly was able to return to her life and her studies after weekly treatment incorporating self-compassion and other forms of therapy.

Befriending the Body Gently

Grounding awareness in the body can in turn help calm the mind, thus decreasing rumination and feelings of numbness after trauma. Since the body lives in the present, gentle awareness of sensations is one of the easiest ways to come into the present moment. Many of us feel disconnected from the body. Novelist James Joyce (1914) put it succinctly, and with wit: "Mr. Duffy lived a short distance from his body."

Many traumatized people may be restless or have trouble sitting still or closing their eyes as it can elicit more anxiety. How do we understand this? van de Kolk (2014) explains and argues that we need to change our assumptions about what is healing in therapy. "If the memory of trauma is encoded in the viscera, in heartbreaking and gut-wrenching emotions . . . and if mind/brain/visceral communication is the royal road to emotion regulation, this demands a radical shift about our therapeutic assumptions" (p. 88).

In fact, van der Kolk (2014) writes that many of his patients report that they cannot feel *whole areas* of their bodies. One way to understand this is as an adaptation to trauma. It is an effort to shut off terrifying sensations. However, it also impacts one's ability to feel fully alive.

The process of self-regulation rests on developing a friendly relationship with your body. This can be a process, as getting in touch with the body often means getting in touch with the experience of trauma and the memories that often arise. The "zone of tolerance" (see Figure 9.1) is one way to develop an awareness of when someone is feeling either numb or overaroused.

Pat Ogden and colleagues (2006), one of the developers of sensorimotor psychotherapy, teaches survivors to activate their *active defenses*, which can be empowering and can help people reexperience strength in the body. I used some of these techniques with Molly (see above). Working side by side, I taught her how to push her arms (palms open) against the wall. Another practice that she enjoyed was stomping her feet on the floor. Doing these practices concurrently, she felt the release of tension and also felt more grounded.

Like other survivors, Molly wasn't able to feel parts of her body. When we talked about this, she reported feeling "numb all over." Very slowly, and step-by-step, I asked her if she could feel her little finger. At first she couldn't, but then after the exercise of pushing her hands against the wall, she was able to reconnect to the sensation in her hands.

From there, we then worked on being able to feel her feet. The exercise of stomping was where we started and then progressed to running in place. She was relieved and felt that she was reclaiming her body. The process is important but should not be rushed and needs to be done slowly and with awareness. van der Kolk (2014) stresses that trauma victims can't recover until they become familiar with the sensations in their bodies. This is difficult if you are constantly on guard.

This is one place where the practices of mindfulness and compassion intersect. In my practice I work with people to notice and then label the feelings in their bodies, a classic and well-researched practice called "labeling" (Pollak et al., 2014, pp. 94–95). It is fine to keep this simple and basic, noticing heat, pressure, tingling, and feeling hollow. It is then helpful to identify the sensations of relaxation. We often explore gestures and movements, noticing subtle shifts in their bodies. While it first can be distressing, strong emotions usually arise. It is important that the clinician knows how to work with strong sensations and emotions so the patient doesn't become retraumatized by accessing past trauma.

It is good to be aware that patients who have been physically or sexually violated often encounter a dilemma. On one hand, they crave comfort and soothing physical touch, but on the other hand, there is often a fear of body contact. Part of the therapy involves a reeducation around sensations. Recent studies of pain, physical disability, and depression are showing that self-compassion is a key factor in healing (van de Kolk, 2014, p. 294). Walking meditation can be another simple way to connect with the body in a gentle way (see Practice K.3, "Anchoring Safely in the Body," in the Appendix).

Jonathan had served in Afghanistan. He was working as a medic and had seen many of his buddies injured in the war. Toward the end of his duty, he was exercising in the gym, one place where the soldiers did not carry guns. Suddenly, there was a loud blast and a blinding light as the building was hit by a suicide bomber. Many of his friends were injured and severely wounded. Jonathan's best friend died in his arms. Working through the night with the doctors and surgeons, they all saved as many lives as they could. Although the event happened years ago, Jonathan was still haunted by loud noises and panicked in enclosed spaces. He has been diagnosed with chronic PTSD, as well as major depression, and drug and alcohol addiction.

When Jonathan entered the tiny, dark, and windowless office in the basement of the clinic, he wasn't able to sit down. "Too much like the gym where we were attacked," he said. So Jonathan and his therapist had their sessions walking around the hospital grounds. At first, Jonathan didn't want to talk fearing that it would make his symptoms worse. However, he was willing to try walking meditation, at first bringing attention to the sensation of the feet touching the ground. Jonathan and his therapist walked together like this for many months, no matter what the weather, often spending a few minutes in silence at the beginning of the session. He was relieved that he didn't have to talk. "I find that talking about what happened makes it worse for me. I'm a physical guy. I like the space and the openness here. I like being able to breathe the fresh air. I don't want to sit still."

Reflecting on what helped, Jonathan took comfort in the feeling of the earth supporting him. As he walked and talked (in spite of his resistance) he began to feel less burdened, and more in the present, rather than living in the horrors of the past. During the course of treatment, he joined a 12-step program, where he found additional help in dealing with his addiction and his PTSD.

Reflections

Many patients wonder if walking practice is really meditation. And is it self-compassion? Absolutely. The Zen master Thich Nhat Hanh (1975) used walking as the basis of his teaching on kindness. He called it the "miracle of walking." While the form is different, the intention is the same. Meditation can be practiced sitting, standing, walking, or lying down. With walking meditation, unlike regular walking, we are not trying to get anywhere. Instead, we are learning to be present with every step, and present with all sensations and discomforts, physical and emotional.

> Jonathan stayed in touch. He began to read about mindfulness and compassion and listen to talks. He was drawn to the meditation teacher Sharon Salzberg, who speaks openly about her traumatic childhood and how meditation helped her stay alive.
>
> "She said something in one talk that I will never forget, and that has made a huge difference for me, especially on those days when it is hard to get out of bed," Jonathan said. "She said that those of us who have experienced trauma have gifts to offer. I was floored. What? This is a gift? I never thought of it that way. She explained that we offer depth, an understanding of how we are all vulnerable, and our personal experience of the power of compassion." Jonathan paused. "I wrote those words down and put them on the mirror in the bathroom. Now, when I look at myself, instead of hating myself and my life I think, 'Because of what I have been through, I have gifts to offer. This is what I need to begin my day.' And I find that I can share this with other people in my life." Jonathan is now working as an addiction counselor.

Self-Compassion for the Clinician

Working with traumatized patients can be exhausting and often overwhelming, especially for a young clinician. When I first began running trauma groups and working with severely traumatized patients, I started having nightmares. There is also literature on what is commonly called secondary trauma. As we delve into exploring the trauma of our patients, our own traumas, often unknown or unacknowledged, may rise to awareness.

Finding balance in our clinical work is essential, as is having excellent supervision with a skilled clinician who is knowledgeable about trauma. Being in our own therapy is an important component of self-care. And having our own mindfulness and compassion practice is an important component of staying grounded and not burning out. It is also useful to pay attention to our own zone of tolerance. Notice when you may become dysregulated after listening to stories of trauma. It is also fine to use a supportive and soothing touch if you are experiencing secondary trauma. Phrases of loving-kindness and compassion can help clinicians in this challenging but rewarding work (see Practice K.4, "Loving-Kindness and Compassion for Yourself," in the Appendix).

Conclusion

The essence of self-compassion in trauma therapy is that we learn to bring kindness and gentle attention to the places in the body and mind where we have been wounded. It is an ongoing process. While some believe that trauma can be healed, psychiatrist Mark Epstein (2013) argues that it is never cured. In fact, Jonathan recently told his therapist that there was a loud noise outside his apartment around the time of the recent July 4 celebrations. He had an immediate startle response, dropped to the floor, and went into a protective fetal position. "This may be with me for a long time," he said. What gave Jonathan comfort was that he could recover quickly, and realize that he was home and safe, and not in a war zone. His mindfulness and self-compassion practice had taught him how to return to the present moment. He has learned to stay with what is painful and what has historically been difficult to feel. In this process, Jonathan learns how to soothe himself and return to the present moment. And to be kind to himself when he is triggered. For many survivors, it is the practice of a lifetime.

Mindfulness and compassion are tools that help trauma survivors stay with a range of experiences, including traumatic stress, as well as anxiety, depression, love, joy, and happiness. Practicing these skills involves a willingness to look at the past as well as our present experience. It helps promote bravery as well as clear seeing.

Mindfulness and compassion are not magic. There is no quick or easy cure for trauma. However, we can learn how to integrate it into our lives, how to practice safety, develop stability, and learn to regulate our day-to-day experience. It is a practice that grows and develops over time. It is also a process of continual practice and growth.

Students often ask where to get trained as mindfulness or compassion-oriented clinicians. The wisest suggestion I have is to become trained broadly as clinicians, working under a trusted supervisor or supervisors. I also suggest developing expertise in many different modalities, including psychodynamic therapy, cognitive-behavioral therapy, EMDR, sensorimotor psychotherapy, and IFS. Developing a sense of when to move someone toward safety or invite them into new unexplored territory requires intuition that is informed by experience. It is also important that the clinician pursue their own mindfulness and compassion practice so they can know, firsthand, the effects of various practices in addition to learning to sit with the intense emotional experiences that come with a history of trauma.

The poet Rumi (1995) put it eloquently: "Don't turn your head. Keep looking at the bandaged place. That's where the Light enters you" (p. 139).

For many, self-compassion can be radical and counterintuitive. And, with effort and practice, it can be profoundly healing. Bringing the tools of mindfulness and self-compassion into therapy is a creative enterprise of adapting these well-researched practices to the unique situation of our patients and incorporating the tools in a safe and supportive therapeutic and interpersonal relationship.

REFERENCES

Epstein, M. (2013). *The trauma of everyday life*. Penguin.

Germer, C. K. (2013). Mindfulness: What is it? What does it matter? In C. K. Germer, R. D. Siegel, & P. R. Fulton (Eds.), *Mindfulness and psychotherapy* (2nd ed., pp. 3–35). Guilford Press.

Hanh, T. N. (1975). *The miracle of mindfulness: An introduction to the practice of meditation*. Beacon Press.

Herman, J. L. (1992). *Trauma and recovery: The aftermath of violence—from domestic abuse to political terror*. Basic Books.

Herman, J. L. (2023). *Truth and repair: How trauma survivors envision justice*. Basic Books.

Joyce, J. (1914). *Dubliners*. Dover.

Ogden, P. (2015). *Sensorimotor psychotherapy: Interventions for trauma and attachment*. Norton.

Ogden, P., Minton, K., & Pain, C. (2006). *Trauma and the body: A sensorimotor approach to psychotherapy*. Norton.

Pollak, S. M., Pedulla, T., & Siegel, R. D. (2014). *Sitting together: Essential skills for mindfulness-based psychotherapy*. Guilford Press.

Rumi, J. (1995). Childhood friends. In *The essential Rumi* (C. Barks, Trans.). HarperCollins.

Scoglio, A. A. J., Rudat, D. A., Garvert, D., Jarmolowski, M., Jackson, C., & Herman, J. L. (2018). Self-compassion and responses to trauma. *Journal of Interpersonal Violence, 33*(13), 2016–2036.

Segal, Z. V., Williams, J. M. G., & Teasdale, J. D. (2012). *Mindfulness-based cognitive therapy for depression* (2nd ed.). Guilford Press.

Siegel, D. (1999). *The developing mind: How relationships and the brain interact to shape who we are*. Guilford Press.

Siegel, D. (2010). *The mindful therapist: A clinician's guide to mindsight and neural integration*. Norton.

van der Kolk, B. A. (2014). *The body keeps the score: Brain, mind, and body in the healing of trauma*. Penguin Books.

Williams, M., Teasdale, J., Segal, Z., & Kabat-Zinn, J. (2007). *The mindful way through depression: Freeing yourself from chronic unhappiness*. Guilford Press.

10

The Inner Process of Inquiry in Psychotherapy

Steven Hickman

The sharing of self-compassion in psychotherapy overlaps considerably with teaching these practices as part of a course or program. The therapist who endeavors to integrate this work into their therapy with clients will find that the wisdom and techniques of teachers of contemplative practice is highly supportive of individual therapeutic work as well.

The overarching intention of this chapter is to draw from the widespread teaching of self-compassion (especially within the mindful self-compassion [MSC] program; Germer & Neff, 2019) to inform therapists who wish to tap into them within a therapeutic context. After establishing the basic tenets of teaching contemplative practice that apply in psychotherapy, we explore the nuanced art of sharing self-compassion in a therapy setting and articulate some of the key "ingredients" in an inquiry-based approach to fostering the resource of self-compassion in clients.

Quite often the most enigmatic and intriguing aspect of this process is inquiry. Inquiry is informally defined and described within mindfulness- and compassion-based programs as the process of helping a person articulate their inner experience in such a way that such exploration supports the development of the capacity of mindfulness or self-compassion itself.

When the therapist asks, "What did you notice?" after the client has described a life experience or engaged in a meditative practice, there is an atmosphere that is pregnant with possibility, and simultaneously, completely unknowable. The therapist has asked the question in a purposefully unstructured way to invite clients into a moment-to-moment recounting of their experience, and until the client speaks, nobody knows what will be shared (sometimes, not even the client themselves!).

For psychotherapists, this territory of the unknown and somewhat unpredictable is perhaps a bit more familiar and a little less terrifying, but nonetheless rich with possibility if handled skillfully.

Ultimately, this process is actually not a mystery because it mirrors almost exactly our own personal experience of contemplative practice. We show up (as a therapist, but also as a practitioner of self-compassion) to whatever is present with a relaxed, observing, and curious presence. We let go of effort and endeavor to meet whatever arises with those same qualities. We watch the arising of mental and emotional activity, we try not to get caught in our stories, we remain as open and accepting as we can be, we ground ourselves in each momentary experience by tuning into the breath and the body, and we may even be mildly entertained by the antics of our active minds.

We try to ask "What?" rather than "Why?," and we aim to radically accept whatever we notice as simply true in the moment but not permanent or even lasting. It is a practice, in that we practice it over and over, we never get it "right" and we never get it "wrong," but it becomes a kind of mental and emotional discipline that we cultivate over time, such that we yield the fruits of this practice through repetition. Whether intrapersonally in our personal practice, or interpersonally in our therapeutic inquiry process, the practice remains the same.

If the therapist is new to sharing self-compassion with clients, there may be an inkling of this openhearted curiosity in mindful inquiry lingering from their personal practice (truly a necessity if a therapist is to genuinely embody the practice in their therapy), but there is often a simultaneous wave of anxiety that washes over them as a result of the uncertainty. "What if I don't know how to respond?," "What if I've never heard this particular kind of response before?," "What if they say something crazy or ridiculous?," or "What if they had a bad experience?" This kind of catastrophic "what-if?" thinking is natural, and yet over time, if the therapist is grounded in the practice, attuned to their own experience in the moment (as they are in their own personal practice), and deeply and openly curious about what the person may say, the process works beautifully, and no answers need to be known upfront. Most often, the way in which one does this is to simply maintain a nonreactive, accepting, and supportive attitude to whatever is shared, which is a re-creation of the therapist's personal practice of self-compassion. By doing so, the therapist is in essence "demonstrating" how the client might be able to take this stance themselves.

There is no place to "get to," so to speak, because it is the experience of being met with presence and compassion that is the "active ingredient" in such an encounter. This way, we can let go of trying to get anywhere at all and instead find a way into a deep resonance with our clients as we accompany them on the journey of practice in a kind, patient, and reassuring way. Appreciating that there is no "right way" to be or nothing to be corrected or fixed, we can instead focus on the client's wholehearted embrace of themselves and their experience as it is. We do not lead or follow on this journey, but we walk beside our clients as they articulate their experience (which is neither "right" nor "wrong" but simply is what it is), perhaps with some confidence and self-assuredness because we have walked here before but still open and embodying humility and openheartedness.

In fact, the equanimity of the therapist (the capacity to be fully present to the unfolding without preference or attachment) is what supports the client in describing the experience in a beautiful dance of sharing, inquiring, further sharing, and reflection that is really what characterizes mindful and compassionate inquiry. When the therapist can be embodied and present, the client gets a direct experience of the practice in the interpersonal space of inquiry that the therapist hopes to foster in the intrapersonal space of the client. In other words, the therapist and client are acting out a relationship between them that the client can then re-create in relation to their internal experiences as they arise in their life over time, long after the therapy has concluded. This process is common in programs like MSC, in which the participants are met with a loving, connected presence and gently supported in bringing that same self-compassionate stance toward their own experiences, and especially themselves. The only thing missing inside the therapy room is the opportunity to observe this process repeatedly in others, as one has in the MSC classroom. However, the core practice and experience are the same.

For most therapists, this is quite familiar territory. The crucible of the therapy room, the corrective emotional experience (Fried, 2002) of a psychotherapeutic relationship and the embodied presence (Geller & Greenberg, 2022) of the therapist are all the consistent "common factors" of psychotherapy (Browne et al., 2021). This is the essence of effective psychotherapy (Bailey & Ogles, 2023), and so the challenge of sharing self-compassion in this setting mainly involves removing some of the elements of therapy that are not conducive to learning the practice. Much as sculptors often say that their process is to chip away all the parts of the stone that are not part of the subject, the therapist teaching self-compassion learns to set aside the various therapy skills and techniques that are familiar but not supportive of the process of practice.

Why Do We Inquire?

We inquire because we wish to support our clients in the development of the resource of self-compassion. In this work with clients, we are supporting the cultivation of a practice or a way of being, not a concept or an idea. To some degree, the analogy is the difference between learning a skill and learning a concept. When learning the *concept* of self-compassion, we might read a book or listen to a lecture, but to develop the *practice* we must actually do it. Thus, we are not teaching *about* mindfulness or self-compassion but sharing the things themselves through our embodied presence (Geller & Greenberg, 2022), cultivated by our personal practice of self-compassion (Germer & Neff, 2019). What happens when the therapist forgets this is that they find themselves lecturing, explaining, or making teaching points within the inquiry process, rather than embodying their practice and letting the client's experience take center stage so that they can develop the resource of self-compassion or mindfulness themselves through self-discovery and self-observation.

Consider the analogous situation of an athletic coach guiding an athlete to refine and improve their performance. In that field, the coach can visually observe the athlete's performance, measure it, and compare it to others. But in the completely private internal experience of mindfulness and compassion, none of this is visible or measurable, and so the therapist must rely on the firsthand account of the participant to understand something of how the practice went and to support them in deepening it. This is not as simple as it might seem at first glance.

At the center of the spotlight here is the *actual* experience that a person had while practicing meditation or being compassionate with themselves in a particular situation. For example, if a client, let's call her Julie,[1] recounts a difficult situation with her partner and at a particular moment noticed a cold, empty feeling in the pit of her stomach, and a wave of fear rolled through her heart as she continued to observe it, and these bodily sensations and emotions prompted her to recall a previous traumatic experience and to have thoughts of needing to escape or stop the feelings, there is a lot in those few moments to try to articulate.

For the therapist who gently inquires into Julie's experience, the task becomes how to help Julie grow from the experience. This could include learning how she actually *did* practice self-compassion as the experience unfolded, how she *might* be able to bring *more* mindfulness or compassion to bear on her experience and herself, and how this experience can generalize for her by equipping her with the capacity to bring the practice to future situations. These three (of many) possibilities could be accomplished with some simple, open-ended questions like "When you became aware of those feelings, how did you respond to yourself in that moment?" or "In looking back on that moment, what do you think you needed?" or even "What do you make of that experience?" In each case, these are gentle but

[1]This and all other case vignettes or examples are fictional amalgams of aspects of many clients used for illustrative purposes only.

pointed inquiries designed to help Julie access her already existent capacity to be more self-compassionate (whether she is aware she possesses it or not), rather than "expert suggestions" by the therapist. This fosters a self-sufficiency that we are hoping the client will develop over time so that the practice is accessible in their daily lives, long after therapy has concluded. All in all, the therapist supports Julie in cultivating a different relationship with such experiences.

But before any of this can happen, Julie's experience needs to be somehow "transmitted" to the therapist. Her experience includes bodily sensations, multiple emotions, painful memories, and perhaps more easily identifiable thoughts. Only the thoughts have a clear verbal component, and yet we are asking Julie to put the whole complex experience into words that are somewhat understandable to her and to us as her therapist. This is not easy and inevitably will fall short of fully capturing the experience that Julie had, but it's the only method we have at our disposal. This verbal expression is further complicated by the limitations of language to describe nonverbal experiences, our habitual patterns of summarizing and labeling experiences rather than literally describing them moment by moment, the inhibiting factor of sharing an intensely personal experience in front of another person, and the impact on our cognitive capacity (like memory) when we are experiencing strong emotions. What Julie finally expresses out loud is only a vague approximation of what she actually experienced at the time.

All of this is to say that the therapist's task is to keep this process in mind and always strive to fully feature Julie's actual moment-to-moment experience by guiding her back, again and again, to what *actually happened* in the situation and away from after-the-fact explanation or interpretation. The intention here is to support Julie in building the resource of self-compassion, experientially rather than intellectually. For example, a therapist could perhaps gently interrupt a storyline to say, "So, in that moment, what was it that you needed?" or "When you became aware of your struggle, how did you respond to that feeling?" The therapist's task is to therefore provide some scaffolding or guidance to facilitate Julie's direct exploration of her practice from the inside, preferably in "real time" or as close to it as possible, by gently but persistently accompanying Julie through her experience moment by moment and encouraging her to stay very close to what actually unfolded, free (as much as possible) from interpretation and evaluation.

Through that process, the therapist engages deeply and kindly with Julie to hear the direct account of her experience and to support staying with that experience mindfully by doing exactly that in the interaction itself. By doing this, the therapist is supporting Julie in engaging this different relationship with arising phenomena (thought, memory, sensation, emotion) by engaging in a compassionate collaborative dialogue between them. Thus, Julie is gently, implicitly, but very powerfully being "coached" to engage in this way with herself and her own experience by "practicing" it in therapy.

If Julie, in the process of recalling it during an inquiry, begins to reexperience any of the emotions, sensations, or thoughts from the original experience, then the therapist's guidance (in essence, the therapist's practice) becomes that of the athletic coach: remaining attentive, supportive, encouraging, and curious. The good therapist, like the good swimming coach (for example), does not do any good by jumping into the pool and rescuing the swimmer but, instead, is most effective by remaining in the supportive coaching role and embodying self-compassion: present, equanimous, and kind (Geller & Greenberg, 2022; Rogers, 2007).

How Might Therapists Miss the Mark in Inquiry?

Having taught literally thousands of people to teach mindfulness and self-compassion over the years, I have had the opportunity to engage with nontherapists as trainees who feel overwhelmed by the specter of inquiry because they feel ill equipped to understand, conceptualize, and theorize about their participants in the way that they imagine therapists do. I like to (somewhat) jokingly tell them that they are actually *lucky* to be free of the burden of conceptualization, diagnosis, treatment planning, and progress reports. These are the chunks of stone that are not the final "sculpture" that I referred to above (at least in the immediate encounter of inquiry). They are extraneous to the learning of self-compassion and mindfulness while also being the standard and necessary tools and processes of traditional psychotherapists.

You might refer to this stance as intellectual humility (Church & Samuelson, 2017). People who are intellectually humble know that their beliefs and opinions are fallible because they recognize that the evidence on which their beliefs are based could be limited or flawed. Intellectual humility means understanding that we can't fully trust what we think about our client because we might be relying on faulty or incomplete information or are unable to appreciate the nuances. As the bumper sticker says, "Don't believe everything you think."

Practicing effective traditional psychotherapy requires a healthy dose of expert knowledge and conceptualization based on assessing available data, balanced against a willingness to be open, flexible, and intellectually humble. In inquiry (as in practice), the less of the former and more of the latter, the better. As therapists sharing contemplative practice and self-compassion, we need to bring a beginner's mind to the encounter with our clients and temporarily suspend the intellectual burden of case conceptualization and diagnostic hypotheses so that we can be genuinely and fully present (Geller & Greenberg, 2022) and compassionate in that encounter. This is far easier said than done.

Much like meditation practice itself, this process of shedding the intellectual baggage of therapeutic practice (while maintaining therapeutic presence) is a continuous process of letting go, moving forward warmly and fully in the present moment with the client, inadvertently returning to the old habit of thinking/conceptualizing/diagnosing, and then letting go again. Over time and with intentional practice, the periods of presence and compassion increase, and the thinking recedes into the background.

Cultivating the Wisdom of Practice in the Space of Inquiry

Within Buddhist psychology, there are four prized emotions or mind states that are said to give us a framework for cultivating positive behaviors and minimizing harmful ones. If we can dwell in these same "divine abodes" as therapists, we can influence the learning process in a similar way and with similar intent: to foster the practice of mindfulness and compassion in our participants. Referred to as the Four Immeasurables (Cheng & Tse, 2015; Mulligan, 2017)—the cultivation of loving-kindness, compassion, empathetic joy, and equanimity—they form a rich suite of practices that open the heart, counter the distortions in our relationships to ourselves, and deepen our relationships to others.

It is particularly fruitful to explore what are referred to as the "enemies" of each of these emotions (Mulligan, 2017) to more easily recognize when we are not teaching from these states of mind and heart. The far enemies are fairly straightforward and easily recognized: Ill will is a far enemy of loving-kindness, cruelty is a far enemy of compassion, jealousy is a far enemy of empathetic joy, and agitation or excitement are far enemies of equanimity.

But the near enemies are much trickier. These are things that look remarkably similar to what you're trying to cultivate but are actually fundamentally different in a dangerous (and often unrecognizable) way.

When we succumb to these enemies (both near and far), there is a kind of rupture in the supporting fabric of the therapeutic relationship that hinders the client from getting all that they might glean from it. When a client feels disdain or distance rather than compassion from a therapist in a moment of sharing, it is a missed opportunity for deepening and may actually inhibit a client from sharing out of a concern for looking bad or weak. These moments of vulnerability and sensitivity are precious and fleeting and are often exquisite opportunities for learning.

When we endeavor to cultivate the Four Immeasurables as we inquire, we find that we actually can't get lost and we can always support people in their journeys of learning and deepening the resources of self-compassion. And when we succumb to their sometimes enticing near enemies as therapists, we can follow the thread of our practice back to solid ground. Needless to say, as we embody these immeasurables in our teaching, they are passed along implicitly to our clients in what Buddhists refer to as "transmission."

Loving-Kindness

Loving-kindness (Wolf & Serpa, 2015; *metta* in Pali) is defined as wishing well toward all beings or "boundless friendliness" and can be seen as the most basic motivation or intention of the therapist. While we would certainly notice ill will (the far enemy of loving-kindness) if it were to arise in our therapy, we may occasionally find ourselves subject to the more subtle arising of the near enemy of selfish or conditional love. This is genuine affection that also surreptitiously includes attachment to a specific therapeutic outcome or a desire to get something beyond the joy of loving itself. There is a quality of conditionality to this state that hinges on the response of the client or an attachment to a particular outcome, rather than an openhearted warmth without grasping.

How might this manifest while we are teaching? It can start innocently enough, perhaps as a moment of silence with a client. These moments can sometimes be disconcerting and we can find ourselves in a problem-solving mode, playing out in our mind the various things we might say to prompt a response from the client, not recognizing that this may simply be a way of lessening their own anxiety or uncertainty. If we can instead step back and say to ourselves, "Ahh, uncertainty is arising. Doubts are here. I notice a sinking feeling in the pit of my stomach," we could maintain our equipoise and encounter the moment with an openhearted goodwill that is expansive enough to hold it all. By trusting our own practice of self-compassion in that moment, we also trust the practice itself for the client in a kind of nonverbal "transmission" that says more than words can ever accomplish.

For Reflection

It is worth considering the more general question of "When does your natural loving-kindness subtly shift into a kind of conditional transaction where you are attached to a particular outcome or response from your client?" A really powerful follow-up question to ask oneself in these moments can be "Is there some underlying need (for me as a person or as a therapist) that needs tending to?" We slip into the near enemy when our practice has not been as strong and regular as it could be or we are experiencing unusual stress in our lives.

Compassion

Compassion (Mulligan, 2017; *karuna* in Pali) is the sensitivity to suffering coupled with the deep desire to alleviate that suffering, without distinction between the suffering of others or of ourselves. Not fully distinct from the goodwill of loving-kindness, compassion concerns itself specifically with suffering.

Again, it is the near enemy of compassion and pity, which is insidious and undermining of our intentions as therapists. When we find ourselves thinking, "Oh, that poor person. I feel sorry for people with such harsh inner critics as they have," we begin to open up the slightest gap between ourselves and the other person that promotes a kind of remoteness from the suffering of another that is gratifying to the self and protective of our own feelings of pain and, again, ruptures the fabric of our work by disconnecting us from clients.

As therapists, we are witnesses to profound, disturbing, inspiring, and heart-wrenching stories of all sorts. And this pain is always embedded in a story: of how it came to be, what it means, how it has changed us, and what we believe about our future as a result. The stories are tender, they are carefully constructed, they are exquisitely detailed and specific, and most dangerous of all for us as therapists, they are incredibly seductive.

But the challenge for the therapist is to "keep our eyes on the prize" of what the story represents and signifies and not the *content* of that story (process over content). What unites us and connects us to the common human experience of suffering is not the content of our story, but the common humanity of the themes that underlie human suffering in general.

The most common pitfall faced by therapists that leads down the road of pity rather than compassion is seeing a hard and firm distinction between ourselves and our clients. Separation does not support compassion, but it certainly supports pity. The key to resolving this separation is to recognize that there is little that separates the client and the therapist in human terms. Beth Mulligan (2017) quotes an aboriginal activist who said, "If you have come here to help me, you are wasting your time. But if you have come because your liberation is bound up with mine, then let us work together." This working together is the work of sharing self-compassion. It is collaborative, egalitarian, and mutually supportive at every turn.

For Reflection

Think back to a recent time when someone shared a touching, compelling, or painful story with you in therapy. Were you able to fully experience the impact of the story? Maybe you can recall feeling the impact of the story in your body as a jolt to the chest or a sinking feeling in the stomach. See if you can rewind back to a moment when a story struck you, viscerally and emotionally.

As a basically compassionate person, you were likely compelled to reach out to them in some way. But reflect a bit more. Was your basic motivation one of wanting to support and comfort them *within* the pain and suffering they were experiencing, or were you motivated more by a desire to find a way to lessen or take away their pain in that moment? In other words, was it possible for you to be with the shared pain of empathic resonance between you and a suffering person, and remain warm and supportive, or was there a pull to fix, lessen, avoid, or mitigate the pain you (or that other person) were feeling? There is nothing inherently "wrong" with wanting to lessen pain (after all, you are a therapist and it's part of your job!) but this may or may not be what a person needs at a particular moment. The self-efficacy fostered by trusting the capacity of your client to access their own compassion in a moment of suffering can be tremendous if one can resist the temptation to fix.

Empathetic Joy

Empathetic joy (Mulligan, 2017; *mudita* in Pali) is rejoicing in the joy of all beings, even if it is not, strictly speaking, our own. As therapists, we recognize empathetic joy when our clients begin to have realizations, insights, and breakthroughs as therapy unfolds. There is a kind of mutuality to the encounter almost as if you are reliving your own discovery of the same thing at some point in your past.

What might disrupt this connecting fabric of empathetic joy? Of course, again, the far enemy of *mudita*, jealousy, is easy to spot. However, a more subtle expression of this separation can be found in the near enemy of blind euphoria or exuberance that is mostly rooted not in shared joy but, instead, in a sense of insufficiency or lack. A therapist might feel a huge sense of relief if they were doubting their own abilities and a client reported a significant breakthrough or insight, and respond effusively or enthusiastically, not out of *mudita* but sheer relief. In the moment, the client might feel a rush of good feelings from the therapist's response, but the lack of mutuality could inhibit that same client from sharing other things unless they were likely to elicit the same response. Thus, such a response can have a chilling effect on the therapy by inhibiting the client from sharing things that they don't see as a "breakthrough" or an "important" insight in order to have their therapist's approval.

Might it be possible instead to think of the space between us and our clients as a kind of semipermeable membrane that is actually a *point of contact* between us? True empathetic joy is the way that we can truly feel their tender beating heart in a moment of joy, and they can feel our heart quiver in resonance with theirs.

For Reflection

Empathetic joy, like all of the Four Immeasurables, is not a rarefied skill practiced only in the sacred space of the meditation hall, therapy office, or retreat center. As humans, we have opportunities to practice it every day. While we might go to the gym to exercise our bodies, the "gym" for practicing the divine abodes is every moment of our lives.

So perhaps your "*mudita* exercise" can be to simply notice joy happening around you (talk about the best homework ever!) and take it in.

And what would it be like to let go of a client being "*my* client," whose joy and overall state of mind are your responsibility as the therapist, and instead allow that person to simply be another human who is walking beside you on this path of life, with joys and sorrows very much like yours? Can you appreciate their virtues and their dreams? You have a role and a responsibility as a therapist, plus a little knowledge and some experience, but you are more *like* your client than you are different. When you both realize that, you both grow.

Equanimity

Equanimity (Wolf & Serpa, 2015; *upekkha* in Pali) is an even-mindedness and serenity in the face of the "fluctuations of worldly fortune." It is this quality of mind and heart that keeps us steady in our seats as practitioners, but also as therapists, and supports us especially when we are engaged in inquiry with our clients.

As you reflect back over the course of this chapter you will see how the common thread running throughout this exploration has been a sense of equanimity in the face of the ups and downs and twists and turns of mindful inquiry and the intimate and unique encounter between the therapist and client.

In the therapy room, equanimity is what allows us to maintain our poise and presence in the face of whatever arises. It is the quality that emerges over time as we begin to trust the practice and the process. There is no "doing" equanimity, as it is more accurately described as a way of "being" instead. There is also no substitute for developing equanimity through continued practice. You can't read a book on equanimity and reading this part of this chapter will not make you more equanimous.

Like with the other near enemies of the immeasurables, indifference or apathy can easily be mistaken for equanimity, especially when simply viewed superficially. The image that comes to mind is the unflappable therapist who can hear accounts of great struggle or joyous breakthroughs and keep their seat through all of it. But look a little closer and you can begin to differentiate true equanimity from indifference or apathy, and it relates to how resonant or attuned that therapist is to what is unfolding versus how disconnected or separate they are. In other words, once again, is the fabric of the mutual interaction intact, or has it been ruptured by indifference?

I am reminded of a poignant moment in a self-compassion workshop I co-led.

One participant, Frank, was quick to raise his hand when we opened up inquiry after practice. He started out calmly but began to sob almost immediately, and between the sobs he said, "For most of my life I have really hated my father. He raised me by himself after my mother left. I would get angry when I thought of him because he was always so angry with me and so critical. It just never stopped day after day, year after year. I really, truly hated him." He paused to collect himself as he had gotten more and more emotionally overwrought as he spoke.

Frank went on to say, "I've always recognized this nasty inner voice as the voice of my father. I literally hear his voice when these thoughts come up," he said, with a trace of bitterness in his voice. "But as we did this exercise and I actually stopped pushing the voice away in anger and actually tried to see how it was trying to help me somehow . . . wow . . . the whole picture changed." He paused to take a breath, and his body relaxed a bit.

"I realized, finally, after all these many years, that my father was actually scared out of his mind about being a parent. He had *no idea* how to be a parent because his parents were totally absent, and there he was, trying to raise me alone, and he was scared shitless! He was afraid of doing it wrong!" With wet cheeks, Frank looked at me and there was such relief in his eyes! We truly felt his pain as well as his revelation and relief, and together we were holding it all with loving-kindness and compassion.

After a brief silence to honor Frank's sharing, I asked the question, "What are you noticing right now as you share this with us?" When I asked that question it was not a rote recounting of "the thing you say when you start inquiry" but, instead, it was a genuine, heartfelt moment of deep curiosity and engagement based on what was present in my heart. I had no agenda other than to invite Frank to stay in the present moment and with himself, just as we were.

This is the true deep role of equanimity in inquiry: to help create a safe space that we hope the client can feel and cultivate over time in their own heart. Held within this space, Frank had the freedom to share, to stop, to cry, to reflect, to slowly put an experience beyond words into words, and to feel the corrective experience of being loved, supported, and encouraged throughout. Creating this kind of safe space is the stock in trade of therapists in general, so it may be second nature for most but appreciating the implications for helping a client foster a self-compassionate response makes it doubly important for the therapist to keep at the forefront.

For Reflection

What can we do when we lose our equanimity? As noted previously, equanimity cannot be rushed, and it is not a skill to be learned intellectually but, instead, a capacity that is cultivated through practice. And as a basic human capacity that we have been cultivating through our ongoing personal practice, it is always available to us if we can find our way back to it.

Begin by asking yourself an incredibly valuable question that Saki Santorelli (2004) once asked a group of mindfulness teachers: "What do you do when you don't know what to do?" In that moment of uncertainty, when your equanimity feels as if it has abandoned you (it actually hasn't, as it is you who have abandoned it) and you are flailing about, slightly panicked, how do you respond? How do you find your feet and your equipoise in moments like this?

My friend and colleague Michelle Becker (personal communication) has informally adapted the work of Paul Gilbert (2009), the developer of compassion-focused therapy, to apply it specifically to teaching mindfulness and compassion (Gilbert & Simos, 2022). Using Gilbert's model of the three emotion regulation systems (threat, drive, and soothing), Becker has suggested a pathway for reregulation that can be quite supportive in moments when we lose our equanimity as therapists. Becker points out that, at any given time, we may find ourselves teaching while predominantly influenced by one of these systems, but only one of them is directly helpful to our participants in inquiry: us being in the drive system.

So, in moments when we have been knocked off-kilter, are surprised, or otherwise lose our equanimity, we have moved into the threat system and we are ready for fight, flight, or freeze. Physiologically, the stress hormones are flowing (Gilbert, 2009), our attention has narrowed on the threat, and equanimity becomes a temporarily distant and unattainable memory. However, if we can notice that we are here in the "threat system" through our mindfulness practice, it can then be possible for us to make our way back to the "soothing system" (perhaps through the practice of self-compassion). From this safe platform of soothing, we are then able to reorient ourselves to the task and intention at hand (the client) and reconnect to our intention from a place of clarity, calm, and equanimity.

The next time you find yourself reeling or out of balance, see if you can find your way back to your "green system" through self-soothing, self-comfort, and self-care and notice what can happen next.

Conclusion

If reading this chapter has raised your anxiety or made inquiry seem even more impossibly complex and unknowable than you thought it was before you started, then I urge you to pause. Take a moment to breathe and to observe the activity of your mind. Soothe yourself however you know how and give yourself a little time to sit with all that you have read and considered here.

When you've had some time with it, you might find it helpful to go back to the beginning and read the chapter again with fresh eyes. My intention was actually to make the process of inquiry more relatable and familiar by exploring the connection it has to personal practice, but anytime a simple concept like this is bound up in multiple pages of words, stories, and concepts, it runs the risk of being obscured. Feel your way into the second reading of the chapter and see that what I invite you to do is to draw upon what you know most intimately already and, as the 15th-century poet Kabir (2004) said, "just throw away all thoughts of imaginary things, and stand firm in that which you are."

This chapter (and this book) can be a trusted map that makes it impossible for you to get lost in the sometimes challenging and emotionally charged experience of teaching powerful practices such as these. It is the best kind of map because it always reminds us "you are here," wherever you happen to be, but wherever that is, you are already home if you are willing to allow yourself to be. In the end, inquiry is nothing more than an encounter with another that reminds us both of our humanity and gives us each a little window into our own experience through the connection with the other.

Perhaps if we take the stance that, most of all, what people need from us is to be seen and to "feel felt," we can let go of all the thinking, fretting, scheming, and theorizing, drop back into our known way of being, and connect human-to-human, heart-to-heart, and walk the journey of mindfulness and compassion with deep intention . . . together. That cooperative endeavor of the embodied therapist relating *inter*personally with the client as a means of fostering the same sort of *intra*personal relationship they wish for that client is the essence of the inquiry-based approach to self-compassion-focused psychotherapy.

REFERENCES

Bailey, R. J., & Ogles, B. M. (2023). *Common factors therapy: A principle-based treatment framework*. American Psychological Association.

Browne, J., Cather, C., & Mueser, K. (2021, February 23). Common factors in psychotherapy. *Oxford Research Encyclopedia of Psychology.* https://oxfordre.com/psychology/view/10.1093/acrefore/9780190236557.001.0001/acrefore-9780190236557-e-79.

Cheng, F., & Tse, S. (2015). Applying the Buddhist Four Immeasurables to mental health care: A critical review. *Journal of Religion and Spirituality in Social Work: Social Thought, 34,* 24–50.

Church, I. M., & Samuelson, P. L. (2017). *Intellectual humility: An introduction to the philosophy and science.* Bloomsbury Academic.

Fried, D. (2002). Corrective emotional experience. In M. Hersen & W. Sledge (Eds.), *Encyclopedia of psychotherapy* (pp. 551–555). Academic Press.

Geller, S., & Greenberg, L. (2022). *Therapeutic presence: A mindful approach to effective therapeutic relationships* (2nd ed.). American Psychological Association.

Germer, C., & Neff, K. (2019). *Teaching the mindful self-compassion program: A guide for professionals.* Guilford Press.

Gilbert, P. (2009). *The compassionate mind.* Constable.

Gilbert, P., & Simos, G. (Eds.). (2022). *Compassion focused therapy: Clinical practice and applications.* Routledge.

Kabir. (2004). I said to the wanting-creature inside me. In *Kabir: Ecstatic poems* (R. Bly, Trans.). Beacon Press.

Mulligan, B. A. (2017). *The dharma of modern mindfulness.* New Harbinger.

Rogers, C. (2007). *On becoming a person.* HarperOne

Santorelli, S. (Performer). (2004, March 4). *What do you do when you don't know what to do?* Presentation at the annual conference of the University of Massachusetts Center for Mindfulness, Worcester, MA.

Wolf, C., & Serpa, J. (2015). *A clinician's guide to teaching mindfulness.* New Harbinger.

PART III

Applications of Self-Compassion in Psychotherapy

11

Self-Compassion for Shame in Psychotherapy

Christopher Germer

Self-compassion is an antidote to shame. Shame is not a formal psychiatric diagnosis, but it is a relevant factor in many mental disorders: anxiety, depression, eating disorders, posttraumatic stress disorder, substance abuse, borderline personality disorder, and even psychosis (Cândea & Szentagotai, 2013; Dearing & Tangney, 2011). Back in 2000, when Paul Gilbert created compassion-focused therapy (CFT), he was specifically looking for a way to treat self-criticism and shame (Gilbert, 2009). Since then, research has shown that shame and self-compassion are inversely correlated, and as people develop the resource of self-compassion in therapy, shame tends to decrease (Germer, 2023). This chapter takes a wide-angle view of how self-compassion-based therapy can be used to alleviate shame. The evidence base is presented first, followed by a case vignette illustrating different aspects of treatment.

What Is Shame?

Shame is a self-conscious emotion characterized by negative self-evaluation. In contrast to guilt, which focuses on *behavior* ("I did something bad"), shame focuses on the *self* ("I *am* bad"; Tangney & Dearing, 2003). Shame also tends to be global: "I'm *all* bad" (Lewis, 1971). Shame can arise when we feel negatively evaluated by others (external shame) or when we negatively evaluate ourselves (internal shame; Ferreira et al., 2022), but the common denominator is that we feel devalued in the minds of others (Gilbert & Irons, 2009).

Shame manifests in a wide variety of ways, including:

- *Inner body sensations*—for example, sinking feeling, muscle tension, nausea
- *External physical expressions*—for example, sweating, flushing, fidgeting
- *Mental signs*—for example, self-criticism, confusion, unworthiness
- *Other emotions*—for example, sadness, anger, fear
- *Behavioral signs*—for example, aggression, withdrawal, submissiveness

To fully experience shame, we need to see "the self-in-the-eyes-of-the-other" (Lewis, 1987, p. 15). This self-conscious capacity begins when a child is about 2 years, 6 months to 3 years of age (Lewis, 2019). However, precursors to shame, such as averted gaze, slumping, and downcast eyes, can be observed in babies as young as 3 months old when they feel disconnected from their caregivers (Tomkins, in Stipek, 1983). *Patterns* of disconnection, such as recurring criticism, neglect, or abuse, can lead to shame-proneness (Claesson & Sohlberg, 2002) and insecure attachment later in life (Gross & Hansen, 2000).

Shame was probably adaptive in human evolution. In order to survive, our hunter-gatherer ancestors needed to live in groups. If one individual broke off from the group, everyone's life was put in jeopardy. Interestingly, violating group norms doesn't necessarily cause shame; shame arises when we feel *devalued* by others (Robertson et al., 2018). Therefore, when an individual broke the rules of the tribe and was devalued for it, shame made them immediately stop what they were doing and everyone lived to see another day.

Shame can be a state or a trait (Sedighimornani, 2018). *State* shame is adaptive and short-lived—shame disappears when we're back in the good graces of our group. *Trait* shame (or shame-proneness) is shame we carry with us everywhere we go. Trait shame develops over time by how we're treated by others, usually through no fault of our own. For example, trait shame can develop in childhood when a caregiver is harsh or abusive, or in adulthood when mainstream culture marginalizes or devalues a person's identities. *Toxic* shame is when shame makes a person unable to function (Stokes & Lewis, 2018). When we refer to shame in psychotherapy, we're usually referring to trait shame.

Shame is probably the most difficult human emotion because it is invisible. Shame is taboo in modern society (Scheff & Mateo, 2016). It's an emotion of denial, as if admitting we feel shame confirms a fatal flaw that renders us unlovable. Shame also makes us want to disappear—go small, go silent, or go away. When shame is intense enough, it can lead to dissociation (Rudy et al., 2022). Behaviorally, we may try to avoid shame by numbing ourselves with food or alcohol or by immersing ourselves in external distractions like binge-watching TV or contributing to interpersonal conflict. None of these reactions allow us to see shame and deal with it, which is why shame is such a difficult emotion.

Self-Compassion and Shame

From a theoretical perspective, self-compassion is the opposite of shame. In Kristin Neff's (2003) three-component model of self-compassion, the opposing factors to self-kindness, common humanity, and mindfulness—self-criticism, self-isolation, and overidentification, respectively—are key aspects of shame.

Research has shown that each of these individual factors are pathogenic, tied to shame, and mitigated by self-compassion. *Self-criticism* is linked to diverse psychopathologies (Werner et al., 2019), it occurs in tandem with shame (Castilho et al., 2017), and a meta-analysis found that compassion-focused therapy was an effective treatment for self-criticism (Vidal & Soldevilla, 2023). *Social isolation* and *loneliness* are linked to many psychological disorders (Meltzer, 2013; Wang et al., 2017), are associated with shame (DeYoung, 2015; Thoresen et al., 2018), and are alleviated by self-compassion (Andel et al., 2021; Xie et al., 2023). Finally, Neff's (2003) notion of *overidentification* overlaps in the research literature with the concepts of *rumination* and *self-absorption*, both of which are linked to psychopathology (Ehring, 2021; Woodruff-Borden et al., 2001) and shame (Joireman, 2004; Milia et al., 2021) and are mitigated by self-compassion (Samaie & Farahani, 2011).

Self-compassion (as a holistic, multicomponent concept) is inversely related to shame in correlational studies among clinical populations. For example, shame is lower among people who are self-compassionate and struggle with anxiety and depression (Callow et al., 2021; Sick et al., 2020), eating disorders (Bellows et al., 2023), body image (Tylka & Huellemann, 2023), and sexual minority stigma (Chan et al., 2020). To explore how self-compassion may be related to less depression, Zhang and colleagues (2018) compared self-worth based on inner support from self-compassion versus self-worth based on external social approval. They found that only self-worth from self-compassion reduced the impact of shame on depression, presumably because self-compassion is a more stable source of self-worth.

Self-compassion and shame are also inversely related in clinical *intervention* studies. As self-compassion increases in therapy, shame decreases in studies on depression (Johnson et al., 2018), posttraumatic stress disorder (Au et al., 2017), narcissistic personality disorder (Kramer et al., 2018), eating disorders (Kelly et al., 2017), and social anxiety disorder (Khoramnia et al., 2020).

Models of Self-Compassion for Shame in Therapy

Increasingly, shame has become a target for self-compassion-based therapies. CFT is the most explicitly self-compassion-based therapy model. Paul Gilbert (2009) had the revolutionary insight that people struggling with shame may cognitively grasp that they are not to blame for their suffering, but they don't feel better because the tone of their inner dialogue remains relentlessly harsh and self-critical. The goal of therapy is to warm up the inner conversation and create a sense of safeness using various methodologies, such as de-shaming shame with psychoeducation, rhythmic breathing to activate the parasympathetic nervous system, developing a compassionate part of oneself, and addressing blocks to self-compassion (Irons & Lad, 2017). Preliminary studies have shown that CFT reduces shame as it alleviates symptoms in different diagnoses, including eating disorders (Carter et al., 2021), depression (Gilbert & Procter, 2006), social anxiety (Boersma et al., 2015), and posttraumatic stress disorder (Au et al., 2017).

Emotion-focused therapy (EFT), originally developed by Leslie Greenberg (2011), shares the view that shame is a pathogenic factor across diagnoses. EFT alleviates shame by activating more adaptive emotions specific to the individual, such as grief, anger, or compassion (Greenberg & Iwakabe, 2011). The first step is helping clients to acknowledge shame, usually by a therapist empathizing with painful emotions associated with shame, such as embarrassment or despair. Clients can't be argued out of shame, so a new experience is created to transform shame, such as listening compassionately to the inner critic and the criticized selves in the two-chair exercise (Shahar, 2020).

Internal family systems (IFS), developed by Richard Schwartz, is another self-compassion-based therapy that directly addresses shame (Schwartz & Sweezy, 2019; Sweezy, 2023). IFS works with parts or subpersonalities. Shame is a burden carried by an "exile"—a child part—stuck in time. Another part—a "manager"—tries to keep shame in check through self-criticism, which usually just increases shame. When shame becomes overwhelming, a "firefighter" might step in with dramatic actions, such as addiction or aggression toward others. Each part has a role to play in helping a person to stay safe and survive, even if their strategies seem counterproductive. All parts are treated with compassion and respect until the exile is unburdened and the "self," who is compassion itself, takes over.

Acceptance and commitment therapy (ACT) is a therapy model that is *implicitly* self-compassionate (Luoma & Platt, 2015). However, recent efforts have been made to explicitly integrate self-compassion into ACT (Neff & Tirch, 2013; see also Chapter 20). For example, in addition to mindfulness and acceptance exercises, Linde and colleagues (2023) taught patients with body dysmorphic disorder to talk self-compassionately to themselves and practice value-guided activities in response to shame, resulting in long-term improvements in shame and increases in self-compassion.

A Mindful Self-Compassion-Based Approach to Shame in Psychotherapy

A general model for self-compassion-based therapy, informed by the mindful self-compassion program, is described in Chapter 1. There are three parts to treating shame in this model of therapy: *mindfulness*, *self-compassion*, and *working with backdraft*. These parts are explained below using the following example (a composite of actual persons):

> Sylvia was a conscientious manager in her state Division of Child Services. During the COVID-19 pandemic, as fewer colleagues showed up for work, Sylvia felt it was her responsibility to fill in and keep things going. She was deeply committed to her work and any lapse was a source of embarrassment to her. Over time, Sylvia's efforts became unsustainable. She started losing sleep, showed up at work exhausted, and found herself snapping at her colleagues and speaking cynically about the work they were trying to do. Eventually, Sylvia was asked by her supervisor to take a leave of absence. When Sylvia arrived in therapy, she reported feeling anxious and depressed.

When clients start therapy, they rarely say they want to alleviate shame, even if shame is a prominent factor in their lives. In Sylvia's case, shame was hiding behind anxiety and depression. Her clinician suspected that Sylvia was struggling with shame for a number of reasons: She was embarrassed about being in therapy ("I can't believe I'm here!"), she seemed ashamed that she couldn't handle her work stress ("I flunked out of work!"), she described moral distress at work ("I was hurting the people I was supposed to help!"), and she worried about returning to work and facing her colleagues again. Sylvia appeared to be a shame-prone person who had tried heroically to manage an impossible work situation.

Mindfulness

The first part of shame treatment is *mindfulness*—knowing that we're feeling shame *while* we're feeling it, with acceptance. Mindfulness helps clients get perspective on what's bothering them, making room for a self-compassionate response. Naming shame is a mindfulness practice but people often feel ashamed to acknowledge that they're feeling shame. In that case, clinicians can help their clients gradually orient toward shame with less-triggering words, such as feeling *embarrassed*, *powerless*, or *not good enough*, or simply *pain*. It isn't necessary to immerse ourselves in shame to trigger a compassionate response; we only need to *touch* shame. However, the more open we can be about shame ("Ah, *this* is shame"), the more naturally self-compassion can flow.

Once shame becomes an acceptable topic in therapy, clinicians can explore with clients how they recognize shame in their lives. As described above, there can be internal signs (e.g., "sinking feeling"), external signs (e.g., sweating), mental signs (e.g., going blank), or behavioral signs (e.g., hiding), or shame can be hiding behind other emotions (e.g., anxiety). When clients are able to identify shame as it arises, they acquire perspective and an opportunity to respond with self-compassion.

> It was a relief for Sylvia to discover that she was feeling shame about her struggles at work. She came to this insight gradually as she and her therapist explored her anguish about leaving work. Sylvia's main expression of shame was self-criticism. Recognizing self-criticism helped Sylvia make sense of her anxiety and depression: Anxiety was her fear of being discovered as "not up to the task" and depression was the result of exhaustion and an inner voice calling her "incompetent" and a "failure." Sylvia also felt validated and shed tears when her therapist described what happened to her as "traumatic." The shame of not being able to keep up with her work made Sylvia doubt who she was as a person.

Sylvia recognized shame most easily as self-criticism, a cognitive aspect of shame. She might have found it even more useful to identify shame as a physical sensation. This is because shame is a threat state that triggers an immediate response in the body. When a person is able to label shame as it arises in the body, they are less likely to slip into self-criticism and rumination.

Self-Compassion

Self-compassion comes after mindfulness. As described in Chapter 1, there are three ways that clinicians can help their clients cultivate self-compassion in therapy: compassionate presence, compassionate alliance, and compassionate interventions.

Compassionate Presence

Compassionate presence refers to a clinician being open and aware of their moment-to-moment experience in therapy. A therapist's presence can have a direct impact on a client's inner experience, even without saying a word (Koole & Tschacher, 2016).

> Sylvia's therapist gave her a lot of uninterrupted time to describe her experience at work. As Sylvia told her story, bouncing between fear, rage, despair, and shame, her therapist was able to feel these emotions resonating in her own body. To stay present, her therapist gently breathed in for herself and out for Sylvia (see Practice B, "Giving and Receiving Compassion," in the Appendix). When Sylvia noticed how calmly and compassionately her therapist was listening, she felt calmer and began to catch glimpses of her old self again—a good person struggling to do the right thing.

In Sylvia's case, her therapist's compassionate presence allowed her to feel safe, which in turn allowed her to see her situation in a new light.

Compassionate Alliance

A compassionate alliance, or compassionate therapeutic relationship, is characterized by radical acceptance, resonance, and resource building (see also Chapter 1).

Radical acceptance is the attitude of self-compassion-based therapy. Radical acceptance is especially important when working with shame because shame is characterized by negative self-evaluation. Our shame-prone clients assume that others (including their therapists) will think negatively about them when they speak, and they're likely to judge themselves whether they speak or not. Therefore, radical acceptance by a clinician is an antidote to shame in psychotherapy. To be radically accepting, therapists should temporarily abandon the effort to "fix" a client, focusing instead on allowing the client to be just as they are while opening to the client's pain and meeting it with kindness and compassion. (Practicing self-compassion helps here; see Chapter 8.) Over time, the voice of a compassionate therapist is likely to be internalized by the client as their own compassionate inner voice.

Radical acceptance is easier said than done. Shame, in particular, is likely to be expressed by clients in therapy by withdrawing emotionally, devaluing the therapist, or becoming overly solicitous. During such challenges, therapists are more likely to maintain radical acceptance and compassion if they can see the motivation underlying shame—namely, the *universal wish to be loved*. When therapists (and their clients) become aware of this tender longing behind shame, shame seems more innocent and the individual becomes more worthy of compassion, as we might feel toward a child or another innocent being.

How does shame arise from the wish to be loved? Human beings are social animals that rely on one another to survive and thrive. At the moment of birth, newborns need to find someone to love them and to provide for all their physical and emotional needs. As we get older, we continue to need love in order to survive and thrive. Not all adults are willing to admit that they need to be loved, but almost everyone can say that they wish to be respected, appreciated, connected, or valued. Shame occurs when we imagine that we're being devalued in the minds of others. This nonpathological view of shame helps clinicians remain compassionate when clients express shame in hurtful and counterproductive ways.

> After about 3 months of therapy, Sylvia started asking pointed questions about her therapist's educational background and treatment methods. Sylvia had hoped to be back at work by then and she felt disappointed with herself—she had a new wave of shame that she tried to manage by blaming her therapist. Her therapist kept a steady eye on Sylvia's shame, especially Sylvia's fear that she would not receive her colleagues' respect when she returned to work. Rather than getting entangled in a conversation about her own competence, her therapist mused aloud about how we all wish to be loved and respected and how shame can arise when we fear the opposite will happen. The connection between shame and the wish to be loved made sense to Sylvia.
>
> Eventually, Sylvia and her therapist discussed how approval from others is an unreliable source of self-worth but Sylvia could do something better: She could learn to love and respect herself in any situation, even in the midst of shame. Sylvia doubted she could do this until her therapist pointed out that Sylvia is already very kind and respectful . . . toward others. She just needs to make a U-turn and include herself in the circle of her compassion.

All three elements of a compassionate therapeutic relationship—radical acceptance, resonance, and resource building—can be found in Sylvia's interaction with her therapist. Her therapist didn't judge Sylvia even as she was being judged, she resonated with Sylvia's fear and shame about returning to work, and she gently introduced Sylvia to the resource of self-compassion. Throughout these interactions, Sylvia's therapist managed to maintain a compassionate attitude, listening and speaking from the heart.

Compassionate Interventions

Home practices are a way of cultivating the resource of self-compassion. Ideally, home practices emerge organically out of the therapeutic conversation and reflect the needs and interests of the client.

> Sylvia was eager to learn more about self-compassion when her therapist pointed out that caring for others without attending to her own needs probably contributed to burnout. Her therapist explained that self-compassion starts with the question "What do I need?" Even when we don't know the answer, simply asking the question gets the ball rolling. Sylvia decided to make "What do I need?" her mantra for the following week. At their next session, Sylvia reported

that she was sleeping better because she gave herself permission to go to bed when she was tired. Sylvia also amazed herself by saying "no" to her sister, who had a habit of borrowing money from Sylvia and not paying her back. With these successes, Sylvia asked her therapist for additional reading material, who recommended *The Mindful Self-Compassion Workbook* (Neff & Germer, 2018). That's where Sylvia learned the "self-compassion break," which became her "go-to" practice after she and her therapist adapted it for shame (see Practice L, "Self-Compassion Break for Shame," in the Appendix).

By the time her therapist had recommended the workbook, Sylvia had experienced the benefit of self-compassion practice and wanted to learn more. However, even before a client is interested in self-compassion, clinicians can suggest self-compassion exercises without mentioning the term *self-compassion*. Self-compassion practice is simply validating suffering and responding with kindness and understanding. Therapists can model this behavior in relationship to their clients and help their clients to do the same for themselves. Home practices like Sylvia's mindfulness of shame in daily life exercise and the "What do I need?" mantra are examples of self-compassion practices that clients can easily integrate into their daily lives. Brief, informal practices are generally preferable to lengthy ones (like meditation), and when practices bring genuine relief, clients are likely to continue practicing them.

Ideally, home practices are designed collaboratively with the client based on the content of the therapy session. They should be a response to a need—a solution to a problem—expressed by the client. Home practices can be tried during the session itself to see if they have the desired effect, such as reducing stress or building courage. In order for therapists to skillfully introduce self-compassion practices to clients, therapists should have direct experience of how self-compassion works from their own practice of self-compassion. A clinician's personal practice is the foundation of self-compassion-based therapy (see Chapter 8 for more on therapists' personal practice).

Backdraft

The third part of self-compassion-based treatment of shame is working with backdraft. *Backdraft* refers to the distress that arises when we give ourselves compassion. As the saying goes, "Love reveals everything unlike itself" or "When we give ourselves unconditional love, we discover the conditions in which we were unloved."

Why does backdraft happen? The only way we know anything is by contrast. If I say to myself, "May I accept myself just as I am," I'm likely to recall when I was treated unacceptably, or I may remember what I consider unacceptable about myself. This process can be confusing to clients because they're in therapy to feel better, not worse. However, backdraft is an intrinsic part of the transformation process and it's a sign that self-compassion is working. Through the mechanism of backdraft, self-compassion reactivates old wounds and makes them accessible for transformation.

Backdraft can take many forms: *mental* (e.g., "I'm defective" or "I'm unlovable"), *emotional* (e.g., shame, fear, anger), *physical* (e.g., aches, pains), or *behavioral* (e.g., withdrawal or aggression). Since shame is a reason that memories get locked out of awareness, when we start practicing self-compassion for shame we're likely to reexperience shame. Furthermore, since shame and trauma are closely linked, old traumas are also likely to arise when we practice self-compassion. Transformation occurs when we respond to backdraft in a manner that we probably needed when our wounds originally occurred: with kindness and compassion. With consistent practice over time, backdraft with a self-compassionate response can even help us reparent ourselves.

> When Sylvia was about 5 years old, her mother started having bouts of depression, which kept her mother in bed for long periods of time while her father was away at work. Sylvia tried in vain to connect and cheer up her mother. Eventually, Sylvia found that by taking over her mother's responsibilities, especially taking care of her younger sister and keeping the house in order, Sylvia felt closer to her mother. Over time, Sylvia became a model child, excelling in school and helpful to a fault.
>
> Burnout stopped Sylvia in her tracks. All her efforts to keep the Division of Child Services going during the pandemic were insufficient and left Sylvia in a state of despair. When Sylvia learned self-compassion, she recognized that her efforts at work were largely driven by her wish to be a "good person." In conversation with her therapist, Sylvia traced that yearning to a 5-year-old girl inside herself who struggled to receive love and connection from her depressed mother. "Tell me I'm good!" was the unrequited longing in Sylvia's heart. Sylvia saw that the shame she felt at work had its roots in feeling "not good enough" as a child. Sylvia was able to return to work soon thereafter, but she stayed in therapy for another year as her childhood longing was compassionately held in the relationship with her therapist. Sylvia also learned to give herself compassion when she needed it, rather than hurling herself into more and more work to prove her worth.

Backdraft can occur anytime we feel compassion, either in interaction with another person (like a therapist) or while practicing self-compassion. Psychotherapy is an ideal environment for clients to learn self-compassion because it's a safe space to recognize and respond compassionately to backdraft.

Safety is an important consideration when working with backdraft. Some clients become overly zealous about self-compassion practice when backdraft occurs, which only leads to more backdraft. This is especially common among clients who experienced childhood trauma and learned to stay safe by doing everything perfectly. Therefore, clients should be encouraged to "go slow" when they practice self-compassion. Clinicians need to monitor and help clients to feel either "safe" or "challenged" while practicing self-compassion, and never "overwhelmed." There is nothing compassionate about harming oneself with self-compassion. If a client feels overwhelmed, therapists can ask, "What do you need to feel safe?" or "How do you care for yourself already?" *Behavioral* self-compassion, such as drinking a cup of tea or taking a walk, is the best form of self-compassion when a client feels overwhelmed. When a client feels safe again, they can practice mental exercises (which are more likely to evoke backdraft), such as the "Self-Compassion Break for Shame" (Practice L in the Appendix), to reprocess and heal shame.

How Does Self-Compassion for Shame Work in Therapy?

It is helpful for clinicians to consider underlying mechanisms of action while working with shame in therapy. There are numerous candidates, such as the transdiagnostic pathogenic mechanisms of *self-criticism*, *isolation*, and *rumination* (described above).

Another putative mechanism of action is *exposure.* This chapter started with the premise that shame is a difficult emotion because it is invisible. Self-compassion has been shown to reduce experiential avoidance of early shame experiences (Farr et al., 2021), and individuals with posttraumatic stress engaged in fewer avoidance strategies following exposure to trauma, which allowed for exposure to happen naturally (Thompson & Waltz, 2008). Self-compassion appears to be a resource that reduces shame by reducing avoidance of shame.

Physiologically, shame is a threat state. Self-compassion appears to deactivate the threat response and generate a sense of *safeness.* Research shows that when people are negatively evaluated by others and feel shame, they produce the stress hormone cortisol (Gruenewald et al., 2004). Research also shows that when people apply self-compassion through a self-soothing touch gesture, cortisol levels decrease (Dreisoerner et al., 2021). Self-compassion, the opposite of shame, is generally associated with increases in parasympathetic nervous system activity (more safety; Kirschner et al., 2019; Svendsen et al., 2020) and decreases in sympathetic nervous system activity (less fear; Arch et al., 2014; Breines et al., 2015).

Finally, shame-proneness is associated with *insecure attachment* in childhood (Park & Shields, 2023) and self-compassion is associated with *secure attachment* (Lathren et al., 2021). Secure attachment is also linked to a wealth of positive mental health indicators (Homan, 2018). In a study on attachment-based compassion therapy, secure attachment increased and self-compassion mediated that change (Navarro-Gil et al., 2020). Therefore, another way that self-compassion probably works in therapy is by enhancing secure attachment.

Conclusion

Shame is an underlying emotion in a host of clinical conditions. Shame is an attack on a person's sense of self, either coming from inside or outside oneself. Self-compassion appears to be an antidote to shame, theoretically, empirically, and clinically. Successful therapy tends to increase self-compassion and decrease shame. Shame can be specifically targeted in self-compassion-based therapy by enhancing mindfulness of shame, responding to shame with self-compassion, and working with backdraft. Therapists can help their clients loosen the grip of shame through their compassionate presence, by fostering a compassionate alliance, and by collaboratively designing self-compassion home practices. A compassionate alliance is characterized by the attitude of radical acceptance, the process of emotional resonance, and the goal of building the resource of self-compassion. While addressing shame in this way, therapists can focus on various mechanisms of change, such as reducing self-criticism, emotional isolation, or rumination; or increasing acceptance of moment-to-moment experience, enhancing the physiology of safeness, or developing secure attachment through the resource of self-compassion. Over the past 20 years, self-compassion-based therapy is increasingly recognized as an effective treatment for shame.

REFERENCES

Andel, S. A., Shen, W., & Arvan, M. L. (2021). Depending on your own kindness: The moderating role of self-compassion on the within-person consequences of work loneliness during the COVID-19 pandemic. *Journal of Occupational Health Psychology, 26*(4), 276–290.

Arch, J. J., Brown, K. W., Dean, D. J., Landy, L. N., Brown, K. D., & Laudenslager, M. L. (2014). Self-compassion training modulates alpha-amylase, heart rate variability, and subjective responses to social evaluative threat in women. *Psychoneuroendocrinology, 42*, 49–58.

Au, T. M., Sauer-Zavala, S., King, M. W., Petrocchi, N., Barlow, D. H., & Litz,

B. T. (2017). Compassion-based therapy for trauma-related shame and posttraumatic stress: Initial evaluation using a multiple baseline design. *Behavior Therapy, 48*(2), 207–221.

Bellows, L. A., Couturier, L. E., Dunn, L. C., & Carter, J. C. (2023). Relational bullying and disordered eating: Testing a moderated mediation model of the role of shame and self-compassion. *Frontiers in Psychology, 14*, 968046.

Boersma, K., Håkanson, A., Salomonsson, E., & Johansson, I. (2015). Compassion focused therapy to counteract shame, self-criticism and isolation: A replicated single case experimental study for individuals with social anxiety. *Journal of Contemporary Psychotherapy, 45*, 89–98.

Breines, J. G., McInnis, C. M., Kuras, Y. I., Thoma, M. V., Gianferante, D., Hanlin, L., et al. (2015). Self-compassionate young adults show lower salivary alpha-amylase responses to repeated psychosocial stress. *Self and Identity, 14*(4), 390–402.

Callow, T. J., Moffitt, R. L., & Neumann, D. L. (2021). External shame and its association with depression and anxiety: The moderating role of self-compassion. *Australian Psychologist, 56*(1), 70–80.

Cândea, D. M., & Szentagotai, A. (2013). Shame and psychopathology: From research to clinical practice. *Journal of Cognitive and Behavioral Psychotherapies, 13*(1), 101–113.

Carter, A., Gilbert, P., & Kirby, J. N. (2021). Compassion focused therapy for body weight shame: A mixed methods pilot trial. *Clinical Psychology and Psychotherapy, 28*(1), 93–108.

Castilho, P., Pinto-Gouveia, J., & Duarte, J. (2017). Two forms of self-criticism mediate differently the shame–psychopathological symptoms link. *Psychology and Psychotherapy: Theory, Research and Practice, 90*(1), 44–54.

Chan, K. K. S., Yung, C. S. W., & Nie, G. M. (2020). Self-compassion buffers the negative psychological impact of stigma stress on sexual minorities. *Mindfulness, 11*, 2338–2348.

Claesson, K., & Sohlberg, S. (2002). Internalized shame and early interactions characterized by indifference, abandonment and rejection: Replicated findings. *Clinical Psychology and Psychotherapy, 9*(4), 277–284.

Dearing, R. L., & Tangney, J. P. E. (2011). *Shame in the therapy hour.* American Psychological Association.

DeYoung, P. A. (2015). *Understanding and treating chronic shame: A relational/neurobiological approach.* Routledge.

Dreisoerner, A., Junker, N. M., Schlotz, W., Heimrich, J., Bloemeke, S., Ditzen, B., & van Dick, R. (2021). Self-soothing touch and being hugged reduce cortisol responses to stress: A randomized controlled trial on stress, physical touch, and social identity. *Comprehensive Psychoneuroendocrinology, 8*, 100091.

Ehring, T. (2021). Thinking too much: Rumination and psychopathology. *World Psychiatry, 20*(3), 441–442.

Farr, J., Ononaiye, M., & Irons, C. (2021). Early shaming experiences and psychological distress: The role of experiential avoidance and self-compassion. *Psychology and Psychotherapy: Theory, Research and Practice, 94*(4), 952–972.

Ferreira, C., Moura-Ramos, M., Matos, M., & Galhardo, A. (2022). A new measure to assess external and internal shame: Development, factor structure and psychometric properties of the external and internal shame scale. *Current Psychology, 41*(4), 1892–1901.

Germer, C. (2023). Self-compassion in psychotherapy: Clinical integration, evidence base, and mechanisms of change. In A. Finlay-Jones, K. Bluth, & K. Neff (Eds.), *Handbook of self-compassion* (pp. 379–415). Springer.

Gilbert, P. (2009). Introducing compassion-focused therapy. *Advances in Psychiatric Treatment, 15*(3), 199–208.

Gilbert, P., & Irons, C. (2009). Shame, self-criticism, and self-compassion in adolescence. In N. Allen & L. Sheeer (Eds.), *Adolescent emotional development and the emergence of depressive disorders* (Vol. 1, pp. 195–214). Cambridge University Press.

Gilbert, P., & Procter, S. (2006). Compassionate mind training for people with high shame and self-criticism: Overview and pilot study of a group therapy approach. *Clinical Psychology and Psychotherapy, 13*(6), 353–379.

Greenberg, L. S. (2011). *Emotion-focused therapy.* American Psychological Association.

Greenberg, L. S., & Iwakabe, S. (2011). Emotion-focused therapy and shame. In R. L. Dearing & J. P. Tangney (Eds.), *Shame in the therapy hour* (pp. 69–90). American Psychological Association.

Gross, C. A., & Hansen, N. E. (2000). Clarifying the experience of shame: The role of attachment style, gender, and investment in relatedness. *Personality and Individual Differences, 28*(5), 897–907.

Gruenewald, T. L., Kemeny, M. E., Aziz, N., & Fahey, J. L. (2004). Acute threat to the social self: Shame, social self-esteem, and cortisol activity. *Psychosomatic Medicine, 66*(6), 915–924.

Homan, K. J. (2018). Secure attachment and eudaimonic well-being in late adulthood: The mediating role of self-compassion. *Aging and Mental Health, 22*(3), 363–370.

Irons, C., & Lad, S. (2017). Using compassion focused therapy to work with shame and self-criticism in complex trauma. *Australian Clinical Psychologist, 3*(1), 1743.

Johnson, S. B., Goodnight, B. L., Zhang, H., Daboin, I., Patterson, B., & Kaslow, N. J. (2018). Compassion-based meditation in African Americans: Self-criticism mediates changes in depression. *Suicide and Life-Threatening Behavior, 48*(2), 160–168.

Joireman, J. (2004). Empathy and the self-absorption paradox II: Self-rumination and self-reflection as mediators between shame, guilt, and empathy. *Self and Identity, 3*(3), 225–238.

Kelly, A. C., Wisniewski, L., Martin-Wagar, C., & Hoffman, E. (2017). Group-based compassion-focused therapy as an adjunct to outpatient treatment for eating disorders: A pilot randomized controlled trial. *Clinical Psychology and Psychotherapy, 24*(2), 475–487.

Khoramnia, S., Bavafa, A., Jaberghaderi, N., Parvizifard, A., Foroughi, A., Ahmadi, M., & Amiri, S. (2020). The effectiveness of acceptance and commitment therapy for social anxiety disorder: A randomized clinical trial. *Trends in Psychiatry and Psychotherapy, 42*(1), 30–38.

Kirschner, H., Kuyken, W., Wright, K., Roberts, H., Brejcha, C., & Karl, A. (2019).

Soothing your heart and feeling connected: A new experimental paradigm to study the benefits of self-compassion. *Clinical Psychological Science, 7*(3), 545–565.

Koole, S. L., & Tschacher, W. (2016). Synchrony in psychotherapy: A review and an integrative framework for the therapeutic alliance. *Frontiers in Psychology, 7*, 862.

Kramer, U., Pascual-Leone, A., Rohde, K. B., & Sachse, R. (2018). The role of shame and self-compassion in psychotherapy for narcissistic personality disorder: An exploratory study. *Clinical Psychology and Psychotherapy, 25*(2), 272–282.

Lathren, C. R., Rao, S. S., Park, J., & Bluth, K. (2021). Self-compassion and current close interpersonal relationships: A scoping literature review. *Mindfulness, 12*, 1078–1093.

Lewis, H. B. (1971). Shame and guilt in neurosis. *Psychoanalytic Review, 58*(3), 419–438.

Lewis, H. B. (1987). Introduction: Shame, the "sleeper" in psychopathology. In H. B. Lewis (Ed.), *The role of shame in symptom formation* (pp. 1–28). Erlbaum.

Lewis, M. (2019). The self-conscious emotions and the role of shame in psychopathology. In V. LoBue, K. Pérez-Edgar, & K. A. Buss (Eds.), *Handbook of emotional development* (pp. 311–350). Springer International.

Linde, J., Luoma, J. B., Rück, C., Ramnerö, J., & Lundgren, T. (2023). Acceptance and compassion-based therapy targeting shame in body dysmorphic disorder: A multiple baseline study. *Behavior Modification, 47*(3), 693–718.

Luoma, J. B., & Platt, M. G. (2015). Shame, self-criticism, self-stigma, and compassion in acceptance and commitment therapy. *Current Opinion in Psychology, 2*, 97–101.

Meltzer, H., Bebbington, P., Dennis, M. S., Jenkins, R., McManus, S., & Brugha, T. S. (2013). Feelings of loneliness among adults with mental disorder. *Social Psychiatry and Psychiatric Epidemiology, 48*, 5–13.

Milia, C., Kolubinski, D. C., & Spada, M. M. (2021). The effects of self-critical rumination on shame and stress: An experimental study. *Behavioural and Cognitive Psychotherapy, 49*(3), 272–286.

Navarro-Gil, M., Lopez-del-Hoyo, Y., Modrego-Alarcón, M., Montero-Marin, J., Van Gordon, W., Shonin, E., & Garcia-Campayo, J. (2020). Effects of attachment-based compassion therapy (ABCT) on self-compassion and attachment style in healthy people. *Mindfulness, 11*(1), 51–62.

Neff, K. (2003). Self-compassion: An alternative conceptualization of a healthy attitude toward oneself. *Self and Identity, 2*(2), 85–101.

Neff, K., & Germer, C. (2018). *The mindful self-compassion workbook: A proven way to accept yourself, build inner strength, and thrive.* Guilford Press.

Neff, K., & Tirch, D. (2013). Self-compassion and ACT. In T. B. Kashdan & J. Ciarrochi (Eds.), *Mindfulness, acceptance, and positive psychology: The seven foundations of well-being* (pp. 78–106). Context Press/New Harbinger.

Park, C. J., & Shields, J. (2023). Childhood attachment insecurity and shame-proneness in adulthood: Implications for clinical social work practice. *Journal of Human Behavior in the Social Environment*, 1–17.

Robertson, T. E., Sznycer, D., Delton, A. W., Tooby, J., & Cosmides, L. (2018). The true trigger of shame: Social devaluation is sufficient, wrongdoing is unnecessary. *Evolution and Human Behavior, 39*(5), 566–573.

Rudy, J. A., McKernan, S., Kouri, N., & D'Andrea, W. (2022). A meta-analysis of the association between shame and dissociation. *Journal of Traumatic Stress, 35*(5), 1318–1333.

Samaie, G., & Farahani, H. A. (2011). Self-compassion as a moderator of the relationship between rumination, self-reflection and stress. *Procedia–Social and Behavioral Sciences, 30*, 978–982.

Scheff, T., & Mateo, S. (2016). The S-word is taboo: Shame is invisible in modern societies. *Journal of General Practice, 4*(1), 1–6.

Schwartz, R. C., & Sweezy, M. (2019). *Internal family systems therapy* (2nd ed.). Guilford Press.

Sedighimornani, N. (2018). Shame and its features: Understanding of shame. *European Journal of Social Sciences Studies, 3*(3), 75–106.

Shahar, B. (2020). New developments in emotion-focused therapy for social anxiety disorder. *Journal of Clinical Medicine, 9*(9), 2918.

Sick, K., Pila, E., Nesbitt, A., & Sabiston, C. M. (2020). Does self-compassion buffer the detrimental effect of body shame on depressive symptoms? *Body Image, 34*, 175–183.

Stipek, D. J. (1983). A developmental analysis of pride and shame. *Human Development, 26*(1), 42–54.

Stokes, S., & Lewis, S. (2018). *The trauma of shame and the making of the self.* Page.

Svendsen, J. L., Schanche, E., Osnes, B., Vøllestad, J., Visted, E., Dundas, I., et al. (2020). Is dispositional self-compassion associated with psychophysiological flexibility beyond mindfulness? An exploratory pilot study. *Frontiers in Psychology, 11*, 614.

Sweezy, M. (2023). *Internal family systems therapy for shame and guilt.* Guilford Press.

Tangney, J. P., & Dearing, R. L. (2003). *Shame and guilt.* Guilford Press.

Thompson, B. L., & Waltz, J. (2008). Self-compassion and PTSD symptom severity. *Journal of Traumatic Stress, 21*(6), 556–558.

Thoresen, S., Aakvaag, H. F., Strøm, I. F., Wentzel-Larsen, T., & Birkeland, M. S. (2018). Loneliness as a mediator of the relationship between shame and health problems in young people exposed to childhood violence. *Social Science and Medicine, 211*, 183–189.

Tylka, T. L., & Huellemann, K. L. (2023). Self-compassion and body image. In A. Finlay-Jones, K. Bluth, & K. Neff (Eds.), *Handbook of self-compassion* (pp. 183–200). Springer International.

Vidal, J., & Soldevilla, J. M. (2023). Effect of compassion-focused therapy on self-criticism and self-soothing: A meta-analysis. *British Journal of Clinical Psychology, 62*(1), 70–81.

Wang, J., Lloyd-Evans, B., Giacco, D., Forsyth, R., Nebo, C., Mann, F., & Johnson, S. (2017). Social isolation in mental health: A conceptual and methodological review. *Social Psychiatry and Psychiatric Epidemiology, 52*, 1451–1461.

Werner, A. M., Tibubos, A. N., Rohrmann, S., & Reiss, N. (2019). The clinical trait self-criticism and its relation to psychopathology: A systematic review—update. *Journal of Affective Disorders, 246*, 530–547.

Woodruff-Borden, J., Brothers, A. J., & Lister, S. C. (2001). Self-focused attention: Commonalities across psychopathologies and predictors. *Behavioural and Cognitive Psychotherapy, 29*(2), 169–178.

Xie, Q., Manova, V., & Khoury, B. (2023). How do dispositional mindfulness and self-compassion alleviate loneliness? The mediating role of rejection sensitivity. *Current Psychology, 42*(27), 23712–23721.

Zhang, H., Carr, E. R., Garcia-Williams, A. G., Siegelman, A. E., Berke, D., Niles-Carnes, L. V., et al. (2018). Shame and depressive symptoms: Self-compassion and contingent self-worth as mediators? *Journal of Clinical Psychology in Medical Settings, 25*(4), 408–419.

12

Alcoholism, Addictions, and Self-Compassion

Alfie Wishart

This chapter is a guide to the therapeutic and clinical application of self-compassion for people recovering from addictions, focusing on foundational principles, clinical context, and clarity of assessment. The terms *alcoholism* and *addiction* are used interchangeably, since research and clinical experience indicate that the etiology and resolution of addictions have much in common, regardless of the substance or process (Shaffer et al., 2004). The variations in treating different addictions are often due to individual factors, such as trauma, family history, and mental health disorders, that affect a person's psychological makeup. Individual differences notwithstanding, this chapter is applicable to alcoholism and a wide range of addictions.

There are several self-compassion exercises mentioned in this chapter. For more information on their format and application, see *The Mindful Self-Compassion Workbook: A Proven Way to Accept Yourself, Build Inner Strength, and Thrive* (Neff & Germer, 2018).

A Quantum Shift in Psychology

Carl Rogers (1986) proposed that the client has

> within him or her self [sic] vast resources for self-understanding, for altering her or his self-concept, attitudes, and self-directed behavior [sic]—and that these resources can be tapped if only a definable climate of facilitative psychological attitudes can be provided. (p. 197)

This was part of a fundamental shift in psychology to focus on mobilizing the client's internal resources. The "facilitative attitudes" Rogers (1986) proposed were empathy, congruence, and unconditional positive regard. Unconditional positive regard with empathy, in the service of facilitating positive change in the client (a reduction in suffering), points to what we have come to recognize and refer to today as compassion.

Clinical and Nonclinical Interventions

This shift, which focuses on the mobilization of clients' internal resources, began to propagate throughout the culture and led to the creation of clinical and nonclinical programs. The clinical programs include positive psychology, founded by Martin Seligman in 1998 (Seligman & Csikszentmihalyi, 2000), and compassion-focused therapy (CFT), founded by Paul Gilbert (2000). The nonclinical programs include mindfulness-based stress reduction (MBSR), founded by Jon Kabat-Zinn in 1979 (Kabat-Zinn, 2013), and mindful self-compassion (MSC), created by Kristen Neff and Christopher Germer in 2010 (Neff & Germer, 2018).

Simultaneous to this shift in mobilizing our innate resources burgeoned as the overall state of mental health in the United States declined (Udupa et al., 2023). The research on mindfulness meditation and compassion accumulated and strongly indicated specific benefits for general well-being and for mental health disorders (Hickey et al., 2017). This opened the door for licensed mental health practitioners to use meditation and compassion exercises with clients.

About Mindfulness

In this chapter, mindfulness receives greater emphasis than what is usually taught with compassion and self-compassion teachings for several reasons. First, mindfulness improves distress tolerance by steadying the mind, which subdues impulsive behavior and habitual responding. Second, the interior focus promotes greater insight, leading to greater self-honesty and therefore, accountability, and is an essential element of recovery and shame mitigation (Goldsmith et al., 2014). Third, it promotes ongoing expansion in awareness of our basic nature, also known as our authentic self, thereby lowering baseline anxiety (Edenfield & Saeed, 2012). It is well-known that if anxiety is present, our compassionate abilities are diminished. Mindfulness creates space for compassion and facilitates learning how to cultivate it and adopt its way. In the contemplative traditions, mindfulness meditation is considered essential for gaining wisdom and is taught as a nondual element of compassion, for simply sitting in meditation, calming and training the mind itself, is an act of compassion.

Initial Considerations

Clients who present with the problematic use of drugs or alcohol vary greatly in length of abstinence, length and quality of recovery, attitudes toward spirituality and/or religion, and motivation. These interlocking factors, once determined, can form the parameters of and the foundation for therapy. The difference between abstinence and recovery is simply whether someone stops on their own (abstinence) or they are actively engaged in overcoming the spiritual malady (recovery; explained below). And knowing the difference between the spiritual malady and a mental health disorder is imperative, in that if someone has a spiritual malady, the psychological approach won't be effective as an initial approach. If the client has this spiritual malady and a mental health disorder, the spiritual malady needs to be addressed first, except when the mental health disorder is too destabilizing. In that case, it is best to treat the spiritual malady and the mental health disorder concurrently.

It may be beneficial to gather collateral information from the family, sponsor, or from previous treatment. I know of no single strategy that could be applied to substance use disorders. Once the basics are ascertained with the assessment suggestions below, the process requires a creative and fluid response to the individual, adjusting each step of the way, if necessary, given the client's development.

The Role of a Sponsor

If the client is in Alcoholics Anonymous (AA) or another 12-step program, it is important to know whether the client has a sponsor. The role of a sponsor is like that of a guide and mentor. If the client is in a 12-step program and does not have a sponsor, they are not fully engaged in their recovery. If the client is actively engaged with a sponsor, it is important to be aware of the sponsor's opinions and directions for the client for several reasons. The sponsor may be aware of things that the client has not yet mentioned or has opted to not reveal to the therapist. Also, knowing what directions the sponsor has given can be supported in therapy. Last, knowing what step the client is working on at the moment can help the therapist tailor the therapeutic approach to support the client's present needs.

Assess for the Client's Attitude toward Compassion

It is useful to have some assessment of the client's level of shame. Shame affects the client's capacity for self-awareness, disclosure, distress tolerance, adherence, change, and more. Shame also affects how the client responds to self-compassion exercises (Bonaz et al., 2021).

High shame-responding clients can find that exercises from the MSC program (see Neff & Germer, 2018), like "Working with Difficult Emotions," can bring forward more emotion than they have the capacity to manage without further training, education, or therapy, whereas an exercise like "Affectionate Breathing" is usually more suitable to start. Then, there are clients who cannot even do the "Affectionate Breathing" exercise without emotional flooding. If that's the case, "Loving-Kindness for Ourselves" may be workable as a beginning.

Assess for Trauma

Trauma has been on the rise in our modern world and is more prevalent in addiction populations (Blanco et al., 2013) and much more prevalent in homes where there is addiction (Huang et al., 2012). To complicate matters, clients sometimes minimize the effects of childhood neglect. This is when a child does not receive proper care, help, attention, comfort, engagement, sustenance, and so on in childhood or later. The presence of trauma does not necessarily preclude the application of mindfulness or self-compassion. However, if there is a history of trauma, mindfulness meditation and self-compassion have the potential to bring traumatic memories to the surface. The process for the resolution of trauma is the same for any habitual pattern with one exception. Traumatic memories are so highly charged with emotion and somatic responses that it is difficult to create an internal space safe enough for them to be processed. Thus, it may be necessary for the client to also seek trauma-focused therapy.

If your client has experienced trauma to the degree it would inhibit therapeutic progress if unprocessed, physical practices may be beneficial. The research on yoga, tai chi, and qigong indicates that they increase interoception (Farb et al., 2015). Simply put, interoception is awareness of the body's internal states, accessing them and assessing them. Interoception plays a direct role in self-regulation and in maintaining physical, mental, and emotional homeostasis. Disruption in the interoception processes has been linked to a number of disorders, including addictions (Farb et al., 2015). Consider such practices if a client appears to stall in their progress with sobriety and/or with therapy for no apparent reason. While the research is scarce, it appears that general aerobic exercise may also have beneficial effects for the relief of trauma symptoms as a result of an increase in interoception (Fetzner & Asmundson, 2015).

Assess for Shame

The presence of shame is directly correlated with addiction, mental health disorders, and posttraumatic stress disorder (PTSD; Patock-Peckham et al., 2018). With addictions, shame is the primary impediment to attaining and maintaining abstinence and the central factor in relapse. A decrease in shame is likely the most accurate predictor for successful recovery (Randles & Tracy, 2013).

Determining the client's level of shame is a key assessment when working with clients who have been in recovery for a long time, particularly when trauma is present. The level of residual shame can help determine where to start with a client and how much caution is appropriate with the self-compassion exercises that tend to tap into deeper emotions. Since self-compassion exercises have the ability to bring suppressed shame to the surface, a useful way to look at the exercises is as a means to access and resolve latent shame.

Assess for the Presence of Alcoholism

The most common approach to determining whether alcoholism is present is the pattern of using and the consequences. This works for extreme cases where someone has been in and out of rehabs and hospitals and has been warned about the perils of their behavior by many. But there are several classes of individuals with problematic substance use, for whom their behavior is not the best predictor for addiction.

The Phenomenon of Craving

If we put people with extreme alcoholic behavior on one side of a spectrum and put those who are not alcoholic on the other, around the midpoint are those people who it may be more difficult to determine whether they are just heavy drinkers or alcoholic. Just to the left of the zero point on the nonalcoholic side are the heavy drinkers, with some problematic consequences. And there are those who find that alcohol can relieve their mental health symptoms. Then, on the right of the zero point, the alcoholic side, are the binge drinkers who can abstain for periods of time, but once they drink, there are severe consequences, and often cannot stop by themselves. Here also are those who have a high degree of self-control and/or are early in their drinking life, managing well enough to avoid severe consequences.

The Spiritual Malady

The notion that alcoholism is a spiritual malady is central to AA recovery.[1] The kernel of this idea began with Carl Jung (Schoen, 2020). The concept was further crystallized as an aspect of methodology in a section of the book *Alcoholics Anonymous* (*The Big Book)* titled "The Doctor's Opinion" (Alcoholics Anonymous, 2002, pp. xxv–xxxii). The need for a spiritual experience became central to recovery in the early days of AA due to the immediate and critical need characteristic of alcoholism. Between 1935 (the official founding of AA) and the publication of *The Big Book* in 1939, the efforts in AA to help alcoholics get sober and remain so was by trial and error. All they had for conceptual confirmation was their experience, and they believed a spiritual experience was necessary to attain and maintain sobriety.

Helping an alcoholic achieve and maintain a spiritual experience, as described in AA, is not usually within the purview of the therapist. However, with a proper understanding of what the spiritual experience is, and the role that shame, trauma, and mental health disorders can play in inhibiting a spiritual experience, the therapist can facilitate the process with both meditation and self-compassion.

Length of Sobriety Is a Secondary Consideration

The length of someone's sobriety is not confirmation of the ongoing stability of sobriety. The same criteria for maintaining abstinence in early sobriety are the same for long-term sobriety. The first signs of a potential relapse usually come in the form of a decrease in social engagement. There may be a decrease in the number of meetings, contact with friends in recovery, a decreased interest in therapy, and an increase in isolation. This is often due to an increase in the presence of shame, or the surfacing of trauma. When these factors are present, it is a strong indication of an impending relapse.

---

[1]This chapter assumes that the reader has some familiarity with 12-step programs in general and with AA in particular. If the reader has little familiarity with the 12-Step experience, it is recommended to listen to speaker recordings (do a general search on "AA speakers") and read the relevant conference-approved literature (*www.aa.org/resources/literature*).

Informal Assessment for Stages of Addiction and Recovery

Morton Jellinek (1890–1963) was an alcoholism researcher, physiologist, and biostatistician. He was managing editor of the *Quarterly Journal of Studies on Alcohol* (now the *Journal of Studies on Alcohol and Drugs*) and instrumental in getting alcoholism classified as a disease. He created what is now called the Jellinek curve, a chart detailing the progressive stages of alcoholism and the progressive stages of recovery (Ward et al., 2016). I have used the chart with clients who were uncertain if they were alcoholic or not, and they identified with nearly every stage of the descent into alcoholism. It can help as a framework for the therapist and the client.

Selecting Self-Compassion Exercises

When selecting which self-compassion exercises to apply initially, there are two main objectives: to avoid backdraft[2] and to assess levels of shame, trauma, and distress tolerance. If there's doubt about the client's emotional stability, it is best to start with the MSC core meditations: "Affectionate Breathing," "Loving-Kindness for Ourselves," and "Giving and Receiving Compassion" (see Neff & Germer, 2018, for descriptions of these practices; see also Practice B, "Giving and Receiving Compasssion," in the Appendix). How the client reacts to these exercises will be a good guide on how to proceed.

Monitoring Progress with Mindfulness Meditation

If the client has a mindfulness meditation practice, it is important to be aware that there are two experiential states that may seem like a successful meditation experience but are not. The first is a type of dissociative state. The person reports that when meditating, there is nothing, it's just blank. This is a nonproductive state and should be avoided since it is a state of dissociation and they will make no progress with meditation and therefore no progress with self-awareness. If a client goes to this space regularly, it is best to work to resolve their general tendency toward dissociation with one of the core self-compassion exercises to begin to build positive feelings toward the self and increase a sense of safety and reduce their tendency to dissociate.

[2]*Backdraft* is a term used by firefighters to describe the phenomenon whereby, if a house is on fire and there is a closed room, the fire will consume the oxygen in the room. Then, if a door or window is breached, the fresh oxygen supply will expand the fire in an explosive manner. A synonymous psychological term is *abreaction*.

The second type is a drug-like state, usually described as a happy place. The client may experience a sense of elation and want to stay there rather than stop meditating. Upon close examination, they are not engaged in the meditation process of identifying and releasing their thoughts but are using that space as an escape. It is the type of false spiritual experience that got them into trouble to begin with, seeking the high rather than a spiritual experience. If this is the case, it can help to put greater emphasis on the here and now, building confidence in the ability to face and work through their immediate problems and addressing unresolved difficulties. The practice here is to help the client further develop the ability to face their life rather than try to escape it.

If neither of the above states are present, monitoring a client's mindfulness meditation can be informative as to their general progress. For instance, if when they first began, they expressed dismay at how hard it is and they feel it won't work for them, then this may indicate shame responding. As they continue, the complaints fade away, and they may begin to report their experience with acceptance—sometimes it is good and peaceful, and sometimes it is not—and a greater awareness of what their mind is doing during meditation. This is a good general indicator of a decrease in shame responding and an increase in metacognition (Hamonniere & Varescon, 2018).

Case Vignettes[3]

Mallory

Mallory is a 38-year-old cisgender White woman. She and her husband have been married for 12 years and have an 8-year-old daughter. Mallory's mother was diagnosed with alcohol dependence, chronic bipolar disorder, and also took an excess of prescription medications. Her mother's symptoms were "extreme" and included verbal and emotional abuse and unpredictable behavior. Mallory's father was passive and there was no other history of alcoholism or addiction on either side of the family. Her parents divorced when she was age 2.

After the divorce, Mallory lived with her mother and spent weekends with her father. When she was 8, her father moved away and then spent weekends with her maternal grandfather. In high school, she went to live with her grandfather after her mother moved away. Mallory flourished in high school academically, socially, and in sports.

[3]Identifying details for each of the individuals mentioned in the case vignettes have been disguised to ensure client confidentiality.

By age 15, Mallory started drinking on weekends and soon was drinking at every opportunity. By senior year, she drank until she blacked out or passed out. She started taking Adderall and occasionally cocaine. Mallory was diagnosed with generalized anxiety disorder, depression at age 18, major depressive disorder, and with chronic PTSD at age 29 from her mother's behavior.

When Mallory met her future husband at age 26, they used cocaine together for about 3 years. When she was 26, they married and she tried to stop drinking but could not. When she was pregnant, she didn't drink during pregnancy but couldn't maintain abstinence afterward. In 2017, Mallory went to AA and has been sober ever since. She got interested in spirituality and meditation (MBSR) and began doing self-compassion exercises, which brought a sense of safety and peace.

In choosing self-compassion exercises for Mallory, initially, the "Compassionate Friend" exercise (Neff & Germer, 2018) seemed best. One of its main functions is to deepen one's connection with their authentic self, but it can bring up strong emotions. And if the person has limited experience with meditative insight, this may limit their ability to benefit from the exercise. Since Mallory hadn't experienced backdraft with the MSC exercises, and had experience with mindfulness meditation, the "Compassionate Friend" exercise was a good place to start (Irons & Beaumont, 2017).

In the exercise, Mallory saw her grandfather but not within the framework of the exercise. She spent time with tender memories, bringing about resolution to some areas of their relationship. Though her experience did not follow the structure of the exercise, I trusted her intuition that what she experienced was right for her at that time. Though Mallory had been able to further connect with her grandfather's compassion for her, it seemed the next step was for her to provide that for herself. The "Compassion for Oneself and Another" exercise was chosen (Neff & Germer, 2018).

In the exercise, Mallory said her father appeared as the "other." Again, following her intuition rather than the form of the exercise, she reported that she was able to resolve her conflict between being hurt by her father's abandonment, wanting to be loved by him, and the shame she had around those feelings. The second time Mallory did the exercise, she said her 3-year-old inner child appeared and felt nurtured. But when it came to connect with the "other," her inner child refused and wanted all the attention for herself.

Going with Mallory's intuition, we worked on loving-kindness for herself and her inner child and moved on to extending compassion when it seemed time. Later, I questioned whether it would have been wiser to start off with loving-kindness exercises or just compassion for herself. But her stages of progress started with her grandfather, which helped her establish a foundation of compassion for herself. Then, with her father with whom there was a deficit of compassion, she was able to nurture herself and bring about some degree of resolution. Then, Mallory was able to reunite with her 3-year-old self where she needed compassion more directly but still with an "avatar." This indicates that she was able to let go of the external sources of compassion and was ready to provide that for herself. Mallory's task now is to include her inner child with the exercises for further resolution and, eventually, once integrated with her inner child, to be able to give herself compassion directly, providing an extra margin of safety against relapse. As stated above, alcoholism is shame based and an increase in shame is a reliable indicator of relapse. Conversely, an increase in self-compassion, an effective antidote to shame, is a reliable indicator of an increase in the stability of recovery.

Mark

Mark is a 64-year-old cisgender White gay male, with a history of mental health and addiction disorders, and recent medical issues. His latest sobriety date is in 2010. Mark was the eldest of four children in a home where his mother was verbally abusive with rapid mood changes and his father was passive and a severe alcoholic. Mark reported that he became aware that he was gay at age 3, for which he felt intense shame and felt he could not go to his parents for his needs. In spite of his high IQ, he was disruptive at school, starting in the fourth grade. Mark started drinking at age 15, which was only on weekends at first but became a daily occurrence. In college, he hadn't come out yet, felt lost, like an imposter, and dropped out after his first year, which are all deeply shame-based responses.

When Mark came out as gay, he was employed at menial jobs and had a relationship of 2 years in spite of his partner's overt and covert cheating. He attended AA at age 23 and stayed sober for 16 years, though he was not diligent about working the AA program. At age 32, he went to nursing school and got an associate's degree. At age 36, Mark developed a herniated disk in his neck and stole opioids from his patients, was caught, and completed the recovery program for nurses. At age 47, he started taking opioids and added benzodiazepines, and after getting caught again, he admitted he was an addict. At age 48, Mark was diagnosed with depression and received 22 electroconvulsive therapy treatments with no discernible effect. At age 52, he went back to AA in earnest and has maintained sobriety since then—in spite of several neck surgeries.

Mindfulness and self-compassion were suggested, and though the practices made sense to him, Mark felt he could not connect. Later, after he weaned off his antidepressant medication, he started taking it again with positive results. He intuitively began to chant "Nam-myoho-renge-kyo" and found a connection with himself he'd never felt before and began to connect with the self-compassion exercises. Both the reboot of his medication and the chanting coincided to facilitate a shift. Mark's negative internal dialogue shifted to "What would I say to a good friend?" When aware of people taking advantage of vulnerable people, compassion for them and himself arose.

Mark had a good response with "Compassion with Equanimity" (see Practice J.2, "The Practice of Self-Compassion with Equanimity," in the Appendix), "Body Scan with Compassion," and "Self-Compassion Break for Shame" (see Practice L, "Self-Compassion Break for Shame," in the Appendix; Neff & Germer, 2018). He focused on the exercises "Working with Shame" and "Working with Difficult Emotions." It was suggested that he alternate between them to build a greater ability to interrupt the automatic shame responding with self-compassion and build distress tolerance with the "Working with Difficult Emotions" exercise. If the shame-based responding became too difficult, it was recommended that Mark switch to the "Loving-Kindness" exercise for oneself to connect positive emotions to his experience of self.

Don

Don is a 53-year-old cisgender White male, in his second marriage, with no children from either marriage. Currently, he's been married 22 years. Don was born with a mild but noticeable birth defect and, because of it, was attacked at age 3 by an older boy. When ridiculed, his response was to beat up the bullies until he was forbidden by his mother to respond with violence. He had to give up his mode of addressing the humiliation and suppressed his anger. Don began to drink at 17 but would limit himself to three beers a night. He didn't like to get drunk but sometimes would lose control and had "only a couple of blackouts." In college, he was diagnosed with an adjustment disorder and given medication for anxiety and depression, which didn't help. His maternal grandfather, with whom he was close, died when he was 26, which exacerbated his anxiety and depression, for which he was again prescribed medication. Again, the medication didn't help. He smoked cannabis socially at age 28 for a couple of years, though lost interest. At age 49, Don's anxiety, depression, and drinking became more prominent and were based on his concern to not "sadden" his parents or have them be "ashamed of or be disappointed" in him. He attended a residential 28-day, non-12-step program, but was treated primarily for anxiety and depression.

Over the years, Don developed the habit of overspending and buying collectibles. His mother had the same pattern. His spending got to the point that he tried to hide money from himself in different accounts but was only moderately successful. He knew his spending was for emotional comfort, but it wasn't until 2022 that he began to limit his habit. His dynamics with money is exactly like some alcoholic behavior. The only significant alcoholism in his family he knew of was with his brother who, at age 55, died of alcohol poisoning with a blood alcohol level eight times the legal limit. Don hasn't yet addressed the grief over his brother's death.

From the beginning of therapy, it was an open discussion as to whether Don was alcoholic or not. The fact that alcohol was a past problem, that he uses alcohol to manage his feelings, that he has problems controlling his drinking, that he spends money for emotional support, and that his brother was severely afflicted with alcoholism all point to the possibility that he is alcoholic. Don's deeply set feelings of not wanting to disappoint his parents, based in shame, drive control over his emotions and behavior.

The first exercise suggested was a basic mindfulness exercise to gauge Don's ability to relax the discursive mind. Though the instructions were clear, he adopted the practice of counting his breaths and was not able to relax. It was suggested he do the meditation without the counting and he found it more helpful at alleviating his anxiety. After he stabilized with meditation, the "Body Scan with Compassion" exercise helped him connect with his body. However, when describing his experiences, he reported only bodily sensations. The "Working with Difficult Emotions" exercise was then recommended for skill building, but his reports consisted only of his physical sensations. After doing the exercise a couple of times, Don decided to limit his drinking by not purchasing any alcohol so he would not drink at home but only socially.

Don has made modest progress learning to pause yet is still highly intellectualized. This may suggest that his suppressed emotional conflicts of many years are at the core of his drinking and that he is self-medicating. However, as noted above, people who do not experience the phenomenon of craving, described above, typically do not have to manage their drinking. At this stage, with Don it would be counterproductive to make a determination of whether he is alcoholic. The plan is to continue with a daily mindfulness practice to increase his insight and distress tolerance and to work regularly with self-compassion exercises to mitigate his shame-based emotional suppression. The hope is that these two skills will eventually bring him to the point that it will become self-evident whether he is alcoholic. Don came to see me a couple months before publication and admitted he was alcoholic, going to AA, and very involved in recovery.

Conclusion

In Western psychology, there persists a tendency to be prescriptive in evaluation and approach, even with mindfulness and self-compassion. The human psyche, however, is often far more mysterious and creative than assumed. Thus, it is vital as clinicians that we ourselves operate from those internal resources. With too little structure (without sufficient emphasis on the exercises and regularity of practice), we can drift off into ineffectuality. With too much form (overemphasizing regular practice and that the client do the exercises in the prescribed way), we can lose our deeper connection with the client. What can keep us in the middle is presence (see Chapter 6 for more on therapeutic presence). Essential to establishing presence is for the clinician to be much farther ahead of the client in their own meditation and self-compassion practices, and have a general and broad understanding of compassion. Without that, we are not too good at translating the literal into the experiential. It allows us to be there and invite the client in.

REFERENCES

Alcoholics Anonymous. (2002). *Alcoholics Anonymous big book* (4th ed.). Alcoholics Anonymous World Services.

Blanco, C., Xu, Y., Brady, K., Pérez-Fuentes, G., Okuda, M., & Wang, S. (2013). Comorbidity of posttraumatic stress disorder with alcohol dependence among US adults: Results from National Epidemiological Survey on Alcohol and Related Conditions. *Drug and Alcohol Dependence, 132*(3), 630–638.

Bonaz, B., Lane, R. D., Oshinsky, M. L., Kenny, P. J., Sinha, R., Mayer, E. A., & Critchley, H. D. (2021). Diseases, disorders, and comorbidities of interoception. *Trends in Neurosciences, 44*(1), 39–51.

Edenfield, T. M., & Saeed, S. A. (2012). An update on mindfulness meditation as a self-help treatment for anxiety and depression. *Psychology Research and Behavior Management, 5,* 131–141.

Farb, N., Daubenmier, J., Price, C. J., Gard, T., Kerr, C., Dunn, B. D., et al. (2015). Interoception, contemplative practice, and health. *Frontiers in Psychology, 6,* 763.

Fetzner, M. G., & Asmundson, G. J. (2015). Aerobic exercise reduces symptoms of posttraumatic stress disorder: A randomized controlled trial. *Cognitive Behaviour Therapy, 44*(4), 301–313.

Gilbert, P. (2000). Social mentalities: Internal "social" conflicts and the role of inner warmth and compassion in cognitive therapy. In P. Gilbert & K. G. Bailey (Eds.), *Genes on the couch: Explorations in evolutionary psychotherapy* (pp. 118–150). Brunner-Routledge.

Goldsmith, R. E., Gerhart, J. I., Chesney, S. A., Burns, J. W., Kleinman, B., & Hood, M. M. (2014). Mindfulness-based stress reduction for posttraumatic stress symptoms: Building acceptance and decreasing shame. *Journal of Evidence-Based Complementary and Alternative Medicine, 19*(4), 227–234.

Hamonniere, T., & Varescon, I. (2018). Metacognitive beliefs in addictive behaviours: A systematic review. *Addictive Behaviors, 85*, 51–63.

Hickey, T., Nelson, B., & Meadows, G. (2017). Application of a mindfulness and compassion-based approach to the at-risk mental state. *Clinical Psychologist, 21*(2), 104–115.

Huang, M. C., Schwandt, M. L., Ramchandani, V. A., George, D. T., & Heilig, M. (2012). Impact of multiple types of childhood trauma exposure on risk of psychiatric comorbidity among alcoholic inpatients. *Alcoholism: Clinical and Experimental Research, 36*(6), 1099–1107.

Irons, C., & Beaumont, E. (2017). *The compassionate mind workbook: A step-by-step guide to developing your compassionate self.* Robinson.

Kabat-Zinn, J. (2013). *Full catastrophe living: Using the wisdom of your body and mind to face stress, pain, and illness* (Rev. ed.). Bantam Books.

Neff, K., & Germer, C. (2018). *The mindful self-compassion workbook: A proven way to accept yourself, build inner strength, and thrive.* Guilford Press.

Patock-Peckham, J. A., Canning, J. R., & Leeman, R. F. (2018). Shame is bad and guilt is good: An examination of the impaired control over drinking pathway to alcohol use and related problems. *Personality and Individual Differences, 121*, 62–66.

Randles, D., & Tracy, J. L. (2013). Nonverbal displays of shame predict relapse and declining health in recovering alcoholics. *Clinical Psychological Science, 1*(2), 149–155.

Rogers, C. (1986). Client-centered approach to therapy. In I. L. Kutash & A. Wolf (Eds.), *Psychotherapist's casebook: Theory and technique in practice* (pp. 197–208). Jossey Bass.

Schoen, D. E. (2020). *The war of the gods in addiction: CG Jung, Alcoholics Anonymous, and archetypal evil.* Chiron.

Seligman, M. E., & Csikszentmihalyi, M. (2000). Positive psychology: An introduction. *American Psychologist, 55*(1), 5–14.

Shaffer, H. J., LaPlante, D. A., LaBrie, R. A., Kidman, R. C., Donato, A. N., & Stanton, M. V. (2004). Toward a syndrome model of addiction: Multiple expressions, common etiology. *Harvard Review of Psychiatry, 12*(6), 367–374.

Udupa, N. S., Joiner, T. E., Twenge, J. M., & McAlliste, C. (2023). Increases in poor mental health, mental distress, and depression symptoms among US adults, 1993–2020. *Journal of Mood and Anxiety Disorders*, 2(5), 100013.

Ward, J. H., Bejarano, W., Babor, T. F., & Allred, N. (2016). Re-introducing Bunky at 125: EM Jellinek's life and contributions to alcohol studies. *Journal of Studies on Alcohol and Drugs, 77*(3), 375–383.

13

Compassion and Self-Compassion for Depression

Paul Gilbert

Chapter 2 discussed an evolution-informed, biopsychosocial approach to compassion and self-compassion. This chapter explores how to use this approach as a guide to help people with depressed states of mind. Although there are many different forms of depression and different symptom clusters, in general, as noted in Figure 13.1, depressed states are seen as a multidimensional syndrome affecting different areas of functioning (Gilbert, 2007).

Some depressions are so severe that people can hardly move, whereas other people with depression can continue with everyday life, but it is a struggle. Some depressions are single episodes but some repeat. Some people recover fully, but some are more chronic. Some people have depression that is also interlaced with episodes of hypomania, called bipolar affective disorder. So, depression is recognized to be a highly heterogeneous process and brain state.

In 2023, the World Health Organization, using standard psychiatric *International Classification of Diseases* classification (which involves various combinations of these symptoms), suggested that:

> an estimated 3.8% of the population experience depression, including 5% of adults (4% among men and 6% among women), and 5.7% of adults older than 60 years. Approximately 280 million people in the world have depression. . . . Depression is about 50% more common among women than among men. Worldwide, more than 10% of pregnant women and women who have just given birth experience depression. . . . More than 700,000 people die due to suicide every year. Suicide is the fourth leading cause of death in 15–29-year-olds.

Some suggest that these are underestimates in some communities and that depression rates and forms vary greatly in different socioeconomic and social groups. There are many different vulnerability factors, triggering factors, maintenance, and recovery factors. Each of these can be linked to biological, psychological, and sociocultural factors. For example, some individuals are more genetically vulnerable to depression, particularly severe and bipolar depressions. Some depressions are linked to physiological changes, such as those that occur during menopause or chronic illness. Depressions have been linked to inflammatory diets and postviral illness (e.g., COVID-19; Mazza et al., 2022). All such processes can interact with life histories, such as early trauma, neglect, and abuse. Some depressions are linked to personality factors and styles of thinking (e.g., perfectionistic, pessimistic, and rejection sensitivity) and attachment styles (Hakulinen et al., 2015). Many depressions are rooted in relational and social contextual problems, such as being in abusive relationships or bad jobs, poverty, and loneliness. Feelings of entrapment and loss of control are common experiences of depression (see Gilbert, 2007; Taylor et al., 2011, for reviews). It is important therefore when applying therapeutic interventions, such as helping people to become more self-compassionate, that we don't apply interventions as manualized forms where one size fits all. Interventions have to be tailored to the specifics of the depression and difficulties.

Interventions

There is now considerable research on how to help people with depression physiologically and with social and psychotherapy. In a recent meta-analysis,

Motivation:	Apathy, loss of energy and interest; things seem pointless, hopeless
Emotional:	Low mood, anhedonia, emptiness, anger or resentment, anxiety, shame, guilt
Cognitive:	Poor concentration, negative ideas about the self, the world, and the future
Behavior:	Lowered activity, social withdrawal, agitation, or retardation
Biological:	Sleep disturbance, loss of appetite, loss of weight, changes in circadian rhythms, hormones, and brain chemicals

FIGURE 13.1. Depression as syndrome. From Gilbert (2022b). Copyright © Paul Gilbert. Reprinted by permission.

Cuijpers et al. (2023) found good evidence for psychological therapies for depression. Many of the studies were with cognitive-behavioral therapies (CBT), although other approaches also have evidence of effectiveness. However, Watkins and Newbold (2020) also note:

> Many patients do not have sustained improvement, and treatments need to scale up to tackle the global burden of mental health. . . . For example, psychological treatments for depression only achieve remission rates of 30%–40% and have limited sustained efficacy (at least 50% relapse and recurrence). . . .

Although psychological therapies are effective to a degree, there is a need to significantly increase effectiveness. As part of that, therapies need to be biopsychosocial focused, ensuring that interventions have physiological and social impacts (Gilbert, 2007). In addition, therapies need to be process focused before moving to outcome studies. For example, what are the interventions for self-criticism and, more specifically, the different types of self-criticism? What are the interventions for trauma, shame, or hopelessness (since these can underpin depression)? It is these, rather than mood directly, that can be the target for interventions. Compassion *focused* therapy (CFT) aims to utilize and develop evidence-based interventions but orientate them through compassion-based motivational systems because these are linked to particular brain and body states that have direct impacts on threat processing (Gilbert, 2020). This is why I did not call it "compassion therapy," because it is bringing compassion motivational processes to a whole range of already well-established evidence-based interventions to try to improve their efficacy by rooting them in specific psychophysiological processes (Gilbert, 2022c).

One of the therapeutic experiences that led me to focus on the importance of generating compassion as the texture for interventions was working with CBT for depression over 35 years ago (Gilbert, 1992, 2022c). In CBT, individuals identify ways of thinking that are linked to depression, such as being a failure and unlovable and the future is hopeless. They are then invited to stand back from that and try to generate more balanced ways of thinking: How would they help a friend? How would they see the situation if they were not depressed? How would they like to deal with the situation if they felt confident? and so forth. For some clients, this was helpful but, for others, it didn't impact mood. For one particular set of clients who were able to identify helpful thoughts but didn't *experience* these as helpful, I asked them to speak them aloud as they experienced them in their minds. My first shock was that the emotional tone was cold, unfriendly, and sometimes hostile, even though the content was trying to be helpful. The obvious solution was to guide clients to generate caring, kind, and supportive tones to their thoughts and focus on empathic motivation to be helpful. The second shock was that many of these clients did not want to do that and thought it would not be helpful or they did not deserve compassion. The third shock was that when clients did begin to engage with compassion, it opened up a Pandora's box of unprocessed distressing memories. This is partly because all motivational systems carry their own trauma. For example, if you enjoy vacations but one day you are badly injured while on vacation, the next time you see an advertisement for a vacation, it may trigger your trauma memory.

Individuals who have experienced neglect and trauma in their attachment and care histories can experience distressing memories being reactivated when they begin compassion training. Therefore, therapy has to detoxify the care system. This often involves working through anger and grief from attachment traumas. It is often through grieving and becoming tolerant and empathically engaged with one's long-lived sense of disconnection that compassion becomes more available to them (see Gilbert & Simos, 2022, for clinical details). This has by others been referred to as backdraft in a fire context, but CFT would advise against that when working with clients because it is a frightening image. Rather, what often can help is the ability to engage with grief (Harris & Ho, 2023). A second focus for generating compassion was my interest in Mahayana Buddhism and its compassion cultivation practices (Gilbert & Choden, 2013). Third, as data on the psychophysiological processes of compassion, neuroplasticity, and the multiple impacts of compassion focusing became more available, CFT worked on evidence-based new ways of understanding how and why compassion cultivation is helpful.

Compassion-Based Formulation

Clinical assessment is linked to an understanding of the specific symptoms and problems of clients. Formulation involves conceptualizing those difficulties within a therapy model, like the CFT model, that points toward intervention. Compassion-based formulations are biopsychosocial and help clients gain insight into our evolved potential for experiencing depressed brain states and how these can be choreographed through developmental and social processes. Therapists guide clients to see depression as a multitextured brain state linked to having a tricky brain that we didn't choose (see Chapter 2). We call it "tricky" because evolution has built into our brain's multiple motive and emotion potentials that were designed for survival and reproduction (Gilbert, 1998). However, these are all contextually sensitive; change the contexts and they can become very harmful. Dispositions to be threat sensitive and anxious can be helpful to animals in a threatening and unsafe context. However, our cognitive competencies for reasoning, anticipating, and ruminating can trigger them, exaggerating and prolonging the sense of threat, causing all kinds of emotional difficulties (LeDoux, 2022). Vengeance is common in various species, but in humans, with our cognitive and reasoning competencies, it can be turned into vicious tribal wars, with horrific weapons. It is for such contexts that compassion motivations can offset threat- and vengeance-based processing systems.

Many of our distressing brain states like depression can be activated involuntarily, against our wishes, and we can desperately try to get out of such states of mind. So, our brain is tricky because it can generate distressing brain states that we don't want but feel controlled by. This is why psychophysiological interventions and psychoeducation become so important in helping people understand some of the early (vulnerability) and later current triggers for these brain states. We can then help people practice mindfulness, compassion, and other psychophysiological interventions that can help switch brain states.

Research shows that both the early and current vulnerability to depression, and recovery from it, are linked to *how we manage* our biopsychosocial minds and relationships. People with depression can have what is called a *negative cognitive triad*: a negative view of the world, the future, and themselves (Beck et al., 1979). People with depression can worry and ruminate on depressive and anxious themes of personal loss and failures, future threats, and feelings of entrapment and defeat. People with depression may withdraw and socially isolate themselves. Shame can make socializing and openness and receiving help from others difficult. So, compassion therapies have to address the social and relational difficulties associated with depression (Foroutan et al., 2018). We also know that there are many psychophysiological changes in depression, some of which relate to genetics, early vulnerability and current trauma, and current difficult social circumstances (Lynch et al., 2024). Hence, various therapies now seek to address the psychophysiological changes of depression by using exercises that support the vagus nerve and affect the frontal cortex (Cozolino, 2017) and impact cognition and social behaviors (Matos et al., 2022; Singer & Engert, 2019). A guided integrative set of practices for working with physiological systems, using imagery and planning behavior, is given in Practice C, "Compassion Practice Sequences to Aid Cultivating Compassion Brain, Body, and Mind States," in the Appendix).

Conceptualizing Compassion

Compassion is a motive that enables us to be sensitive to our distress and empathically validate and commit to try to do what is helpful. While people with mental health problems may be sensitive to their distress, they may find it difficult to tolerate or know what to do. So, they disengage and close down around it. Importantly, when we are hit by any major trauma, such as getting cancer, losing somebody we love, or being abused, we often have to cope with three major emotion systems: anger that it has happened, fear of the consequences, and grief for the loss it entails. It is not uncommon for depressed people to feel overwhelmed and frightened by these emerging states (Gilbert et al., 2014). Hence, compassion involves *building the courage* that supports emotional tolerance to many different and at times intense emotions as well as trying to work through the underlying causes of depressed states. Examples from clients include the following (clinical examples represent a typical kind of process rather than any specific person):

- Sally came from a neglectful background. She found it very difficult to work through her extensive and intense grief and yearning to be loved. If she touched on these feelings, an intense sense of loneliness could feel overwhelming to her. She also felt them to be signs of weakness.
- Kevin used alcohol to manage his depression, for which he was ashamed. He did not want to face (was frightened of) feelings of rage toward his early life abuse and the perpetrators. He felt such feelings were dangerous and made him feel unlovable, out of control, and isolated.
- Anne did not want to face the fact that her relationship with her partner was toxic and she needed to find the courage to leave, fearing being alone.
- Tim clung to harsh self-criticism, believing it would drive him to success, but it drove him into depression.

As for most therapies, the first movement of CFT is to gain clarity on what the key issues are for any particular client. Helping clients tell their stories and experience validation from the therapist helps them to "make sense" of their mental states. This can open to discussions on formulation and how the process of the therapy might unfold. At some point, the therapist engages in a brief exploration of the nature and value of compassion (see Chapter 2), highlighting the roles of courage, wisdom, and commitment in working on and through difficulties. Without courage, individuals become avoidant. Without wisdom, they can become reckless, flounder, or try to help themselves in ways that can make things worse. Like courage and wisdom, commitment can be low to begin with and develops through the course of the therapy. There are many processes that support commitment, such as feeling safe, small short-term gains, insight, clarity on tasks, feeling competent to perform tasks, and therapists that are encouraging and supportive of the journey and difficulties faced.

The Therapy Relationship

The therapeutic relationship operates like an attachment relationship in that it provides both a secure base and safe haven functions (H. Gilbert, 2022; Holmes & Slade, 2017). As provided by the therapist, these empathic-guided interactions begin the process of enabling the client to find the courage and wisdom within themselves to engage with their sources of suffering. A diagram for these functions is given in Figure 2.1 in Chapter 2.

The secure base provides the context for the client to experience being validated, empathically understood, and cared for. That in turn provides the basis for the client to trust the therapist and enables the therapist to engage the client in guided exploration, encouragement, and risk taking, which underpins the development of courage, confidence, and wisdom. Crucially too, a secure base provides the context for experiencing positive affect, for play, and the joy of social relationships. Neglected children can struggle with the ability to play and find joy in the world and relationships. In helping clients experience an encouraging, playful secure base, clients become able to develop their inner secure base. Hence, CFT seeks to help clients with validation and encouragement and explore ways in which they can bring more playful and enjoyable activities into their lives.

Developing trust in a secure base also allows the therapy to provide a safe haven, which is the regulation of emotion and distress. We are soothed and calmed by the signals of caring partly because they trigger psychophysiological systems, such as the vagus nerve, oxytocin, and various neuro circuits that down-regulate threat processing and up-regulate positive effects of connectedness. Overall, based on the attachment system and psychological functions of care, CFT has two fundamental properties. First, a secure base helps clients develop the courage to face difficulties, tolerate difficult emotions, and develop wisdom and confidence. Second, a safe haven is linked to the ability to down-regulate aversive affect, primarily by stimulating care-based psychophysiological systems, such as the vagus nerve. *Crucially, compassion helps clients establish these relationships within themselves so that when confronted by life difficulties they can access their inner secure base and thus self-empathize, self-validate, self-reassure, and provide encouragement, as well as self-soothe and settle where appropriate.*

Building a (Self-)Compassionate Mind

As noted above, there are many psychotherapies that have been specifically developed to help people with depression (Cuijpers et al., 2023). There is an increasing number of studies that are indicative of CFT's effectiveness for depression as outlined in recent meta-analyses (Millard et al., 2023; Petrocchi et al., 2024) and for the more complex cases, such as people with bipolar disorder (Gilbert et al., 2022) and with chronic and treatment-resistant depressions (Asano et al., 2022).

Various interventions can focus on helping people with how they think about situations, problem solving, resolving relational issues, processing avoided emotions, and stimulating positive emotion and positive rewardable behaviors, to name the most common. Many of these interventions are also core to CFT but are contextualized within a compassion motivational system. The biopsychosocial approach identifies biological, psychological, and social processes that can be cultivated and will support a compassionate mind in alleviating depression.

It is useful to invite clients to discuss their ideas of compassion, what they like and don't like about it, how they think it could be helpful or unhelpful for them, and why they think they wouldn't be able to do it or don't deserve it.

Practice: Building a (Self-)Compassionate Mind

Over the years, CFT developed a specific example of asking the client to imagine a friend they like, to prime that feeling by thinking about what it is they like about them. Then, invite the client to imagine that their friend phones them up in a distressed state because they have to go to the hospital but are frightened of hospitals. The therapist invites the client to reflect on how they would be with their friend. Typically, the client notes that they would be very sensitive to their friend and concerned about their friend (the psychology of engagement and concern) but, in addition, would try to work out what would be helpful to their friend (what actions to take). Commonly, clients acknowledge that they would go with their friend. They are then able to reflect that when one is frightened or distressed, having somebody with you who cares about you has a soothing courage-giving quality. The therapist is then able to highlight the two aspects of compassion as sensitive engagement plus action and to indicate that the client has intuitive wisdom and understanding about compassion. Helping clients recognize that therapy will help them build the courage and wisdom to be sensitive to, and work out how to act on, what will be helpful to them, sets a helpful framework.

> Deborah was a new mother with depression who had lost feelings for her baby and viewed herself negatively. She did not like the idea of kindness to herself. However, when invited to think about if she were not depressed and was at her compassionate best, how would *she like to be* with her baby, she was quite able to articulate a range of helpful and caring behaviors. The therapist was

able to help her see that she had compassion and motivation as a mother, but the depression had knocked out her energy and ability to feel connected or act on her motives. Recognizing that she could perform small compassionate behaviors was the beginning of help. Sometimes (as in behavioral approaches), helpful behavior can be seen as compassionate behavior and can be a crucial beginning. Later, Deborah was able to grieve her loss of feeling and connect to her own history. Helping clients see this as courageous and wise compassionate behavior, even if it lacks feeling, can be helpful.

Cultivating compassion motivation has a range of psychophysiological properties that the client may not be aware of but they can learn to tap into. All interventions are textured and patterned within a compassion-focused therapeutic *journey* (that some therapies may do automatically without necessarily naming it). Interventions should not be taken out of the context of the unfolding of that journey, for example, randomly teaching clients soothing rhythm breathing or compassion imagery when they're not ready or motivated means they may not be engaged, thus this is not helpful.

The Biological

CFT is informed by growing research on the psychophysiological systems underpinning compassion and how to recruit them as therapy targets (see Chapter 2). This is important because, as noted, caring evolved partly to help regulate threat processing and have a calming as well as encouraging effect on recipients (Gilbert, 2022b). There is good evidence that a caring, empathic therapeutic relationship itself has physiological effects (Cozolino, 2017). Therapists who are empathic, caring, and compassionate have better outcomes than therapists who are nonempathic, cold, and detached (Vivino et al., 2009).

CFT's compassionate mind training exercises, such as breathing, imagery/visualizations, and behavioral practices, produce significant changes in heart rate variability in the general population (Matos et al., 2022). Measures of heart rate variability indicate how balanced the autonomic nervous system is. Low heart rate variability tends to indicate high stress. Steffen et al. (2020) found that in a group of students with depression, CFT induced changes in heart rate variability that predicted self-compassion changes. The reverse is true: Changes in self-compassion also predicted changes in heart rate variability to self-critical and self-compassion writing tasks. Gilbert and colleagues (2022) found that CFT produces changes in heart rate variability in individuals with a diagnosis of bipolar disorder. Keeping these two-way relationships in mind directs attention to the ways heart rate variability can be directly trained and thus have an impact on compassion and mental health. Importantly, Singer and Engert (2019) outline how different practices, such as empathy versus compassion versus mindfulness, impact neurophysiological systems in overlapping but also in different ways, indicating the importance of specificity of training.

As part of a biopsychosocial approach to compassion, the therapist is concerned with helping "the body support the mind." There are many ways to do this, one of which can be to nurture the self with diet and exercise. In addition, we can practice particular ways of using posture and breathing that affect compassion-linked psychophysiological systems, such as the vagus nerve, immune system, and frontal cortex. Various patterns of breathing can balance the autonomic nervous system and other physiological systems. These normally involve deepening and slowing the breath, creating a rhythm for the breath, and paying particular attention to the out-breath, which is the part of the breath that stimulates the vagus nerve. CFT also focuses on using facial muscles to stimulate a feeling of compassion, for example, creating a slight smile and imagining helping a friend.

As noted above, CFT seeks to help people think about the emotional textures of their thoughts and actions because when individuals with depression are trying to generate helpful thoughts or behaviors, their emotional tones and textures can be cold or angry. Hence, clients practice generating *compassionate emotion-textured* thought tones and compare them with neutral or hostile ones. For example, suppose that you are feeling worried about going for a job interview and you have a series of thoughts about if you mess up the interview, for example, "I will get too anxious to answer properly" or "I might not know the answers to questions they ask." Ruminating on those fears can undermine your confidence. So, suppose that you can stand back from those fears and generate some more helpful and supportive ideas. Here are some examples:

"Yes, interviews are anxiety provoking, so my anxiety is perfectly understandable [validation], so what is helpful for me [encouragement]?"

"Maybe slowing my breathing and remembering to slow down and try to settle my body when I sit in the interview chair [coping]."

"I can practice my interview by thinking through things they might ask me; I know the information because I have experience in this type of job [positive recall and self-reassurance]."

"They must see that, otherwise, they wouldn't have short-listed me [evidence]."

"I can express a friendly style and I have been successful at interviews before [positive recall and self-reassurance]."

"It will be a disappointment if I don't make it, but I can deal with disappointments and can move on from here [realism and acceptance tolerance]."

Indeed, the importance of being able to deal with disappointments without being harsh on oneself is an important life skill (Gilbert, 2022b).

On a logical level, these self-supporting thoughts may be helpful and give us a more balanced supportive perspective.

Exercise: Exploring the Hostile versus Helpful Emotional Tones of Self-Focused Thinking

It is not just the content of our thoughts but the emotion textures and motivations of our thoughts that are crucial as to how helpful they are. To explore this, give yourself a moment and just think how helpful that kind of more balanced self-supportive thinking is. Now imagine that you hear those thoughts in your mind but in a somewhat frustrated or even contemptuous way, as if you are trying to tell yourself to "pull yourself together; stop being so anxious and just get on with it!" You could try that now. Read them through but this time with the irritated and annoyed voice tone in your head. How helpful are they now? Not much! Next, spend a few moments deliberately grounding yourself in your body with your breathing techniques of slower, deeper breathing and your focus on the motivation to be helpful, maybe bringing to mind somebody who you would help in a similar situation. Then, focus on the emotional textures for these helpful thoughts. The inner tone of one's thoughts should be one of empathic friendliness, kindness, and warmth where possible. Note how helpful they "feel" this time.

The point of this exercise is to indicate that many interventions can help people with depression (Cuijpers et al., 2023). However, in CFT, they are textured with compassion, emotions, and motivations that seek to stimulate care-linked psychophysiological systems that can help regulate the self.

Imagery

CFT uses imagery but helps clients understand what imagery is and isn't and also that some clients struggle with imagery. Imagery can be used to help clients focus on the experience of receiving compassion. Examples here can be imagining being in a safe place and the place welcoming you, taking pleasure in your being there. A sense of connectedness to nature or place can be powerful for some people. In addition, we can practice this while being in places such as a pleasant field or forest, looking over a lake or mountain, and practicing feeling part of and connected to the landscape. Safe place imagery can also act as a secure base to explore and have fun. Indeed, a client many years ago said that if she could create a safe place, she wouldn't want to just sit and become relaxed and quiet but have fun and play. This resonated with me because play is a very important part of developing positive emotion and confidence, and one of the functions of a secure base is to provide the context for it. Since then, I've always combined the concept of a safe place with the importance of feeling safe, connected, and supported in and by the place, and also noted to clients that one can either be calm and meditative or active and playful. Some clients have imagined themselves simply being at peace and others imagined themselves as flying over forests and lakes or dancing; whatever creates a sense of connectedness and engagement can be helpful.

Imagery Exercise: Taking In Compassion

Another visualization can be breathing in white or colored light as a healing light. This is tapping into the body-based feeling of receiving or taking in caring. Again, the focus is not so much on the strength of the visualization but on how individuals experience the visualization in their body, tuning into the issues of being cared for and about. In some Buddhist visualizations, one can imagine the Buddha at the center of the universe, emanating these colors of healing energy, and therefore being a recipient of the Buddha's motivation that all beings (including oneself) be free of suffering and the causes of suffering.

In CFT, clients can create their own "imaginary other," which they then relate to. This visualization involves imagining a compassionate other having all of the ideal qualities they would like from a caring, helpful other (Lee, 2005). The process of thinking about what it is they would want from an ideal caring other can in itself be revealing and therapeutic. Clients at times activate archetypal imagery. Because the mind is designed for social relationships, with social mentalities, it can sometimes be easier to stimulate compassion systems through imagining being related to compassionately (Gilbert, 2022c). In other words, like a sexually arousing fantasy, the client imagines a compassionate other talking to them or supporting them but tries to feel into a bodily connection to the image. Since this is imaginary, the client is also working out what it is they would find helpful or need from the support of another: What would they want to hear and how would they want to feel validated? If the client suggests qualities such as voice tone and empathic response from the image, the therapist asks them to hold that and see what it feels like in the body.

Compassionate Imagery: Compassionate Coach

Brown and colleagues (2020) offered an excellent example of using compassionate images as used in CFT, in vivo for those with paranoid fears. They used the virtual reality of entering a lift [elevator] and tube train [subway] while imagining being accompanied by their imagined compassionate coach. As for CFT, they indicate:

> The aim is to harness the experience of being nurtured and eventually internalize it so that a new and distinctive memory is created that can be easily accessed. A compassionate coach can have any identity but must embody all the qualities of compassion, including strength, warmth, wisdom, and kindness, and should encourage the individual to be kind toward themselves. (p. 2)

This indicates how images of a "compassionate coach or other mind" can be used for imagining a "mentalizing other mind" being focused on caring and supporting the self. We are imagining ourselves as existing in the mind of another as empathically cared about, valued, and dedicated to addressing our suffering and growth. We are mentalizing them mentalizing us (see Gilbert, 2022a).

Building the Skills of the Compassionate Self and Mind

Having an image of the kind of self that one wants to become can be central to guiding our behavior. For example, if we want to become a musician, a tennis player, or a slim person, we practice the skills associated with moving toward that version of ourselves. Creative imagination of a version of oneself, and exploring the impact that has on coping, has been explored in other paradigms. For example, there is evidence that imagining oneself as one's "best possible self" and thinking about engaging in various life issues from that experience of self is related to emotional change and increased optimism (Meevissen et al., 2011). Giving oneself counseling while imagining oneself as Sigmund Freud, compared with just oneself, reduced depressed feelings significantly more than as self (Osimo et al., 2015). CFT utilizes such creative imagination and guides people to think about their own version of *their compassionate self*.

In Buddhism, this is called *bodhicitta*. For example, it may be the compassionate self that has more patience, tolerance, and empathy, and is able to listen and has a specific motive to be helpful, not harmful. People are guided to use breathing and then to enter into the version of the character of their compassionate self very much like an actor taking on a particular role. There is good evidence that focusing one's thinking by creating a version of the self that one wants to become impacts how one thinks about life difficulties. Arimitsu and Hofmann (2017) utilized aspects of CFT's compassionate mind training (Gilbert & Choden, 2013) and compared it with cognitive reappraisal and responsibility reattribution training. The instructions for compassion thinking were:

> Let's make an alternative thought in a compassionate way rather than in a self-critical way. Think about the qualities you value in compassion and become them as you imagine yourself in the role. Please imagine and try to hear kind voices from the perspective of a compassionate self who is understandable, supportive, kind, and encouraging to you. (p. 3)

They found that compassionate thinking reduced levels of negative emotions more so than responsibility reattribution and control conditions.

Developing a compassionate self can be of tremendous value for people with depression because it helps them to shift brain states. Gilbert and Basran (2018) invited participants in a training workshop to form dyads. Each participant in a dyad spent around 2 minutes talking about a life difficulty in the emotion of the difficulty to the partner who listened in silence. They were then instructed to engage the "Compassionate Self-Induction with Breathing" exercise, "Body Grounding" (focusing on the compassionate wisdom of the tricky brain), and the "Desire to Be Helpful." Then, they talked about their life difficulty again from the compassionate mind perspective. We found that participants experienced the switch as being significantly helpful. In the compassionate version of themselves, they felt more empathic to themselves, had more insight into the difficulty, felt better able to cope, and were more encouraged for the future. These types of intervention have proved very helpful in depression (e.g., Gilbert et al., 2022).

Compassion focusing can also be developed through compassionate letter writing to oneself and creating compassionate reappraisals and reframes. The compassionate self can be used to support a client's exploration of trauma and complex emotional conflicts. CFT also guides clients to practice at least one compassion-focused behavior a week. These can be different behaviors chosen collaboratively for depression. They might be tolerance, patience, friendliness, assertiveness, empathic interest in others, or behaviors that support physical well-being. For all of these interventions, the key is to texture the intervention by deliberately bringing the wish to be compassionate to self to mind and then engaging imagery and the body in a compassionate brain state. Crucial, therefore, is how individuals are able to do that and for some clients, it can take some time. As noted above, it may involve working through traumas associated with giving and receiving care. Hence, before clients can do this, they may need to work through the anger and grief associated with previous experiences of caring.

Evidence

CFT was developed for and with clients who struggled with other therapies and who came from difficult backgrounds. It integrates many interventions from other therapies. Thus, intervention studies need to explore not only the effectiveness of the therapy but also whether it does indeed add value over other approaches, such as standard CBT. These are complex studies to undertake, especially requiring appropriately qualified therapists. Nonetheless, an increasing number of studies are indicative of CFT's effectiveness as outlined in recent meta-analyses where depression is a common target for the interventions (Millard et al., 2023; Petrocchi et al., 2024).

Conclusion

CFT seeks to help individuals with depression become compassionate and supportive of themselves and, in this way, recruit psychophysiological systems that evolved for affect regulation. There are now different approaches to self-compassion as a personal support and psychotherapy, which require ongoing evaluation of effectiveness. Developing a therapy for depression, however, can be tricky because it's underpinned by many different types of difficulty, and in the long term it's probably more helpful to develop interventions for the underlying difficulties rather than just focus on the symptom–syndrome itself. Crucial, too, is helping people change their social circumstances because if they continue to live in hostile and toxic relationships, they stay vulnerable to relapse, which can be a challenge.

REFERENCES

Arimitsu, K., & Hofmann, S. G. (2017). Effects of compassionate thinking on negative emotions. *Cognition and Emotion, 31,* 160–167.

Asano, K., Tsuchiya, M., Okamoto, Y., Ohtani, T., Sensui, T., Masuyama, A., et al. (2022). Benefits of group compassion-focused therapy for treatment-resistant depression: A pilot randomized controlled trial. *Frontiers in Psychology, 13,* 903842.

Beck, A. T., Rush, A. J., Shaw, B. F., & Emery, G. (1979). *Cognitive therapy of depression.* Guilford Press.

Brown, P., Waite, F., Rovira, A., Nickless, A., & Freeman, D. (2020). Virtual reality clinical-experimental tests of compassion treatment techniques to reduce paranoia. *Scientific Reports, 10*(1), 1–9.

Cozolino, L. (2017). *The neuroscience of psychotherapy: Healing the social brain* (2nd ed.). Norton.

Cuijpers, P., Miguel, C., Harrer, M., Plessen, C. Y., Ciharova, M., Papola, D., et al. (2023). Psychological treatment of depression: A systematic overview of a "meta-analytic research domain." *Journal of Affective Disorders, 335,* 141–151.

Foroutan, S., Heidary, A., Askary, P., Nadery, F., & Ebrahimi Moghaddam, H. (2018). The effect of functional analytic psychotherapy on improving depression and communication skill in patients with obsessive compulsive disorder. *Journal of Psychological Science, 17*(69), 611–617.

Gilbert, H. (2022). The therapeutic relationship in compassion-focused therapy. In P. Gilbert & G. Simos (Eds.), *Compassion focused therapy: Clinical practice and applications.* (pp. 385–400). Routledge.

Gilbert, P. (1992). *Counselling for depression: A cognitive-interpersonal approach.* Sage.

Gilbert, P. (1998). Evolutionary psychopathology: Why isn't the mind better designed than it is? *British Journal of Medical Psychology, 71*, 353–373.

Gilbert, P. (2007). *Psychotherapy and counselling for depression* (3rd ed.). Sage.

Gilbert, P. (2020). Compassion: From its evolution to a psychotherapy. *Frontiers in Psychology, 11.*

Gilbert, P. (2022a). Compassionate mind training: Key themes. In P. Gilbert & G. Simos (Eds.), *Compassion focused therapy: Clinical practice and applications* (pp. 273–312). Routledge.

Gilbert, P. (2022b). The evolved functions of caring connections as a basis for compassion. In P. Gilbert & G. Simos (Eds.), *Compassion focused therapy: Clinical practice and applications* (pp. 90–121). Routledge.

Gilbert, P. (2022c). Setting the scene: Psychotherapy at a crossroads and a compassionate way forward. In P. Gilbert & G. Simos (Eds.), *Compassion focused therapy: Clinical practice and applications* (pp. 3–23). Routledge.

Gilbert, P., & Basran, J. (2018). Imagining one's compassionate self and coping with life difficulties. *EC Psychology and Psychiatry, 7*(12), 971–978.

Gilbert, P., Basran, J. K., Raven, J., Gilbert, H., Petrocchi, N., Cheli, S., et al. (2022). Compassion-focused group therapy for people with a diagnosis of bipolar affective disorder: A feasibility study. *Frontiers in Psychology*, 1297.

Gilbert, P., & Choden. (2013). *Mindful compassion.* Constable Robinson.

Gilbert, P., McEwan, K., Catarino, F., & Baião, R. (2014). Fears of negative emotions in relation to fears of happiness, compassion, alexithymia and psychopathology in a depressed population: A preliminary study. *Journal of Depression and Anxiety.*

Gilbert, P., & Simos, G. (Eds.). (2022). *Compassion focused therapy: Clinical practice and applications.* Routledge.

Hakulinen, C., Elovainio, M., Pulkki-Råback, L., Virtanen, M., Kivimäki, M., & Jokela, M. (2015). Personality and depressive symptoms: Individual participant meta-analysis of 10 cohort studies. *Depression and Anxiety, 32*(7), 461–470.

Harris, D. L., & Ho, A. H. (Eds.). (2023). *Compassion-based approaches in loss and grief.* Taylor & Francis.

Holmes, J., & Slade, A. (2017). *Attachment in therapeutic practice.* Sage.

LeDoux, J. E. (2022). As soon as there was life, there was danger: The deep history of survival behaviours and the shallower history of consciousness. *Philosophical Transactions of the Royal Society B, 377*, 20210292.

Lee, D. (2005). The perfect nurturer: A model to develop a compassionate mind within the context of cognitive therapy. In P. Gilbert (Ed.), *Compassion: Conceptualisations, research and use in psychotherapy* (pp. 326–351). Routledge.

Lynch, C. J., Elbau, I. G., Ng, T., Ayaz, A., Zhu, S., Wolk, D., et al. (2024).

Frontostriatal salience network expansion in individuals in depression. *Nature, 633*, 624–633.

Matos, M., Duarte, C., Duarte, J., Pinto-Gouveia, J., Petrocchi, N., & Gilbert, P. (2022). Cultivating the compassionate self: An exploration of the mechanisms of change in compassionate mind training. *Mindfulness*, 1–14.

Mazza, M. G., Palladini, M., Poletti, S., & Benedetti, F. (2022). Post-COVID-19 depressive symptoms: Epidemiology, pathophysiology, and pharmacological treatment. *CNS Drugs, 36*(7), 681–702.

Meevissen, Y. M., Peters, M. L., & Alberts, H. J. (2011). Become more optimistic by imagining the best possible self: Effects of a two-week intervention. *Journal of Behavior Therapy and Experimental Psychiatry, 42*(3), 371–378.

Millard, L. A., Wan, M. W., Smith, D. M., & Wittkowski, A. (2023). The effectiveness of compassion focused therapy with clinical populations: A systematic review and meta-analysis. *Journal of Affective Disorders, 325,* 168–192.

Osimo, S. A., Pizarro, R., Spanlang, B., & Slater, M. (2015). Conversations between self and self as Sigmund Freud—a virtual body ownership paradigm for self-counselling. *Nature Scientific Reports, 5,* 13899.

Petrocchi, N., Ottaviani, C., Cheli, S., Matos, M., Baldi, B., Basran, J. K., & Gilbert, P. (2024). The impact of compassion-focused therapy on positive and negative mental health outcomes: Results of a series of meta-analyses. *Clinical Psychology: Science and Practice, 31*(2), 230–247.

Singer, T., & Engert, V. (2019). It matters what you practice: Differential training effects on subjective experience, behavior, brain, and body in the ReSource Project. *Current Opinion in Psychology, 28,* 151–158.

Steffen, P. R., Foxx, J., Cattani, K., Alldredge, C., Austin, T., & Burlingame, G. M. (2020). Impact of a 12-week group-based compassion-focused therapy intervention on heart rate variability. *Applied Psychophysiology and Biofeedback, 46,* 61–68.

Taylor, P. J., Gooding, P., Wood, A. M., & Tarrier, N. (2011). The role of defeat and entrapment in depression, anxiety, and suicide. *Psychological Bulletin, 137*(3), 391–420.

Vivino, B. L., Thompson, B. J., Hill, C. E., & Ladany, N. (2009). Compassion in psychotherapy: The perspective of therapists nominated as compassionate. *Psychotherapy Research, 19*(2), 157–171.

Watkins, E. R., & Newbold, A. (2020). Factorial designs help to understand how psychological therapy works. *Frontiers in Psychiatry, 11,* 429.

World Health Organization. (2023). *Depression.* www.who.int/news-room/fact-sheets/detail/depression.

14

Implementing Self-Compassion in the Treatment of Borderline Personality Disorder

Christian Stiglmayr

For a long time, the treatment of patients diagnosed with borderline personality disorder (BPD) was considered to be unpromising, exhausting, and frustrating for therapists. In the 1990s, I worked at a university psychiatric clinic in the south of Germany, and this clinic was also reluctant to admit patients with BPD for these reasons. When we started to establish dialectical behavior therapy (DBT) for the treatment of patients with BPD in the clinic in 1994, it greatly facilitated our work. For me, DBT was the boat that offered the possibility to stay and work together with people with BPD in a rough and uncontrollable sea. DBT is packed full of skills for the patients as well as for the therapists, enabling each other to survive under these bad conditions and even find a way out to a life worth living. Despite this excellent method, however, dealing with the enormous suffering of the patients remained unsatisfactory for me. In addition to all the skills, I lacked another level of dealing with the agonizing suffering of the patients. In 2012, I came in contact with mindful self-compassion (MSC). For me, it was *the* answer in dealing with unchangeable pain. It was *the* answer to how to communicate radical acceptance without being abstract, only confronting and direct, without being heartless. In the beginning, when I first learned about self-compassion, I thought Christopher Germer and Kristin Neff had developed this specifically for patients diagnosed with BPD.

In this chapter, I explore the integration of self-compassion into DBT, highlighted with real-world examples.

Diagnostic Criteria, Comorbidity, and Differential Diagnostics

BPD is a severe mental illness that causes a great deal of incomprehension and excessive demands, not only on the part of those persons affected but also on the part of their social environment and treatment providers. For this reason, it was and is not uncommon for patients diagnosed with BPD to be denied psychotherapy, especially on an outpatient basis; in their distress, patients often seek inpatient facilities where they receive inadequate treatment due to a lack of disorder-specific services.

Diagnostic Criteria

The symptoms and experiences of patients diagnosed with BPD can be allocated to three psychopathological dimensions: (1) disorders of affect regulation, (2) disorders of identity, and (3) disorders of social interaction.

Disorders of Affect Regulation

Disorders of affect regulation are characterized by rapidly triggered, excessively strong, and long-lasting emotional states. Depending on the extent, these emotional states can no longer be perceived by the person who is affected in a differentiated manner; a diffuse feeling of inner tension remains, which is often accompanied by dissociative experiences (Stiglmayr et al., 2005). These states of tension and dissociation, which are experienced as uncontrollable and highly unpleasant, are attempted to be ended as quickly as possible with the help of immediately effective but, in the long term, dysfunctional behaviors, such as self-injury or suicide attempts. Impulsive behavior in the form of binge eating, increased alcohol or drug use, or high-risk behavior (e.g., climbing construction cranes, or subway surfing) is also a result of impaired affect regulation. Some persons who are affected have violent outbursts of anger; others, on the other hand, are completely unfamiliar with outward feelings of anger toward others and direct their anger inwardly at themselves.

Disorders of Identity

Disorders of identity in patients diagnosed with BPD are characterized by the absence of a clear sense of self. Instead, patients report highly fluctuating ideas about themselves, permanently changing life goals and preferences, and may modify their physical appearance frequently. The consequence of this lack of identity is a chronic feeling of inner emptiness, which can be extremely agonizing for many persons who are affected.

Disorders of Social Interaction

Disorders of social interaction are characterized by a rapid alternation between idealization and devaluation of the counterpart. This is accompanied by inappropriate proximity–distance regulation. The relationship behavior of patients diagnosed with BPD is in many cases similar to that of pubescents. For this reason, patients diagnosed with BPD are often referred to as "chronic pubescents at a high level."

Comorbidities and Differential Diagnosis

Comorbid disorders can significantly influence the extent and course of BPD. Consideration should be given to posttraumatic stress disorder (PTSD), alcohol and drug abuse or dependence, eating disorders, anxiety and obsessive–compulsive disorders, affective disorders, attention-deficit/hyperactivity disorder, dissociative disorders, and nonorganic sleep disorders. Additional personality disorders are also frequently observed.

Psychotherapeutic Methods for the Treatment of BPD

Currently, five main therapeutic methods for treating patients with BPD have been investigated in randomized controlled trials: DBT (Linehan, 1993a, 1993b, 2015a, 2015b) and schema-focused therapy (Arntz & van Gendersen, 2021) are considered therapy concepts close to behavioral therapy; mentalization-based therapy (MBT; Bateman & Fonagy, 2011) and transference-focused psychotherapy (Yeomans et al., 2015) belong to the psychodynamic methods; and a therapeutic approach according to the guidelines of the American Psychiatric Association has also shown to be effective (McMain et al., 2009).

The most comprehensive overview of the data on the efficacy of individual treatments for BPD is provided by the Cochrane Review (Storebø et al., 2020). MBT as well as DBT are the methods with the most evidence of effectiveness and are therefore explicitly recommended by experts for the treatment of patients diagnosed with BPD.

The following is a brief description of DBT, as the practice of self-compassion has already been extensively incorporated in this book.

DBT for the Treatment of BPD

DBT is a manual-based, behaviorally oriented therapy. In addition to the established cognitive-behavioral methods, DBT integrates a variety of other strategies and techniques, especially conversational psychotherapy, Gestalt therapy, hypnotherapy, and Zen Buddhism.

The Worldview in DBT

If the "behavioral" in the title of the method refers to its basic behavioral therapeutic orientation, "dialectical" stands for the underlying worldview. Linehan (1993a) refers to the Hegelian understanding of dialectics: The thesis is incomplete in itself and thus demands its negation—the antithesis. This conflict finds its resolution in the synthesis. The synthesis subsequently forms the new thesis, which in turn calls for a new antithesis. According to Hegel (1968), the goal of this process is the unity of man in love. In his view, when people seek help (e.g., in the form of therapy), they are stuck in this process, unable to find a resolution of thesis and antithesis in synthesis. This is exactly where DBT comes in: Contradictory truths (e.g., "Life is not worth living as it is" vs. "Any change feels existentially threatening") are juxtaposed to restart the process of synthesis with the resulting tension (e.g., "I can move even when I am very afraid"). At the same time, the therapist constantly makes sure that the patient remains in a position to face this process—that is, whenever the patient finds themselves in a state in which they cannot think or act clearly (dissociation, high states of tension), they apply the skills that were taught to them explicitly to become capable of acting and working. As soon as the patient can participate in the process again, the therapist is left with the task of benevolently and warmly accompanying the individual process while teaching further skills necessary for a life worth living. The dissolution of dichotomous ways of looking at things and, thus, a deep inner acceptance of oneself and one's environment, represents the attractive final goal of DBT.

Linehan (1993a, 1993b, 2015a, 2015b) describes the concept of "Wise Mind" as the most effective skill for resolving two conflicting poles. Wise Mind describes the synthesis of a "rational" and "emotional" mind. Linehan uses it to refer to the place of inner wisdom—a place that every living being possesses. Wise Mind, therefore, contains the intuitive knowledge of what is the right decision for a living being in which situation. Occasionally, however, access to Wise Mind is blocked by strong emotions or basic assumptions (e.g., "I must not be weak"); then, the therapeutic task is to (re)activate this connection to ensure that the patient takes the path that applies to them personally (e.g., "If you listen to yourself, what does your Wise Mind recommend to you about this situation?").

Goals of DBT

Within the context of DBT, it is assumed that an emotion regulation disorder underlies patients diagnosed with BPD. Based on a biosocial etiology model, Linehan (1993a, 1993b) concludes, on the one hand, that a *biological* disposition leads to (1) an increased sensitivity to emotional stimuli, (2) an increased emotional arousal level, and (3) a slowed return to the emotional baseline level. Phenomenologically, these abnormalities are manifested by an average ninefold increase in emotional arousal compared with psychologically healthy control subjects, which is triggered far more frequently, rises more rapidly, and lasts about twice as long (Stiglmayr et al., 2005). On the other hand, due to unfavorable, often traumatizing social conditions (i.e., "invalidating environment"), patients do not learn sufficient skills to regulate their emotional response.

For this reason, patients diagnosed with BPD usually experience their emotions as uncontrollable, and a very deep-rooted problem arises: Persons who are affected try, as far as possible, to avoid their emotions (i.e., patients with BPD are usually very emotion phobic). This concerns almost all distinct emotions, such as shame, guilt, anger, and fear, but also pleasant emotions, such as love or joy. However, since emotions cannot be permanently avoided, those affected persons develop regulatory strategies, such as nonsuicidal self-injurious behavior, alcohol or drug use, high-risk behavior, or suicide attempts. These are effective in the short term but very harmful in the long term.

The overriding goal of DBT treatment is thus to develop access to one's own emotions and the needs behind them. Since emotions and needs are always an expression of the self, DBT is nothing other than a constant journey to oneself through the eye of the needle of emotions.

The implementation of this treatment goal is divided into two subgoals (Linehan, 1993a):

1. The first step is to teach patients diagnosed with BPD to change extreme emotionality and reduce maladaptive mood-dependent behaviors. The skills required for this are taught within a skills-training program (Linehan, 2015a, 2015b).
2. In the second step, patients with BPD should be taught to allow their own feelings, thoughts, and activities to be justified and to trust them.

Structure of Therapy

The duration of outpatient therapy is designed to be 1–3 years and, in rare cases, even longer. The course of therapy is clearly structured and can be divided into three therapy phases. While therapy Phase 1 focuses on reducing dysfunctional behavior, therapy Phase 2 focuses on the processes that have so far been suppressed by the dysfunctional behavior: first and foremost, the emotions and needs that have so far been avoided. If virulent comorbid PTSD exists, it is necessary to address the existing trauma during this second therapy phase. In recent years, DBT-PTSD has been developed for this purpose (Bohus et al., 2020). The procedure is based on trauma exposure; in addition, the procedure includes numerous techniques for building and enhancing the practice of self-compassion for dealing with trauma-specific suffering. The final third phase of therapy serves to shape a meaningful life, as well as the deep inner acceptance of one's own person as they are. In addition to the skills already taught, techniques and attitudes of self-compassion in particular are used in this therapy phase (Germer & Neff, 2019; Gilbert & Simos, 2022).

The Practice of Self-Compassion in the Treatment of Patients Diagnosed with BPD

Self-compassion is an essential component in working with patients diagnosed with BPD in light of the suffering they experience. As shown in the study by Salgó and colleagues (2021), patients with BPD practice significantly less self-compassion. Keng and Wong (2017) were able to show that childhood parental invalidation and lack of self-compassion are both strongly associated with BPD symptoms. Linehan (1993a) already assumed that the invalidating environment is a negative predictor for the development of self-compassion. Concurrently, it could be shown that loving-kindness and self-compassion lower self-criticism and improve self-kindness and acceptance in patients with BPD (Feliu-Soler et al., 2016). Therefore, it cannot be started early enough with its teaching and practice.

Since the perception of emotions is a central therapeutic focus of DBT, there is always a confrontation with pain, which is accompanied by many emotions. Self-compassion is therefore also an essential component in DBT to enable the patient to deal constructively with their pain.

At the same time, the confronting of a patient's enormous suffering can cause the therapist to feel empathic pain for their patient. In addition, patients' high emotionality, as well as confrontation with their own difficult experiences, can cause suffering in the therapist. Therefore, the practice of self-compassion is also helpful for us as therapists.

Definition of Self-Compassion

"Self-compassion" is the competence to be acquired to transform moments of suffering into something helpful and positive. Self-compassion is the ability to meet oneself in a crisis in a benevolent and friendly way—instead of devaluing, insulting, rejecting, or even hurting oneself.

According to Germer and Neff (2019), self-compassion is defined by

- Mindfulness ("To respond to my perceived distress, I need to know that this is a moment of suffering").
- Self-kindness ("I meet myself in a situation of suffering with the greatest possible kindness, care, and understanding").
- Common humanity ("I am not alone with my misery").

Self-compassion is thus a state of "loving, connected presence" (Germer & Neff, 2019, p. 30). The practice of self-compassion is not aimed at making the pain go away but is practiced because this is a painful and suffering moment.

Background to Consider When Teaching Self-Compassion to Patients with BPD

Most patients with BPD grow up with the conviction that they are wrong and inappropriate. That means they look for the causes of the problems they have to deal with exclusively in their own person ("If I were different, I would have fewer problems"). A basic feeling of existential shame accompanied by the basic conviction that "I am wrong" is the immediate consequence. Particularly in situations of suffering, a judgmental, insulting, unkind, and condemning way of dealing with oneself takes place. This leads to further reinforcement of the painful experience and the resulting devaluation of one's own person—a vicious circle. Of course, this cycle does not lead to a change in behavior or to an improvement in people's relationships with themselves.

Since the persons who are affected are also used to being treated like this by others in their environment (invalidating environment), a treatment defined by self-compassion can initially often trigger fierce resistance and thus bring additional suffering with it. Germer and Neff (2019) call this phenomenon "backdraft": "When we feel loved and the doors of our hearts open, the love goes in and the pain comes out" or "Love reveals everything unlike itself" (p. 197). Many patients with BPD are not able to be compassionate toward themselves when beginning therapy for fear of this unfamiliar experience and are often not even able to physically touch themselves with benevolent intent. This is especially true for patients who are severely traumatized. Most patients cannot express this in an emotionally adequate way but react with anger toward themselves or the therapist with distraction maneuvers or dissociation. Thus, the patient's reaction to self-compassionate interventions is often a good diagnostic tool: If the patient cannot practice self-compassion, or even experiences it as threatening, then the therapeutic process is still very much at the beginning (therapy Phase 1). If, on the other hand, the patient shows some capacity to treat themselves with kindness, to physically touch themselves benevolently, then the patient has made significant progress in the therapeutic process (therapy Phase 2 or 3).

Requirements That Help Teach Self-Compassion

To be able to apply the practice of self-compassion, patients with BPD need to cultivate certain skills. These include distress tolerance skills, which enable the patient to regain control over themselves in the event of an experienced loss of control. After regaining control, the patient should stop using the distress tolerance skills. Since there is always an underlying reason for this hyperstress, it is then necessary to identify the triggering situation. Then, the patient has to identify the emotions involved in the triggering situation. Otherwise, tension would arise again because the triggering problem remains unsolved. To implement this, the patient needs emotion regulation skills. And finally, the patient needs mindfulness skills. Mindfulness skills are necessary to help the patient identify all of the components involved in the triggering situation, in addition to getting distance from their emotional arousal. An overview of the skills to be taught can be found in Linehan (2015a, 2015b).

Based on my own clinical experience, I suggest the following recommendations:

- In the case of persistent and serious suicidal or self-injurious behavior, I do not recommend teaching self-compassion; or, if it appears responsible, only a minimal amount of it.
- The patients should be able to detect and regulate their emotions.
- The patients should live in a reasonably safe environment. This also includes at least one stable relationship.
- It would be helpful if the patient had some basic understanding of mindfulness.

Practical Exercises for Teaching Self-Compassion to Patients with BPD

For patients with BPD for whom a confrontation with the practice of self-compassion is still very anxiety provoking, it can be helpful to first approach the topic theoretically. In this case, the therapist can explain the physiological aspects of self-compassion. This is also possible when dysfunctional emotion regulation behaviors are still present. Most patients are very interested in physiological processes.

Case Vignette[1]

THERAPIST: Are you interested in what happens physiologically when you have negative thoughts about yourself?

PATIENT: Hmm, can't do any harm.

THERAPIST: Well, your brain can't distinguish whether you're being attacked from the outside or the inside—that is, when you say to yourself what a failure and useless person you are, your brain behaves like it would if a tiger attacked you. Adrenaline and cortisol are released, your heart rate goes up, and your muscles tense up. Your brain goes into fight-or-flight mode. For example, every time you berate yourself, you put a lot of stress on your brain and body. Is that what you want?

PATIENT: No, not really. But I don't have any other choice.

THERAPIST: You mean that happens automatically?

PATIENT: Yes. Besides, that's true. I'm a failure.

THERAPIST: Would you like me to tell you a little more about that?

PATIENT: Yes, why not. It sounds interesting.

THERAPIST: Let me ask you a question: What do you think is man's mission in evolutionary terms?

PATIENT: Survival—and reproduction.

THERAPIST: That's exactly it! For example, we are not originally in the world to be happy. But we are in the world to survive. The idea of being happy is a relatively new idea that has only existed since humans stopped fighting constantly for their survival.

PATIENT: Well, then I'm not doing anything other than what we were actually developed for.

THERAPIST: Yes, that's right. And that's something we humans are really good at, which quickly becomes automatic. Attacking or fleeing. Or in your case, freezing if neither of those is possible. (*Pause*) Now, my question to you, though, is whether that's also a goal for your life, to be in a state like that all the time. Does that feel good to you?

PATIENT: No, of course not. That's what I'm here to change, isn't it?

THERAPIST: Well, then, I'm reassured. Because I really couldn't have taught you anything more about attacking yourself. Shall I now tell you what you can do instead to achieve your goal?

PATIENT: Go ahead.

THERAPIST: But before that, I'd like to explain to you how that works.

---

[1] All case vignettes are fictional but are based on real cases.

Then, it will be easier to understand what you can or should be doing instead. Okay?

PATIENT: Okay.

THERAPIST: As we have already established, we are actually built for survival—that is, we have a very well-developed threat system. But now we humans also have something that is also very well trained, which is the counterpart to that threat system. (*Pause*) Have you ever noticed that we humans come into the world much too early? That we are actually still completely incapable of surviving without our parents' care.

PATIENT: Yes, that's true. We can't actually do anything.

THERAPIST: Exactly! Actually, we arrive in the world before we can take care of ourselves. However, the fact that we are born before we are fully developed has also given humans an advantage in evolutionary terms. Do you have any idea which one?

PATIENT: Hmm . . . maybe it makes us even more moldable?

THERAPIST: Exactly! We are already starting to learn while other mammals are still in their mother's womb. That makes us humans very adaptable and flexible. (*Pause*) However, we do have a problem. In order for us to survive, we have to adapt to our environment, but this only works if we get certain things from our environment. Do you have any idea what that might be?

PATIENT: Hmm . . . love?

THERAPIST: Yes, exactly. Love is a big concept there, of course. Broken down, it means that we need care; for this, there is a so-called care system in our brain, which is as strongly developed as our threat system. Have you ever observed how mothers and possibly fathers behave toward their newborns?

PATIENT: Yes, they talk so funny.

THERAPIST: Yes, that's exactly how it is. There are three things they do to help the baby mature: You give them warmth, contact—for example, touch—and then you talk so funny to the baby. Besides the content, it is especially the tone of voice that matters. There is something nurturing about it. And it is precisely these three components that make our care system kick in: Contact, warmth, and a caring, nurturing voice. (*Pause*) Do you have any idea why I'm telling you this in such detail?

PATIENT: Well, maybe I'm supposed to be more caring with myself?

THERAPIST: Yes, that's the point. And how can you do that?

PATIENT: I don't know.

THERAPIST: Just like the mother or father does with their baby: by giving warmth, contact, and vocal attention. (*Pause*) Sounds weird, doesn't it?

PATIENT: You want me to touch myself. Caring?

THERAPIST: Do I see panic in your eyes?

PATIENT: You can see that, right? I can't do that at all.

THERAPIST: Okay, it's important that you first understand the background. The point is that whenever you apply this care to yourself, your care system automatically kicks in and oxytocin and endorphins are released. At the same time, the threat system calms down. So, this gives you the opportunity to counter your threat system. But whether you actually implement this is, of course, your decision.

A very simple but effective exercise could bring patients even closer to practicing self-compassion. In this exercise, the patient should imagine how they would treat a good friend who is in a bad situation. They should then ask themselves how they would treat themselves if they were suffering. This exercise is often a good opportunity to talk about the different ways of dealing with suffering and its effects. Practice M.1, "How Would I Treat a Friend?," in the Appendix, contains a description of this exercise.

The next step is to develop self-compassion for oneself. For this, the patient must perceive and accept their distress and suffering. For example, you can ask, "Do you see how much you are suffering at this moment?" This process can take a long time; therefore, it makes sense to let the patient set their own pace. A good exercise that can be done with the patient at this point is the "Self-Compassion Break" (Germer & Neff, 2019; see Practice M.2 in the Appendix for a description of this exercise).

If the patient is already able to perceive and regulate emotions, they are unavoidably also confronted with the painful components of emotional experience. It is precisely at this point that the use of self-compassion is recommended for dealing with these painful experiences. A good and helpful exercise is "Being with Difficult Emotions" (Germer & Neff, 2019; see Practice M.3 in the Appendix for a description of this exercise). Below is a conversation excerpt based on a shortened version of this exercise.

Case Vignette

THERAPIST: Do I understand you correctly that the breakup with your girlfriend makes you sad and desperate?

PATIENT: Yes. It's almost unbearable! And it is so unfair!

THERAPIST: Yes, that's painful, isn't it?

PATIENT: Yes. I don't even know what to do with it.

THERAPIST: How have you dealt with this pain so far?

PATIENT: I didn't want it to be there at all. And when it was there, I hurt myself and had suicidal thoughts.

THERAPIST: And how do you think you should deal with it now?

PATIENT: Differently. But there is no solution for it.

THERAPIST: Yes, there is. Would you like to try the solution together with me?

PATIENT: Hmm . . . do I have another option?

THERAPIST: Not really. Okay. Can you tell me where exactly you perceive this pain?

PATIENT: Here, in the chest.

THERAPIST: Can you take an inner journey to this place? What does this place look like from the inside? Big, small? Hard, soft? Hot, cold?

PATIENT: Big and hot. And very hard, dark.

THERAPIST: Okay. Can you bring your attention to this spot inside you? Maybe you can imagine running warm water over that spot or giving it a massage?

PATIENT: This feels very unfamiliar. . . .

THERAPIST: Yes, I believe you. Is there anything else that you feel?

PATIENT: Maybe the place will soften a little. . . .

THERAPIST: Great. And is it possible for you to bring your attention to this place on the outside of your body? Perhaps by placing a hand on this spot?

PATIENT: (*Puts his hand on his chest.*)

THERAPIST: And what do you feel now?

PATIENT: Hmm . . . it feels like I care about this place a little bit. I wish my girlfriend had been there for me like that.

THERAPIST: I believe that. But now you are there for yourself instead. . . .

THERAPIST: Can you perhaps add a few caring and comforting words to say to yourself? Perhaps like when you comfort a child in a similar situation? It is enough if you say it to yourself in your mind.

PATIENT: That feels strange. Foreign and unfamiliar. And somehow also wrong.

THERAPIST: Yes, of course, it is exactly the opposite of how you experienced it when you were a little boy—and you're not used to talking to yourself kindly. What else does it feel like?

PATIENT: It somehow becomes more bearable.

THERAPIST: See if it is possible for you to just allow the feeling and the pain that comes with it—without wanting or needing to change anything. Instead, you are simply there for yourself, at least right now in this moment.

To summarize, components of the exercise "Being with Difficult Emotions" include the following:

- Naming the emotional pain.
- Localizing emotional pain in the body.
- Soothing touch on this area; thereby warmth and body contact.
- Gentle vocalization.
- Accepting the emotional pain.

This exercise can be done whenever painful emotions arise. Finally, at an advanced stage, it can also be used to confront the childhood experience of not belonging and being unloved.

First Results on the Use of the MSC Program for Patients with BPD

In 2018, my colleagues and I conducted a randomized controlled study (Ledenig et al., 2018) where we compared MSC (Germer & Neff, 2019) with a waiting list. Thirty-one patients diagnosed with BPD participated: 15 persons within the MSC group and 16 within the waiting list. Eighty-one percent of the participants were female. Among many other aspects, we assessed self-criticism and shame. There were three evaluation stages: once before the MSC program started, another one after the MSC program, and finally a follow-up 3 months after the program. In patients with BPD, a significant reduction in the level of self-criticism and self-hate and a significant increase in self-soothing were observed. This effect even increased over the follow-up period. These results are consistent with the findings of Feliu-Soler and colleagues (2016).

Due to the positive effect of self-compassion for patients diagnosed with BPD, it seems to make sense to teach self-compassion on a larger scale. For this purpose, a program is currently being developed in which self-compassion will be taught in a group for 6 months in 20 sessions. This is a combination of the DBT skills training by Linehan (2015a, 2015b) and the MSC program by Germer and Neff (2019).

Conclusion

Especially for patients who experience a great deal of suffering, self-compassion is a necessary therapeutic component. In general, its teaching and practice cannot begin early enough. Since many patients diagnosed with BPD are overwhelmed with the confrontation of loving aspects of themselves, especially at the beginning of therapy, a theoretical approach to the topic is recommended as a first step. A deeper practical introduction should take place only when the patient no longer exhibits serious dysfunctional behavior and can deal with their emotions appropriately. In any case, the practice of self-compassion is a very helpful and necessary therapeutic tool, especially for patients who experience as much suffering as patients diagnosed with BPD. Furthermore, self-compassion is also a necessary component for us therapists. Again and again, I find it helpful to pause briefly in therapeutically stressful and challenging situations in order to apply a moment of self-compassion. It is not uncommon for situations to arise in which I practice self-compassion together with the patient and thereby serve as an example of a helpful approach to self-compassion.

REFERENCES

Arntz, A., & van Genderen, H. (2021). *Schema therapy for borderline personality disorder* (2nd ed.). Wiley.

Bateman, A. W., & Fonagy, P. (Eds.). (2011). *Handbook of mentalizing in mental health practice.* American Psychiatric.

Bohus, M., Kleindienst, N., Hahn, C., Müller-Engelmann, M., Ludäscher, P., Steil, R., et al. (2020). Dialectical behavioral therapy for posttraumatic stress disorder (DBT-PTSD) compared with cognitive processing therapy (CPT) in complex presentations of PTSD in women survivors of childhood abuse: A randomized clinical trial. *JAMA Psychiatry 77,* 1235–1245.

Feliu-Soler, A., Pascual, J. C., Elices, M., Martin-Blanco, A., Carmona, C., Cebolla, A., et al. (2016). Fostering self-compassion and loving-kindness in patients with borderline personality disorder: A randomized pilot study. *Clinical Psychology and Psychotherapy, 24,* 278–286.

Germer, C., & Neff, K. (2019). *Teaching the mindful self-compassion program: A guide for professionals.* Guilford Press.

Gilbert, P., & Simos, G. (Eds.). (2022). *Compassion focused therapy: Clinical practice and applications.* Routledge.

Hegel, G. W. F. (1968). *Gesammelte werke.* Meiner.

Keng, S. L., & Wong, Y. Y. (2017). Association among self-compassion, childhood invalidation, and borderline personality disorder symptomatology in a Singaporean sample. *Borderline Personality Disorder and Emotion Dysregulation,* 4, 24.

Ledenig, N., Thürmann, A., Mundle, G., Jacoby, E., Günther, M., Kemmer, M., et al. (2018). *Effectiveness of mindful self compassion (MSC) on self-criticism and shame in patients with borderline personality disorder: A new treatment for BPD?* Poster presentation at the International Congress on Borderline Personality Disorder, Sitges, Spain.

Linehan, M. M. (1993a). *Cognitive-behavioral treatment of borderline personality disorder.* Guilford Press.

Linehan, M. M. (1993b). *Skills training manual for treating borderline personality disorder.* Guilford Press.

Linehan, M. M. (2015a). *DBT skills training handouts and worksheets.* Guilford Press.

Linehan, M. M. (2015b). *DBT skills training manual* (2nd ed.). Guilford Press.

McMain, S. F., Links, P. S., Gnam, W. H., Guimond, T., Cardish R. J., Korman, L., & Steiner, D. L. (2009) A randomized trial of dialectical behavior therapy versus general psychiatric management for borderline personality disorder. *American Journal of Psychiatry, 166,* 1365–1374.

Salgó, E., Szeghalmi, L., Bajzát, B., Berán, E., & Unoka, Z. (2021). Emotion regulation, mindfulness, and self-compassion among patients with borderline personality disorder, compared to healthy control subjects. *PLoS One, 16*(3), e0248409.

Stiglmayr, C. E., Grathwol, T., Linehan, M. M., Ihorst, G., Fahrenberg, J., & Bohus, M. (2005). Aversive tension in patients with borderline personality disorder: A computer-based controlled field study. *Acta Psychiatrica Scandinavica, 111,* 372–379.

Storebø, O., Stoffers-Winterling, J. M., Völlm, B. A., Kongerslev, M. T., Mattivi, J. T., Jørgensen, M. S., et al. (2020). Psychological therapies for people with borderline personality disorder. *Cochrane Database of Systematic Reviews, 5,* CD012955.

Yeomans, F. E., Clarkin, J. F., & Kernberg, O. F. (2015). *Transference-focused psychotherapy for borderline personality disorder. A clinical guide.* American Psychiatric.

15

Cultivating Self-Compassion in Response to Anxiety

Lizabeth Roemer
Gerson F. Borrero
Molly Sawdy
Jessica R. LoPresti

In this chapter, we focus on how self-compassion can be beneficial in response to experiences of anxiety. First, we describe the nature of anxiety, including its relation to environmental and structural factors. Next, we share a conceptualization of how anxiety arises and is maintained that forms the underpinning for our therapeutic approaches to treating anxiety, including the cultivation of self-compassion. We then briefly review the main elements of treatment and their relation to self-compassion. Finally, we conclude with some examples of challenges to cultivating self-compassion and how to address them.

Understanding the Nature of Anxiety

Humans naturally experience anxiety across a range of contexts and in a variety of ways. It is evolutionarily adaptive to attend to potential threats to our safety, physical integrity, and social inclusion; to experience a cascade of physical sensations like a racing heart, sweaty palms, and shortness of breath when we perceive a threat; and to prepare to fight, flee, or freeze in these contexts. And yet, in our modern lives, we often encounter threats that cannot be effectively addressed by fighting, fleeing, or freezing. We also can imagine threats, recall them, or view them on media platforms so that our bodies and minds respond as though the situation is present, even when it is not. The threats (e.g., traumatic events, oppression) we encounter throughout our lives can lead us to learn to respond to both external and internal reminders of these experiences (e.g., an angry voice, our own racing hearts, exclusion) with fear and anxiety, leading to new learning experiences that increase the scope of our anxious responding. We can also use our minds to try to prepare for threats (worry), and this cognitive activity can interfere with our ability to be present in our lives as they unfold. Fearing our own emotional reactions can naturally lead us to try to push those reactions (thoughts, feelings, sensations) away, which can further intensify them, creating a cycle of anxiety and distress. Fear and anxiety naturally evoke behavioral avoidance and constriction, which sometimes function to keep us safe and avoid harm, but often restrict our lives and sense of satisfaction and meaning, creating increased distress and anxiety, and furthering the cycle of anxiety.

Environmental, Societal, and Structural Contributions to Anxiety

While Western psychiatry and psychology conceptualize anxiety disorders in terms of individualistic, person-centered models, we must acknowledge the environmental, societal, and structural sources of threat that humans face that naturally lead to anxiety (e.g., see Graham-LoPresti et al., 2020). Increased weather-related threats tied to the climate crisis; COVID-19, and other diseases that spread without consistent public health responses; extractive capitalistic messages regarding the need for endless productivity and minimization of worth and care for workers and their families; fraying of social networks; and systemic marginalization of individuals based on race, gender identity, sexual orientation, disability, class, and other social identities all contribute to reasonable experiences of anxiety and distress. Messages that stigmatize mental health struggles further this cycle by leading us to criticize our own responses, thus intensifying them.

Although structural, social, and environmental problems require systemic solutions that directly target these contexts, as clinicians we also work to help individuals who are experiencing the consequences of these contextual stressors. To be effective, we develop an understanding of the individual and relational factors that maintain and intensify anxiety, as well as the strategies and experiences that can reverse this cycle and help individuals thrive despite these anxiety-provoking contexts.

Conceptualization of Anxiety That Guides Our Interventions

We conceptualize difficulties with anxiety as stemming from three interrelated natural human processes (Roemer & Orsillo, 2020). The first process is the development of a *problematic relationship with one's internal experiences*. Specifically, people can learn to narrowly focus on threatening internal experiences; to criticize and judge these experiences; and to overidentify, fuse, or become entangled with these experiences. For instance, Sara, who experiences physical tension and arousal, along with negative thoughts about herself and a sense of unease when she is being mistreated by a coworker, may focus in on these sensations, view them as a sign of her own weakness or lack of competence, and see them as self-defining, perhaps with a thought like "I'm oversensitive." These natural human reactions then lead to the second process of *rigid experiential avoidance* (i.e., rigid attempts to control or eliminate distressing internal experiences). When thoughts, feelings, and sensations are viewed as problematic, signs of weakness, or dangerous, it is natural to try to get rid of them. However, pushing them away, particularly with a rigid attachment to eliminating them, is often unsuccessful and can, in fact, paradoxically increase them, and make them even more aversive, increasing the first process. So, Sara may find that she feels even more tension and her critical thoughts are even more intrusive. The final process involves *nonengagement in personally meaningful behaviors*. One way to experientially avoid is to remove oneself from contexts that can elicit uncomfortable internal experiences. While this can lead to immediate relief, it also maintains dissatisfaction and can feed negative views of oneself as life becomes more constrained and contains fewer experiences of meaning and connection. Sara may withdraw at work by starting to arrive late, not speaking up in meetings as often, or no longer seeking contact with coworkers. While this diminishes the intense discomfort at the moment, it likely leads to even more thoughts about not being competent or being oversensitive.

Integrating Self-Compassion into Acceptance-Based Behavioral Treatment for Anxiety

We present comprehensive approaches to addressing this cycle elsewhere (Graham-LoPresti et al., 2020; Roemer & Orsillo, 2020); here we focus specifically on how self-compassion is integrated into our clinical approach. Cultivation of self-compassion can effectively counter the self-criticism and self-judgment that characterize the problematic relationship with internal experiences, helping clients to disentangle from internal experiences and allow thoughts and feelings to rise and fall naturally without taking them as indicators of permanent truth or self-worth. Sara, mentioned above, might develop practices and habits that allow her to notice her physical sensations and critical thoughts and bring compassion to them, perhaps adding the thoughts, "It's hurtful to be treated this way when I am trying hard in this position. I have the thought that I'm oversensitive because

I've received that message in many contexts, but this is an understandable reaction to a difficult situation." Interrupting the cycle with care and compassion for herself can diminish her attempts to suppress her thoughts and feelings (i.e., experiential avoidance) and open space for her to consider what action she wants to choose in this situation, rather than automatically avoiding (i.e., nonengagement in personally meaningful actions). Sara might then find ways to address her coworker's mistreatment, make other connections at work that are rewarding, or realize that her work situation is unhealthy and needs to be changed.

Self-compassion may also be useful in ameliorating the impact of various factors that affect anxiety symptoms, such as internalized racism. Internalized racism refers to the acceptance and adoption of negative stereotypes, ideologies, and beliefs about people in communities of color by people of color. Existing research suggests that there are many risk factors associated with internalized racism, including experiences of racism (Graham et al., 2016; Sosoo et al., 2020). This same line of research suggests that internalized racism may be one mechanism through which experiences of racism and oppression are associated with more severe anxiety symptoms.

Cultivation of self-compassion may target anxiety related to internalized racism. Specifically, internalized racism can be characterized as a form of self-criticism, as individuals endorsing internalized racism are inherently operating under the assumption that negative beliefs of themselves and the community are justified or truthful (Graham et al., 2016). Internalized racism is associated with lower degrees of self-esteem and greater degrees of psychological distress (Syzmanski & Gupta, 2009). For instance, a client of color may begin to internalize messages that they hold inferior intellect as compared with their White counterparts in school, which leads to heightened anxiety while engaged in academic pursuits (e.g., studying, taking an exam, contributing to class discussions). This student might say to themselves, "It makes sense that I'm feeling anxiety in this class because of all the messages I've received from society that I'm not smart. That doesn't mean it's true and doesn't mean it's not worth trying." If self-criticism plays a role in internalized racism's associations with anxiety, self-compassion may help ameliorate the associated anxiety and stress (Graham et al., 2016; LoPresti et al., 2023).

Strategies to Cultivate Self-Compassion in Response to Anxiety

In our clinical work, we use many strategies to help clients live fuller and more rewarding lives during their natural, human anxious responses. We briefly overview these and provide in-depth descriptions, examples, and practices that explicitly target self-compassion.

The Therapeutic Relationship

The therapeutic relationship is a central context for helping clients cultivate self-compassion that allows them to disentangle from anxious responses and engage meaningfully in their lives. The therapist's own practices of self-compassion and compassion, coupled with the model of how clients' responses make sense and are natural, form a foundation for conveying understanding, validation, and care to the client, which helps a client to develop their own sense of self-compassion and compassion for others. Treating clients as inherently worthy and their responses as natural has a powerful impact on their understanding of themselves. Clients often vulnerably describe painful experiences and emotions in response to their environment. It is imperative for us, as clinicians, to model compassion in these circumstances by validating the humanness of emotional responses to painful experiences. For instance, a transgender man of color might disclose stress after being misgendered by their boss in a staff meeting and shame around having this emotional reaction. In this situation, a clinician might spend time validating the emotions (e.g., "Of course you're feeling distressed; this is a human response to having your identity ignored and not feeling seen and respected"). Similarly, a client describing a panic attack while not initially finding their child when picking them up from day care might describe self-criticism and feeling "silly" about their response. A clinician could respond that the client's deep care for their child's well-being is understandable, and sensations of panic are a natural response to this perceived threat to their child. This validation can counter the cycle that self-criticism and shame can exacerbate.

Psychoeducation

Across various intervention contexts (individual therapy, structured group interventions, mental health promotion workshops, digital mental health approaches), we have found that psychoeducation can have several important psychological effects, including facilitating self-compassion. Even in assessment contexts, clients often comment that learning that their anxious symptoms "make sense" and naturally arise from their lived experiences and the nature of being human, rather than being indicators of something wrong or weak in them, decreases their self-critical thoughts. Acknowledging the naturally anxiety-provoking effects of childhood experiences, traumatic exposure, ongoing structural oppression, and interpersonal stressors can naturally combat the harmful internalization that often results from these contexts. Increasing self-compassion through psychoeducation, especially as it relates to oppressive experiences, may also be a catalyst for cultivating self-compassion by sharing knowledge learned in session with others who also experience identity-related oppression (e.g., race-based stress and trauma, misogynoir). Thus, self-compassion learned through psychoeducation may facilitate self-empowerment for the client as well as the client empowering others within their social network.

Formal or informal psychoeducation about self-compassion itself can also be beneficial, as clients often come to therapy with misconceptions. Therapists can direct them to Kristin Neff's website (*https://self-compassion.org/what-self-compassion-is-not-2*), which includes clear descriptions of these common misconceptions and a link to a longer article, for clients who are interested in additional reading. Or it may be helpful to develop handouts or share some of these clarifications in discussions of barriers to self-compassion. We also find it helpful to include Shelly Harrell's (2021) perspective on the ways that the terms *self-compassion* or *self-care* can mistakenly perpetuate an individualistic view of self, while a more interconnected view acknowledges that caring for ourselves allows us to care for others and vice versa.

> Mabel, a middle-aged White woman, reported chronic, uncontrollable worry that she had experienced throughout her life. When her therapist introduced the concept of self-compassion, Mabel shared that she did not want to "let [herself] off the hook" for her mistakes and shortcomings and that it was important to her to take responsibility and be accountable to others for her actions. The therapist acknowledged Mabel's concerns and reflected on the value Mabel had shared of being responsible for her behavior and its impact on others. The therapist shared that self-compassion means recognizing one's humanness and fallibility, and not adding criticism to the pain of natural imperfection (which can further exacerbate cycles of worry). The therapist shared research that shows that self-compassion actually allows people to acknowledge and learn from their mistakes and therefore enhances, rather than undermines, accountability. In addition, because self-compassion can help to interrupt the cycle of worry, it can allow for more attentional capacity to attend to one's actions and to repair after one's mistakes.

Mindfulness Practices

Neff (2012) conceptualizes mindfulness as a component of self-compassion, noting the importance of observing emotions as they arise, rather than pushing them away or overidentifying with them. In our work, we conceptualize self-monitoring, formal practice (i.e., setting aside time to practice observing with curiosity and openness), and informal practice (i.e., bringing curiosity, openness, and awareness to activities in our lives) as three ways to cultivate mindfulness. In all of these practices, clients (and we) are developing an ability to notice experiences as they arise, notice reactions to these experiences, notice how we become entangled in these reactions, and then perhaps notice how we can disentangle from them. This process of observation naturally elicits feelings of self-compassion (e.g., "Look how busy my mind is!" "It's hard to be in my body today"). As such, we consider all of these practices to be practices of self-compassion. The *mindfulway-throughanxiety.com* website contains recordings of several formal practices we have found helpful. *Inviting a difficulty in and working it through our bodies*, a practice adapted from mindfulness-based cognitive therapy (Segal et al., 2002), involves recalling a difficult moment and noticing how it feels in one's body and then practicing allowing it to be there, rather than pushing it away. This embodiment of acceptance can help clients develop an ability to enact self-compassion when anxiety and distress arrive in their lives.

Self-Compassion Exercises

Specific practices that target self-compassion can also be helpful when working with clients struggling with anxiety. Clinicians may want to adapt many of the exercises presented in this volume to meet specific clients' challenges. Practice N, "Adaptation of 'How Would You Treat Your Friend?,' " in the Appendix, is based on a self-compassion exercise (Neff & Germer, 2018) to use with a client who is struggling with their anxious response to discrimination.

Another exercise that can be helpful for clients who experience a lot of anxious arousal (either panic or situation-specific anxiety responses, like social anxiety) is physically soothing themselves while acknowledging their emotions (adapted from Neff & Germer, 2018):

- "Begin by noticing where you feel anxiety or discomfort in your body."
- "Also, notice your breath."
- "If you wish, put your hand on the part of your body where you feel the distress, or put your hand on your heart or your hand or arm."
- "Notice the feel of your touch."
- "You might imagine warmth and kindness flowing from your hand to your body."
- "If you feel like it, you can add words that you find soothing, like 'I know this is a hard time,' or 'This feels important and that's stressful,' or 'I can be kind to myself.' "
- "Allow yourself to feel whatever you're feeling, simply adding in this physical care for yourself."

Values Clarification and Values-Based Actions

A central component of our work with clients struggling with anxiety is helping them to identify what matters to them or how they want to be in their lives and then helping them take actions that are consistent with what matters to them. Values-based actions disrupt the cycle of restricting one's life due to anxiety and begin the process of acting in ways that are rewarding and meaningful, even when thoughts, sensations, and feelings of anxiety arise. An important first step to engaging in values-based action is to identify a client's values. There are various ways to help a client identify these values (see Orsillo & Roemer, 2016; Roemer & Orsillo, 2020, for explicit forms and values-identification skills). Once a client can start identifying their values, the clinician can underscore the importance of learning how to flexibly live by the identified values. Self-compassion can be helpful here because the rigid implementation of values-based action may potentially turn into distress due to values clashing. In other words, inflexibly engaging in the values one has may result in unwanted distress from one value seemingly contradicting another value a client may hold. Thus, it is helpful to view values-based action through the lens of self-compassion and by prioritizing one's physical, emotional, and psychological safety.

When clients begin to explore the ways their lives have become constrained, critical thoughts and feelings often arise, and they may blame themselves for not engaging more in important areas of their lives. Clinicians can help clients see how their lived experiences, including messages they have received and external barriers they have faced (e.g., oppression), have naturally inhibited their ability to do everything that matters to them. As clients begin to try out new actions, they can also practice self-compassion when they miss opportunities or fall back into old habits of avoidance or inattention. Further, they may compassionately recognize that there are some contexts in which avoidance or withdrawal makes sense and is warranted by the hostile situation they are in.

The following dialogue provides an example of how values-based actions and self-compassion can be effective tools for working with clients who carry minoritized identities and also experience anxiety. The vignette includes a brief practice that is informed by Neff's (2012) "Identifying What We Really Want" self-compassion exercise applied using a case example with a transgender Asian American woman in her mid-20s after the client has clarified their values:

CLIENT: I still feel really anxious. I keep worrying that I'm a failure as a person and in my career. I keep thinking that I'm not good enough at my job and that I'm not distinguishing myself enough from my coworkers. I think that part of it may have to do with my job environment, given that a few times coworkers and others mixed me up with the other Asian American woman in the office. However, not receiving a promotion or substantial bonus recently makes me worry that I'm just not good at my job. I find it hard to control these worries and I just shut down sometimes because of them, which makes doing my job even harder.

THERAPIST: It sounds like you've been going through a really tough time lately. The worries that come with these experiences of discrimination would be a lot for anyone to handle and these feelings are perfectly understandable. I can imagine that these feelings and the situation must be especially painful for you since you identified working hard in your career as a value.

CLIENT: Yes, it's very important to me. I feel like not being able to act consistently with that value when I shut down is making me feel even more anxious about everything.

THERAPIST: In that case, maybe we should talk about some methods to help you work toward that value, even when you're not feeling your best. How does that sound?

CLIENT: That sounds like a good idea.

THERAPIST: First, let's talk about how people sometimes try to use self-criticism as a motivator for action. Can you think of any ways that you may criticize yourself, with some intention that doing this criticizing will help you perform well in your career?

CLIENT: Well, I tell myself that I'm a failure or that I'm incompetent when I don't complete a task on time, fail to meet the expectations that I set, or see a coworker get the promotion that I want.

THERAPIST: Does this cause you any emotional pain?

CLIENT: It does a lot, actually. I feel incredibly anxious and bad about myself when I think these things and then I shut down. My work is then affected negatively.

THERAPIST: That's understandable. Others would likely feel terrible if they thought these things about themselves. Try to give yourself compassion in feeling the emotional pain these judgments cause. Now, bring a loved one or someone else who you are close with and would consider nurturing to mind. What type of supportive things do you think they would say about whether thinking these thoughts are beneficial for your well-being and behavior?

CLIENT: Well, my best friend would probably tell me that being so hard on myself makes it harder for me to work in ways that I value and that thinking these things about myself is making me more anxious and making it harder for me to do my job in meaningful ways. They would probably also say that the discrimination that other people in my office show me is more of a reflection of them than of my own capabilities. They might remind me that Asian American individuals often feel the need to outperform their peers due to the model minority myth and that I can be proud of my job performance without burning myself out or getting promoted as quickly as I hoped.

THERAPIST: That sounds like an insightful thing that your friend may say. Now, could you try to notice each time you find yourself making these negative judgments about yourself and the pain they cause you? And try to give yourself compassion for experiencing this pain, as it is human and understandable. Then, think about what your friend would say to you, to deepen your self-compassion. This self-compassion may help guide you to more clearly choose how to engage in tasks to work toward your value of working hard in your career. How does this sound?

CLIENT: I like this, I would like to try it out for the next time that we meet.

In this vignette, the therapist affirms the injustice and pain that the client experiences and normalizes these outcomes. The therapist goes on to identify how accepting the pain of these experiences and thoughts can be mitigated by supportive dialogue meant to foster self-compassion. This dialogue and subsequent engagement of self-compassion may then facilitate the client's ability to identify actionable items to engage in valued living.

Ending Therapy

When clients are preparing to leave therapy, clinicians can encourage them to practice self-compassion, using all of the methods learned throughout treatment, when they notice that some of their old habits of anxious responding reemerge. They can reengage with their practices, with care and kindness, and continue to develop and strengthen their new habits of responding.

Navigating Specific Challenges with Self-Compassion Practices

Practicing Grace and Care for Self

One challenge that can arise for clients with anxiety who try to practice self-compassion is that it can feel like the instruction is to feel other than they feel. When they feel worried about their competence or critical of their failures, cultivating self-compassion can seem like a criticism of the experience they are currently having and might sound like messages people receive, like "Don't worry, be happy" or "Don't criticize, be kind to yourself." Instead, it can be helpful to suggest that clients *act* with care for themselves, while they feel whatever they are feeling.

The following dialogue illustrates how we might introduce this to a client with generalized anxiety:

CLIENT: I tried to bring self-compassion to my experiences this week, but I'm really bad at it.

THERAPIST: Can you say more about what happened that made you have the thought that you're bad at it? [Identifying thoughts as thoughts to help with disentangling from them.]

CLIENT: I was working on an assignment for class, and I kept getting distracted from what I was reading, and I was thinking about how bad I am at school and that I'm going to fail. And then I noticed I was being critical of myself, so I tried to think about how to be kind to myself. But I still felt anxious about the work and bad about what I was doing, so it felt fake to imagine kind words. So, then I just thought about how bad I am at self-compassion.

THERAPIST: First, nice job noticing that you were having critical thoughts! That's such an important first step. And it makes a lot of sense that even though you wanted to think and feel differently, that didn't automatically change these habitual thoughts. And then it sounds like you started to feel critical of yourself for having critical thoughts! That can be a hard cycle to get out of.

CLIENT: Yes! That's exactly how it felt. Like this is another thing I'm bad at.

THERAPIST: (*Nodding*) That is so understandable and I'm so glad you noticed this stuck point and shared it here. I can get caught in that kind of cycle too. One thing that can help is to switch focus to *doing* something kind and caring for ourselves, instead of trying to *feel* a certain way. As we talked about before, we can't always change how we feel or the thoughts that arise, but we can more easily change what we do. What if instead of trying to *feel* compassion for yourself in a moment like that, you shifted to *doing* something that feels kind or caring? You could play some music you like, light a candle, take a break to stretch or walk, or do something else that you find caring.

CLIENT: I just had the thought that I don't deserve something caring when I haven't done my work yet, but I remember that we talked about kindness as something we all deserve and that isn't based on a particular outcome. I guess maybe I could try to do something like that.

THERAPIST: Yes! That's such an important thing to remember. We get lots of messages that we have to earn kindness and care, but we all deserve care and we can meet our goals more easily when we are getting that care. Another thing you might try is to develop some habits of doing caring things for yourself each day so that you get more used to giving yourself care. And you can bring any kind of mood or thoughts to your caring actions—there's no wrong way to feel while you engage in actions of care for yourself. Let's talk through some specific actions you might try this week.

Therapists can develop lists of caring actions with clients or can give them general lists of different actions and let clients choose which activities resonate with them.

Challenging Stereotypes and Expectations by Practicing Self-Compassion

Practices of caring for oneself may become complicated for folks who experience various forms of oppression and develop certain expectations for themselves based on stereotypical archetypes. One example of this is the "strong Black woman" archetype, which is characterized by societal expectations that Black women remain psychologically, emotionally, and physically strong, despite various stressors that they may experience in their lives (Romero, 2000). Embedded in this archetype is the expectation that Black women can continually serve as caretakers for others in perpetuity. The adoption of this archetype is associated with anxiety and other negative mental health outcomes among Black women (Donovan & West, 2015). Self-compassion exercises for caretakers may aid in alleviating the distress that Black women experience due to the adoption of the strong Black woman archetype.

The following example uses the imagined case of a Black bisexual mother:

CLIENT: Recently, I just feel so overwhelmed with everything going on. I need to be there for my daughter to help her get ready for school, help her with her homework, teach her about life, cook, and do the laundry, all while balancing my job and caring for my ailing mother. Recently, it's just been so difficult. My partner is able to help financially with her job, though she works longer hours than I do, and can't be there to help with the housework and much of the parenting. I just feel like I've been dropping the ball lately because I find myself becoming really anxious regarding my finances, whether I'm being a good mother, partner, and daughter, and worrying about the future in general. I just shut down. Sometimes, I freeze and stop whatever I am doing and start crying because of the anxiety I feel. I also find myself aimlessly scrolling through social media to try and avoid facing my responsibilities. I'm such a failure; I need to be better.

THERAPIST: First, it's great that you're able to identify what you're feeling and possible causes for the anxiety and thoughts of being a failure that you're having. It seems like you have a lot on your plate and are a caregiver for many people in your life, along with your work responsibilities. I think many people may feel overwhelmed in your position. Knowing that others would feel the same way as you in your position, you could try to show yourself some compassion for feeling anxious and overwhelmed, instead of being critical.

CLIENT: You're probably right. It's just that I need to be strong for my family. I can't afford to be the person they worry about. They need me. I'm supposed to be able to handle everything.

THERAPIST: You're likely right. Your family probably does need you to be there and care for them at times. However, do you think that you can care for them if you yourself aren't being taken care of?

CLIENT: Well, it is certainly hard to do so right now.

THERAPIST: Exactly. Just like the batteries on a phone, there are times when we are depleted of our energy and our resources and we can't give anymore. It's important to find time to do things to recharge our batteries, even if these are small and quick activities. Caring for ourselves is sometimes the best way to care for others.

CLIENT: That makes sense: I never thought about how it would be hard to support my family if I'm not taking care of myself first and making sure my batteries are charged.

THERAPIST: Why don't we discuss some ways in which you can do things that would be taking care of yourself and refilling your batteries?

The clinician highlights to the client that an important component of being a caregiver for others is being a caregiver to oneself. This allows for a degree of vulnerability and tenderness that is counter to the strong Black woman archetype. Self-compassion and activities to care for oneself can be applied to a range of presenting concerns for people who carry marginalized identities and experience ongoing distress from existing oppressive systems.

Conclusion

Because criticism and invalidation naturally create and intensify anxiety, self-compassion can interrupt this cycle and help to lessen anxiety and contribute to an increased ability to engage more fully in personally meaningful actions. When therapists validate clients' habitual reactions and convey compassion for their experiences, including recognizing related external and systemic contexts, clients can begin to interrupt the self-critical cycle that drives anxiety with some moments of compassion toward themselves. Clinicians can also provide psychoeducation that helps clients to better understand the ways that their physiological arousal, tension, and anxious thoughts/worries are natural and human responses, further deepening their self-compassion. Describing the ways that external contexts like chronic invalidation, loss, and systemic oppression contribute to the cycle of anxiety can further enhance self-compassion and reduce the self-criticism clients often have of their own anxiety responses. Clinicians can also introduce general mindfulness exercises to help clients relate differently to their thoughts, feelings, and sensations. Being able to see reactions clearly in these exercises, with kindness and without becoming entangled with them, naturally promotes self-compassion and reduces criticism and judgment. In addition, therapists can use specific self-compassion exercises to more directly develop this skill for clients. These exercises can be adapted so that they acknowledge clients' contexts. Finally, therapists can work with clients to help them clarify what's important to them and to engage in meaningful, values-based actions. Self-compassion skills help clients see what matters to them more clearly and also to take action, even when anxious thoughts or sensations arise while doing so. Increased values-based living reduces the disruption of anxious symptoms and enhances quality of life. It also empowers clients to find meaning in their lives even in the face of external barriers and harm.

REFERENCES

Donovan, R. A., & West, L. M. (2015). Stress and mental health: Moderating role of the strong Black woman stereotype. *Journal of Black Psychology, 41*(4), 384–396.

Graham, J., West, L., Martinez, J., & Roemer, L. (2016). The mediating role of internalized racism in the relationship between racist experiences and anxiety symptoms in a Black American sample. *Cultural Diversity and Ethnic Minority Psychology, 22*, 369–376.

Graham-LoPresti, J. R., Abdullah, T., & Calloway, A. (2020). Culturally responsive assessment and treatment of generalized anxiety disorder. In L. T. Benuto, F. R. Gonzalez, & J. Singer (Eds.), *Handbook of cultural factors in behavioral health: A guide for the helping professional* (pp. 231–245). Springer Nature.

Harrell, S. (2021, May 22). *Weekend wisdom: Self-love and self-care*. www.thesoulfulnesscenter.com/post/weekend-wisdom-self-love-and-self-care.

LoPresti, J. R., Abdullah-Swain, T., Borrero, G., & Scott, D. (2023). Racial microaggressions and trauma symptoms in a Black American sample: The moderating role of self-compassion. *Journal of Contextual Behavioral Science, 29*, 209–218.

Neff, K. D. (2012). The science of self-compassion. In C. K. Germer & R. D. Siegel (Eds.), *Wisdom and compassion in psychotherapy: Deepening mindfulness in clinical practice* (pp. 79–92). Guilford Press.

Neff, K. D., & Germer, C. (2018). *The mindful self-compassion workbook: A proven way to accept yourself, build inner strength, and thrive*. Guilford Press.

Orsillo, S. M., & Roemer, L. (2016). *Worry less, live more: The mindful way through anxiety workbook*. Guilford Press.

Roemer, L., & Orsillo, S. M. (2020), *Acceptance-based behavioral therapy: Treating anxiety and related challenges*. Guilford Press.

Romero, R. E. (2000). The icon of the strong Black woman: The paradox of strength. In L. C. Jackson & B. Greene (Eds.), *Psychotherapy with African American women: Innovations in psychodynamic perspective and practice* (pp. 225–238). Guilford Press.

Segal, Z. V., Williams, J. M., & Teasdale, J. D. (2002). *Mindfulness-based cognitive therapy for depression: A new approach to preventing relapse*. Guilford Press.

Sosoo, E. E., Bernard, D. L., & Neblett, E. W. (2020). The influence of internalized racism on the relationship between discrimination and anxiety. *Cultural Diversity and Ethnic Minority Psychology, 26*(4), 570–580.

Szymanski, D. M., & Gupta, A. R. (2009). Examining the relationship between multiple internalized oppressions and African American lesbian, gay, bisexual, and questioning persons' self-esteem and psychological distress. *Journal of Counseling Psychology, 56*(1), 110–118.

16

The Process of Self-Compassion in Eating Disorder Recovery

Ann Saffi Biasetti

Self-compassion is a life-giving skill for those suffering from an eating disorder, as well as for the clinicians who work with them. This chapter explores learning how to deliver and apply the skill of self-compassion for people with eating disorders to bring forth resiliency and action-oriented steps toward self and body protection, as well as fostering emotion and nervous system regulation necessary to sustain recovery.

Anyone who has worked with this population understands that self-compassion is often out of reach for those whose self-harming behaviors present as quite contrary to self-compassion, leaving clients stuck in cycles of despair, grief, self-hatred, shame, and blame toward themselves and their bodies. As clinicians longing to help and meet their suffering, we can also be left feeling helpless and hopeless in how to offer self-compassion so that it can be received and held to grow the life-giving protection and safety our clients are longing for the most.

The Struggle of Eating Disorders: Some Statistics

As a clinician and certified eating disorder specialist, I have been treating those with eating disorders for over 30 years. I have witnessed the cycle of harm and despair, as well as the loss of self-agency that exists in one's body and self that develops after years of body hatred and self-harm. Whereas the prevalence of the disorders has always been high, since the COVID-19 pandemic the spike in eating disorder diagnoses, especially in young adults, has been staggering. It is estimated that currently upward of 30 million people in the United States, and approximately 73 million worldwide, alone are suffering from anorexia, bulimia, and binge-eating disorder, among others (Association of Anorexia Nervosa and Associated Disorders [ANAD], 2023). The threat to life caused by eating disorders places them in the category of being one of the most prevalent and life-threatening mental health disorders in the United States today, second only to opioid overdose (Arcelus et al., 2011).

Women continue to be afflicted with eating disorders at higher rates than men (Hudson et al., 2007). Rates among lesbian, gay, bisexual, transgender, queer, and diverse folks point to alarming statistics (ANAD, 2023). Transgender college students experience disordered eating at approximately four times the rate of their cisgender classmates and transgender people report using their eating disorder to modify their body without hormones (ANAD, 2023). Gender dysphoria and body dissatisfaction in transgender people are often cited as the key link to eating disorders (ANAD, 2023). Black, indigenous, and people of color are significantly less likely than White people to have been asked by a doctor about eating disorder symptoms and are half as likely to be diagnosed or to receive treatment.

The Challenge to Define Recovery

Recovery from an eating disorder is poorly defined in the literature and therefore, conceptualizing a clear understanding of what constitutes recovery is still poorly understood (Hower et al., 2022). Recovery currently focuses on physical and behavioral changes, emphasizing behavioral and symptom management, through cognitive-based treatments and exposure therapy (American Psychiatric Association, 2023). Unfortunately, statistics show clients still meet diagnostic criteria 5 years or longer after treatment, with only 50% of patients showing significant improvement (Polivy & Herman, 2002).

If you work with this population, you will find, as I do, that clients attest to recovery being so much more than physical change. There is a great deal to heal beyond behavioral recovery and a great deal that behavioral recovery does not address, including the lived experience of being in a body, or embodiment. Living in a cultural paradigm that upholds mind/body duality disregards the inherent knowledge that one's body could provide and has manifested into sociocultural norms that marginalize and oppress bodies that do not fit the standards and ideals set and leave clients continuing to feel disembodied, even after symptoms and behaviors have been managed. Clients are left struggling, disembodied, and in attempts to find a way to reconnect with their bodies, and those who are treating them are left hearing continued disconnection expressed through body hatred, nonacceptance, criticism, and the longing and wish to change the body they are in. Often, even when self-harming behaviors have lessened or are "controlled," many clients report that they still do not feel free from critical thoughts and in their relationship with their bodies (Steindl et al., 2017).

Perpetual Disembodiment: The Sociocultural Influence

Clients with eating disorders long to heal a whole "self," and to do that requires us as clinicians to move beyond reductionist treatment modalities that hold a higher regard for mind over body, or cognition over the felt, internal sense of a body. To help our clients heal their whole selves, we must guide them in learning and practicing *embodiment.* French philosopher Merleau-Ponty (1962) defined embodiment as "becoming a consciousness and being an experience" (p. 96). When self-compassion is integrated into treatment, we create a holistic recovery, which addresses the felt sense of the internal body, meets one's self-critical cognitive ruminations in a new way, and meets not just their individual histories but also the systemic harms that one's body has met out in the world, and allows our clients to eventually move toward shifting away from harm to their body to befriending their body. However, this is not easy to do. Those suffering from these self-harming behaviors are a population that, despite needing self-compassion and embodiment, often feel little to none of it, and may even report, due to not feeling deserving of it, that self-compassion leaves them feeling more dysregulated within, rather than the ease and softening that we know self-compassion may bring to our other clients and that we experience for ourselves.

Chronic dieting, instigated by diet culture and the diet industry, is a multimillion-dollar system that promotes fat phobia and the marginalization, oppression, and stigmatization of those in larger bodies. It is a system of body oppression that worships thinness and the promotion of weight loss as a means of attaining higher status and value, equates size to health and moral virtue (Harrison, 2019), and is a form of disordered eating that is often overlooked due to its popularity and acceptability in our culture. Recent statistics report that 42% of adults from general populations are in attempts to lose weight through dieting at some point in their lifetime (Santos et al., 2017), despite there being a 95% failure rate among them (ANAD, 2023). Dieting that is established in childhood and/or young adulthood has a 35% rate of turning into pathological dieting throughout one's lifetime and 25% advance to full-blown eating disorders (Neumark-Sztainer et al., 2007).

The idea of a certain body size having greater value and worth not only further marginalizes already marginalized groups but also has racist origins at its roots. In her book *Fearing the Black Body: The Racial Origins of Fat Phobia*, professor and author Sabrina Strings (2019) discusses the "racial origins of fat phobia," shedding light on fat phobia's roots developing during the transatlantic slave trade when colonists placed superiority, morality, and value upon the White body and upheld restraint of desire, and thinness to be an expression of this superiority. Fat became seen not just as a sign of immorality but also as racial inferiority.

Healing the Self: From Disembodiment to Embodiment

Diet culture invites one far away from embodiment. Embodiment stands in sharp contrast to diet culture, which invites people out and away from their bodies and their internal communication, as well as continues to set standards on what bodies deserve to embody and what bodies do not. Embodiment is an inherent human right as we all come into the world as embodied beings, and although our culture separates us from our bodies, we can choose to reconnect with them. Re-embodying involves learning to listen to the internal, sensory communication from one's body, attending to what we sense. The more we embody, the more we feel at one with the body so that it is no longer viewed and lived in from an objective place, but rather is *lived in* through a connected, subjective knowledge that continues to build trust, inner communication, and connection.

A primary result of an ongoing eating disorder is feeling separate, alone, and different, both out in the world and with oneself. It is through embodied knowledge that our clients begin to take ownership of their bodies and ownership of their recovery process. Embodiment is the grounding in the recovery process that supports the first steps in the growth of self-compassion.

During my doctoral studies, I embarked on a constructivist-grounded theory study that explored the role self-compassion played in both recovery and sustainment of recovery. I was interested in understanding why my clients with eating disorders were having such a difficult time accepting and integrating self-compassion, as well as in understanding the process of self-compassion in recovery—exactly what did it "do," and what was its action? The grounded theory unfolded a mechanism of delivery that I now use with my clients that allows this life-giving skill of embodiment and self-compassion to unfold and become integrated into one's recovery and life (Saffi Biasetti, 2015).

Stage I of Recovery: Grounding in the Body

The late, great, spiritual master Thich Nhat Hanh beautifully expressed how self-compassion is inherent to one's body if we pay attention. He stated that if walking along we step on a nail, the hand immediately reaches down to comfort the foot. Without thought, the body's inherent reaction is one of wishing to comfort, care, and alleviate the suffering from one part of the body to the next. This passage speaks to the interplay between the body and self-compassion during a period of recovery when little to no self-compassion is found.

The beginning stage of recovery is where one's body becomes the *grounding* of the recovery process and is the foundation for the development of self-compassion and beginning reconnection to oneself. However, it is also the hardest. In my research, I found this was a time defined as feeling "broken." Broken is indicative of body and mind feeling separate, and a time when self-compassion is least present. Rather, self-loathing, self-hatred, self-criticism, and shame are felt the most. As clinicians this is a period when we hear clients reporting everything opposite to embodiment and self-compassion. Self-harming behaviors are at their highest, as well as reports of body image struggles, nonacceptance, and often body hatred. One's body is not just perceived through the image to be an enemy but is also felt and sensed as one.

Ongoing self-harming behavior unfortunately impacts both the body and the brain. When behaviors such as starvation, chronic dieting, binge-ing, and purging, including overexercising, to name a few, are part of daily lives, there is an impact on one's body and brain that leads to autonomic nervous system dysfunction, and limbic system structure dysregulation and state change (Skowron et al., 2020). This leaves clients with an inability to properly perceive body image, as well as the inability to correctly access, assess, perceive, or interpret internal sensations.

The ability to be aware, access, and appraise bodily sensations is called "interoceptive awareness" (IA; Price & Hooven, 2018, p. 2). IA helps us gain awareness of the internal signals from our body. When we lose the ability to register and interpret our bodily signals, our autonomic nervous system becomes challenged and dysregulated in its ability to properly represent our internal world. The more autonomic dysfunction takes place, the further we lose our ability to sense and integrate the information we receive from the inner state of our bodies (Chen et al., 2021). A client's inability to sense and feel a proper, consistent, and ongoing register of hunger and fullness cues is one of the first signs of IA disruption. When clients are experiencing this loss of sensory register, it is imperative to "bring the body back," and the way we do this is to honor and name one's body as a central focus or what I call an "informant" in treatment from the start.

Focusing on body information is a way to develop the *yang side* of self-compassion, now known as *fierce self-compassion*. In *Fierce Self-Compassion: How Women Can Harness Kindness to Speak Up, Claim Their Power and Thrive*, Kristin Neff (2021) describes three expressions of fierce self-compassion, each of which serves a specific focus:

(1) protection—experienced as bravery, empowerment, and clarity; (2) providing—experienced as fulfillment, balance, and authenticity; and (3) motivation—experienced as encouragement, wisdom, and vision.

During the beginning stage, the focus is on protection and reconnection with the inner experience of one's body for the safety of the body and self. Therapists can introduce this concept by telling clients that their role is to both help them and their bodies stay safe and protected. Centering the body as a living, knowledgeable entity and modeling self-compassion toward it not only creates great respect for one's body but also helps to move the client toward a subjective experience of their body and away from the objective reality they have been living in. Body information, such as what they are noticing inside day-to-day: hunger/fullness cues, pain/discomfort, and energy levels can be presented through compassion expressed for one's body. Below are some examples of what I hear from my clients and how I support grounding through body reconnection:

CLIENT: What is happening to my body?

THERAPIST: Your body is trying to tell you something very important. Part of what we will be doing in treatment is trying to figure out your body's internal messages since you have felt disconnected from them for so long.

CLIENT: I can't eat because I have pain/nausea in my stomach every time I do!

THERAPIST: Yes, that's happening because your poor stomach and intestinal tract are not used to having regular, consistent food given to them. That pain you feel is these organs trying to talk to you and tell you they need some more nourishment to work properly.

CLIENT: I no longer menstruate.

THERAPIST: I see your endocrine system is sending you a message that something is out of balance. You and I will try to figure out what that may be and how we may reestablish balance.

CLIENT: My mind and body feel separate.

THERAPIST: Yes, of course they do. Out of fairness, we all live in a culture that invites us to be divided this way. Unfortunately, the more we move away from internal knowledge, the more we stop listening and feel disembodied and disempowered. By learning to listen in, you will begin to feel safer, clearer, and empowered.

When acknowledged and approached by slowing down the session and gently directing the client's attention to mindfully observe their bodily experience at the moment, one's body becomes a source of knowledge and discovery. Clients become curious and often want to know more, rather than move back into criticism and judgment. All disordered eating behavior may be framed through this curiosity now. Through internal knowledge, clients come to observe that all behavior was there in service of adaptation and help and this creates a softening into opening and understanding that they never meant to harm themselves or their bodies. Rather, they were just trying to feel safe and protected within, and behavior was one of the ways they attempted to do this. This self-compassionate reframe is of utmost importance. It allows disidentification from the disorder and a release from the idea of "broken" as comprising their entire identity and allows space and separation from the disorder to take place. They can experience that not all parts of them are broken, they never meant to cause harm, and there is a way out of the current suffering (see Practice O.1, "Feet, Spine, and Seat: Welcoming the Body into the Room," in the Appendix).

Stage II of Recovery: Listening and Responding to the Body

The middle stage of recovery is one framed by authenticity and truth that stems from listening to body signals, and, most importantly, *responding* to these signals. Responding means that clients are beginning to take *responsibility* and ownership of their recovery. This phase can be called *power and independence*, and it is a pivotal point in recovery where denial lessens, mindfulness increases, and suffering is acknowledged. They begin to get more curious as to what they may need to do or stop doing to take charge of their body's well-being. Self-compassion continues to be fierce, in how it shows up—in this phase, in a way that corresponds to Neff's (2021) *providing.* Reconnecting with the internal will to survive creates a need and wish to create a path of recovery that one can feel ownership of. This is not "resistant" or "willful," as it is sometimes mistakenly labeled—rather, this is the expression of the need to "take back" one's body; own it, learn from it, and care for it now in a new way forward in embodied connection, rather than separation.

During this middle stage, self-compassion is established first and foremost through the relational field. Through continued modeling of kindness and hope from clinician to client, we begin to invite a new belief. I call this the *outside influence*, whereby the client experiences self-compassion by receiving compassion offered from an external source and turning it inward. It is the self-reflective ability to be able to shine light on what is possible, rather than what is broken. During this phase, the reframing of symptoms and oneself can greatly influence the steps toward one's ability to turn the connection into self-compassion. A case vignette of this reframing of symptoms is below. (All client names and identifying information have been changed to maintain confidentiality.)

> Betty came to me for treatment of a long-standing binge-eating disorder. She had made great strides in therapy during the first phase. She learned to structure meals three times a day as well as added-in snacks. She recognized how restriction and diet mentality had been her biggest instigators of self-harm, both toward her body and mind. Her level of wishing and wanting to be self-protective was indicative of her internal self-compassionate growth. I pointed this out to her in each session, despite her lack of belief in it. The importance of seeing and believing in what the client cannot yet see and believe in is of utmost importance.
>
> Betty came to see me one session after a particularly challenging weekend where she felt body shame sparked by body image comparison while attending a family event. Despite knowing this would be a challenging time, she expected that she would be able to "manage" it without the return of behavior creeping in. When binge episodes returned over the weekend, she found herself in a downward "spiral," stating to me, "I totally regressed!" She felt shameful and embarrassed by her "letting it all go," as well as self-loathing and criticism returning both toward self and body.

My reframe in Betty's session began with reframing her symptoms and then acknowledging her embodied experience of this event. I offered the following:

> "I'm sorry this weekend was so difficult on so many levels. I noticed that it was hard for you to come here today and tell me about it. I saw how your body caved into the couch as you told me. I am wondering if you still are noticing the shame inside as we sit here together and, if so, where do you feel it the most inside? (*Betty is crying, noticing the shame located the most in her belly.*) I know it's hard for you to place a hand there [from my experience, many clients are often not yet ready to touch "triggering" body parts], but perhaps you can just place the pillow there as a way of meeting this feeling and sensation exactly where it is and how it is. (*She holds a couch pillow close to her center.*) Let's just take a few breaths here and notice what it's like to meet this space inside right here, right now. Notice the sensation that the pillow brings to this internal space, as well as your breath. What do you notice? (*She reports a softening as tears flow.*) Yes, I can see that softening in your face and body and through the tears. Let's remain here for a few more breaths just being with this softness inside. I invite you to just rest here a little longer."

I have not focused on Betty's shameful event, behavior, or *any part* of her story yet. Not until her body, which initially was in nervous system dysregulation, has calmed. Once calm, I apply what I call the *self-compassionate reframe.* A self-compassionate reframe is applied once an internal felt shift of calming is experienced and verified by the client. At that point in time, I offer a reframe of the experience the client has shared through modeling what a self-compassionate response sounds like. There is an emphasis on self-compassion through self-understanding and gentle relearning. Here is what I said to Betty:

> "Take a couple more deep breaths and when you are ready you can slowly come back into the space with me. Yes, this weekend was hard, very hard, and I am sorry you have been carrying around this internal feeling of shame both within your mind and in your body. I'm sure you could notice how that feeling showed up inside from the moment the body comparison began. (*Betty strongly agrees, crying.*) Out of fairness, your internal system responded the only way it is used to responding. You shut down and went into collapse. That's the internal state you know well. The one you have known for so long since you were a little girl! (*She strongly nods and agrees.*) It's also the state where these binge behaviors show up the most! So, *of course, these behaviors happened*! We could not have expected anything else right now. You are not relapsing—rather, right now, you are just *relearning.* And that is part of this recovery and healing journey. We will always be relearning. Let's look back on the weekend now with fresh eyes and see what can possibly be learned."

When self-compassion comes in *from the outside*, through the therapist's presentation of what was happening *inside*, *over behavior*, it can offer protection against reshaming and allows self-compassion to be felt in a coregulated state together. In this example, Betty and I carefully went back to look at that upsetting weekend through the lens of self-compassion. We searched for the moments when critical thoughts were showing up long before the weekend in anticipation of the weekend; we searched for slight changes in behavior, such as restriction, that she realized was happening for many days before her binge behavior; and we searched for ways she could now be more protective in thoughts and body going forward.

During this middle stage, self-care, self-compassion, and self-love may still be buried somewhere within. What is most important is that our clients feel that their worth, ability, and potential are seen by us, even when they cannot see it. Reframing tough behavioral moments into compassionate, caring, protective moments of embodied learning allows the client to continue to have hope and belief in oneself and plants the seeds for self-compassion to grow.

Stage III of Recovery: Integrating Self-Compassion and the Body into Life

The later stage of recovery is where therapists begin to hear the action of self-compassion take place. Compassion shows up fiercely through what can be labeled a *holding*, which is often felt as an internal protector and, in turn, supports motivation and moving forward in the recovery process. As self-compassion grows, it allows for a different way to hold oneself during challenging moments and creates the safety needed for clients to develop and maintain motivation, determination, and commitment to go forward. The constant soothing and returning to safety are essential to take the next steps during recovery, which is filled with unknowns about what life, self, and body will be like and look like if they continue forward.

The following is a case vignette of a client in the third stage of recovery exhibiting self-compassionate safety and protection. The following is a case example of a client who is in the third stage of recovery.

Case Vignettes

"Terry" expresses how the action and holding of self-compassion keep her moving forward now, despite years of dieting and body image struggles:

> "I have my moments, like the other day when I felt ashamed to eat at work in front of the others when they were all eating salads and smoothies and I brought my leftover dinner. I was about not to eat because I felt too anxious to eat with them. But I remembered that I had to protect my body. It's not fair to deny my body because I feel anxious now. So, instead, I just took my food in the car and ate in peace. Eventually, I'd like to get to the place where I just don't give a s—t! But, for now, I figured it was better to be kind to my body and do what I did."

My client "Laura" expresses this holding in a fierce way now:

> "Yeah, since I stopped the restriction and dieting, my body has changed. I don't fit into things the same this summer. I noticed thoughts of wanting and wishing for a different body. I remember us discussing that, in this world, how can I not wish that? I quickly calmed, took a breath, and held compassion for myself and my body, knowing I may always

feel this way, but I don't have to *do* anything about it but continue to take care of myself. It's just not an option to harm myself anymore!"

These examples show how self-compassion and viewing one's body through a subjective, embodied lens increased mindfulness, protection, self-awareness, and self-growth, even in difficult moments. A recovery that is supported by and through self-compassion keeps returning our clients, as it did for Terry and Laura, safely back to a self that is less harsh, less critical, and more accepting. From this internal feeling of safety, clients can begin, during this later phase, to explore the tough stuff, such as past trauma, and a deeper understanding of what impacted disembodiment from the start. Many intersections may impact one's ability to safely be in their body. Questions for clients to reflect on include "What has my body been subjected to out in the world all these years?"; "What harm/s have I done to my body to keep it disembodied?"; "How can I stay with its messages and communication now?"; and "How may I no longer leave my body behind?" These questions touch upon a crucial step during this phase, which I call *body forgiveness* (Saffi Biasetti, 2023).

Body Forgiveness

Body forgiveness (Saffi Biasetti, 2024) is a research project I have embarked on this year, to discover the interwoven process of self-compassion and embodiment. It entails forgiving oneself for harm, criticism, and hatred toward one's body *and* forgiving the body for it being what one has not wanted it to be. It is a process of grieving and mourning what was and what will be. Clients need to grieve and let go of what they hoped their body would look like and the many years they spent harming it if they were to grow into full and protective embodied living. Body forgiveness favors body neutrality over positivity and honors and allows for the suffering that may continue to be felt living in a body that one and/or the world wishes were different. "Alex" expressed this forgiveness during one of my groups:

> "I blamed my body for everything wrong in my life. I'm now realizing, for all it's been through, how can I not be kinder? My body was teased, abused, rejected, and still is at times, and all I was doing to it was the same. I am now realizing I never meant to harm myself or my body and my body never meant to cause me any harm either. We were both just trying to survive."

When clients embody self-compassion, we begin to hear perfectionism soften and a greater acceptance of oneself and one's human qualities emerge. Clients surrender and soften into understanding and accepting that recovery held in self-compassion may mean a never-ending arc of return to the various phases of recovery along the way. With self-compassion present, it mediates disappointments and shame, allowing higher levels of self-development, awareness, and self-connection, with each return, rather than becoming fixed or regressive in that phase. When self-compassion is embodied, it sets the stage for an understanding of recovery that is no longer dualistic and determined by or contingent upon behavior alone. Rather, recovery becomes inclusive of felt, embodied moments of shifts, cognitive reframes, and movement forward in life and relationships, sometimes despite behaviors being present (see Practice O.2, "Body Forgiveness Practice," in the Appendix).

Conclusion

Self-compassion, when carefully unfolded into treatment for those struggling with reconnection to their body, food, and self, allows for the gentle unfolding of body reconnection to occur shifting our clients from disembodiment and unsafety within to safety and a return to embodiment. Self-compassion allows a new nonbinary view and understanding of recovery to emerge, one that is inclusive and allows for the possibility of embodied growth to take place even during behaviorally regressive points. It allows for hope and faith to build and carry one forward and helps clients connect to the limitless possibilities they possess when they see and hold themselves in compassion.

REFERENCES

American Psychiatric Association. (2023). *The American Psychiatric Association practice guideline for the treatment of patients with eating disorders* (4th ed.). Author.

Arcelus, J., Mitchell, A. J., Wales, J., & Nielson, S. (2011). Mortality rates in patients with anorexia nervosa and other eating disorders: A meta-analysis of 36 studies. *Archives of General Psychiatry 68*(7), 724–731.

Association of Anorexia Nervosa and Associated Disorders. (2023). *Eating disorder statistics.* https://anad.org/eating-disorders-statistics.

Chen, W. G., Schloesser, D., Arensdorf, A. M., Simmons, J. M., Cui, C., Valentino, R., et al. (2021). The emerging science of interoception: Sensing, integrating, interpreting, and regulating signals within the self. *Trends in Neurosciences, 44*(1), 3–16.

Harrison, C. (2019). *Anti-diet: Reclaim your time, money, well-being and happiness through intuitive eating.* Little, Brown.

Hower, H., LaMarre, A., Bachner-Melman, R., Harrop, E. N., McGilley, B., & Kenny, T. E. (2022). Conceptualizing eating disorder recovery research: Current perspectives and future research directions. *Journal of Eating Disorders, 10*, 165.

Hudson, J. I., Hiripi, E., Pope, H. G., Jr., & Kessler, R. C. (2007). The prevalence and correlates of eating disorders in the National Comorbidity Survey Replication. *Biological Psychiatry, 61*, 348–358.

Merleau-Ponty, M. (1962). *The phenomenology of perception* (C. Smith, Trans.). Humanities Press.

Neff, K. (2021). *Fierce self-compassion: How women can harness kindness to speak up, claim their power and thrive.* Harper Wave.

Neumark-Sztainer, D., Wall, M., Haines, J., Story, M., & Eisenberg, M. E. (2007). Why does dieting predict weight gain in adolescents? Findings from project EAT-II: A 5-year longitudinal study. *Journal of the American Dietetic Association, 107*(3), 448–455.

Polivy, J., & Herman, C. P. (2002). Causes of eating disorders. *Annual Review of Psychology, 53*, 187–213.

Price, C. J., & Hooven, C. (2018). Interoceptive awareness skills for emotion regulation: Theory and approach of mindful awareness in body-oriented therapy (MABT). *Frontiers in Psychology, 9*, 798.

Saffi Biasetti, A. (2015). *Broken into life: A grounded theory on the role of self-compassion in eating disorder recovery.* Unpublished doctoral dissertation, Sofia University.

Saffi Biasetti, A. (2023). *Body forgiveness: The role of forgiveness in the development of embodiment.* Unpublished manuscript.

Santos, I., Sniehotta, F. F., Marques, M. M., Carraça, E. V., & Teixeira, P. J. (2017). Prevalence of personal weight control attempts in adults: A systematic review and meta-analysis. *Obesity Reviews, 18*(1), 32–50.

Skowron, K., Kurnik-Łucka, M., Dadański, E., Bętkowska-Korpała, B., & Gil, K. (2020). Backstage of eating disorder: About the biological mechanisms behind the symptoms of anorexia nervosa. *Nutrients, 12*(9), 2604.

Steindl, S. R., Buchanan, K., Goss, K., & Allan, S. (2017). Compassion focused therapy for eating disorders: A qualitative review and recommendations for further applications. *Clinical Psychologist, 21*(2), 62–73.

Strings, S. (2019). *Fearing the Black body: The racial origins of fat phobia.* New York University Press.

17

Couple and Relationship Distress

The Power of Self-Compassion Training in Therapy

Michelle Becker

As a licensed marriage and family therapist for over two decades, I've been keenly aware of the power of relationships to harm and to heal. Relational pain showed up everywhere in couple, family, and individual sessions. It showed up in play therapy sessions with 4-year-old children, in mother–daughter sessions with a 72-year-old daughter and her 95-year-old mother, in preschool through high school settings, in senior centers, in domestic violence programs, and in my private practice working with individuals, families, and couples of all ages and stages. It also showed up across all socioeconomic and cultural variables and differing psychopathologies. Whether relational pain was a cause or contributing factor in the presenting problem, or the presenting problem was causing relational problems, I could see the effects of relationships gone awry.

I also saw the healing that healthy relationships can foster. When people understand the suffering underneath unskillful relational behaviors and learn to relate to each other with more kindness, profound changes can positively affect their relationships. The psychotherapeutic relationship forged in compassion is itself a major factor in the effectiveness of psychotherapy (Geller, 2017, p. 3). As humans, we are interdependent. None of us has reached adulthood without having been cared for, even at the most basic level, by others. We are wired for belonging. When we are connected to safe others, we can feel content and have a sense of nonwanting (Gilbert & Choden, 2015, p. 56). When we have had enough experiences of being safely connected to others, we develop a secure attachment style in which we have confidence that others will be there for us when we need them.

People who have secure attachment styles tend to have healthier relationships (Shaver et al., 2016).

Most couples that come in for therapy struggle to create a bond that is characterized by secure attachment. Because of their own prior life experience, especially where something was lacking in the response from their primary caregiver, individuals don't experience relationships as a safe place where they can be themselves and also be accepted (Bolt et al., 2019). Instead, they develop strategies to cope with the insecurities in their primary relationships. These strategies include the clinging and co-dependent tendencies of people who are anxiously attached, the self-reliance and avoidance of emotional intimacy in people who are avoidantly attached, and the mix of both in the disorganized attachment style (Bolt et al., 2019). Self-compassion can provide the "reparenting" that can help patients heal these attachment wounds of anxious and disorganized attachment styles so that ultimately a secure attachment with their partner can develop (Lathren et al., 2021). People with avoidant attachment styles may benefit from compassion training (Bolt et al., 2019). The good news is that self-compassion skills training in the context of couple therapy can foster both self-compassion and compassion.

I have been training others in self-compassion, training teachers of self-compassion, and training therapists in how to integrate self-compassion training into psychotherapy for over a decade now. I have seen firsthand the power of self-compassion to heal relational pain in individuals. I have also had a front-row seat to the power of self-compassion to shepherd patients through relationship distress in a way that fosters both greater self-actualization and deeper connection in their relationships. Impressed with the power of self-compassion to spill over into relationships, I developed a program to bring compassion into couple relationships, much of which is also available in my book *Compassion for Couples: Building the Skills of Loving Connection* (Becker, 2023).

My intention in this chapter is to bring together theory, research, and clinical examples to illustrate how the clinical application of self-compassion skills training can be used to foster greater compassion, acceptance, and intimacy in couple relationships. Although I focus here more on couple relationships, these skills can be practically applied to any close relationship, as the therapist deems appropriate.

Research on Self-Compassion and Relational Effects

Although it is common for people to fear that self-compassion training will make them more selfish and negatively impact their relationships, research indicates the opposite is true. Some of the important points that may be reassuring to therapists and patients alike include the following:

Self-Compassion Is Associated with Improved Health and Emotional and Interpersonal Well-Being

Researchers noted decreased negative states, like anxiety and depression, and increases in positive states, such as life satisfaction. Also, people who are high in self-compassion tend to be high in secure attachment and low in insecure attachment (Lathren et al., 2021; Neff & Beretvas, 2012; Neff & Pommier, 2013; Yarnell & Neff, 2013).

Self-Compassion May Be Contagious

A study by Miller and Kelly (2020) had college students watch a video of another student practicing self-compassion around an academic failure and noted that those who watched the intervention video were more self-compassionate around their academic failure than those in the control group who watched a control video. Thus, when we witness others practicing self-compassion, it may increase our tendency toward self-compassion.

Self-Compassion as a Mediator between Insecure Attachment and Relationship Quality

Self-compassion was a stronger predictor of positive relationship behavior than attachment style. Higher levels of self-compassion were associated with greater relationship satisfaction both for the individual and for their partner. High self-compassion was associated with secure attachment. Low self-compassion was associated with preoccupied and fearful attachment styles, and there was no significant correlation with the dismissive style (Neff & Beretvas, 2012). Another study also found that self-compassion was a mediator between insecure attachment and relationship quality (but notably not relationship satisfaction), and the authors suggest that individuals who are anxiously attached may benefit from strengthening the flow of compassion to the self, whereas individuals who are avoidantly attached might benefit from strengthening the flow of compassion to others (Bolt et al., 2019).

Self-Compassion and Relationship Skills

Among other effects, self-compassion increased perspective taking, supporting the autonomy needs of one's partner, conflict resolution, forgiveness, and increased compromise while, at the same time, decreased self-sacrificing (Lathren et al., 2021; Neff & Beretvas, 2012; Neff & Pommier, 2013; Yarnell & Neff, 2013).

Self-Compassion Training in Couple Therapy

As a therapist, you may be thinking that it's a good idea to incorporate self-compassion training into your work with couples but also wondering how you might go about it. The following discussion illustrates a pathway clinicians can take in helping couples train in the skills of self-compassion while simultaneously increasing compassion in the relationship.

The Role of the Therapist

The way the therapist shows up is a model for how couples can begin to show up for each other. When the therapist embodies compassion while interacting with each partner, especially concerning relational patterns, partners begin to glimpse new ways of relating to each other. When the therapist demonstrates a nonjudgmental warmth, understanding, and acceptance toward each person while simultaneously firmly interrupting unhelpful couple behavior patterns, couples witness new ways to relate to each other. Rather than sit back and watch how the relationship patterns play out, the therapist actively intervenes when unhelpful patterns emerge in situ, helps the couple understand their pattern (more on that later), and offers suggested alternatives. The therapist embodies both the soft front of compassion by validating, comforting, and soothing, and the strong back of compassion by protecting the couple from harming each other in session, motivating them to try a new approach, and providing them with skillful alternatives. Through it all, the therapist demonstrates humility along with the attitudes of curiosity and flexibility, helping couples find their unique path to self-compassion rather than trying to fit them into some self-compassion formula. Accordingly, the exercises and examples in this chapter are intended to inspire possibilities for working with couples, rather than a rigid prescription.

The Role of Self-Compassion in Couples Work

One advantage to self-compassion training in the context of couple therapy is that it doesn't allow for a fixation solely on one's suffering. While true self-compassion always includes others through the component of common humanity, individuals in couple therapy can become fixated on their suffering to the exclusion of their partner's suffering. When we train in self-compassion in the context of couple therapy, the partner's suffering is always present and equally validated, and common humanity is experienced directly.

Self-compassion "dissolves the self," as my colleague, Chris Germer, often says (personal communication, July 27, 2021). This is because when we open fully to our suffering, we begin to understand the nature of suffering itself. Suffering isn't about "me" anymore. Rather, as in Rumi's *Guest House* poem (as cited in Germer & Neff, 2019), suffering is a visitor. And we begin to see that suffering visits everyone from time to time, including our partners. Being more familiar with the nature of suffering, it becomes easier to spot it in others and having trained in self-compassion we begin to have some notion of the types of things that may help to relieve suffering in others. In this way, self-compassion helps us build a foundation for compassion in our relationships. Importantly, self-compassion also provides the resiliency needed to engage in a relationship and take the risk of being vulnerable.

Learning self-compassion, however, is also a vulnerable endeavor. Not everyone is willing to engage in the process of learning self-compassion. Germer and Neff (2019), founders of the mindful self-compassion (MSC) program, note several blocks to learning and practicing self-compassion. Couples are often more willing to engage in treatment to enhance their relationship than they are to learn self-compassion directly. A recent study on the compassion for couples (CFC) program (which trains compassion at the systems level, as described later in this chapter) found that training-group participants experienced an increase in self-compassion that is statistically significant relative to a control group. Furthermore, the majority of males in the sample reported being invited to the program by, attending fewer previous trainings than, and being significantly less familiar with self-compassion than their female partners. These differences between partners may suggest that couple-based trainings can successfully train self-compassion in individuals who might not be personally motivated to seek out an education on self-compassion (Welch, 2023). Just as an increase in self-compassion can have a positive impact on the family system, an increase in compassion in the family system may have a positive impact on one's self-compassion. The following reflects a systems approach to training compassion in psychotherapy, thereby increasing self-compassion in both partners.

Compassion-Focused Therapy Sets the Stage

Therapists can introduce self-compassion skills training to couples, by first helping them understand the way human brains are wired to respond to stress, care for each other, and achieve their goals (see Chapter 2). Paul Gilbert (2015), the developer of compassion-focused therapy, discusses the evolutionary development of three emotion regulation systems: threat/defense, care/soothing, and drive. Threat/defense is the system that gets activated when we perceive danger. We move into fight–flight–freeze mode to restore safety. However, these actions don't usually foster more safety in our relationships. Alternately, we move into the drive system to fix ourselves, our partners, and our relationships. However, people don't generally appreciate being "fixed" by their partners (which implies they are broken). Rather, we want to feel safe and connected, which happens in the care/soothing system. The model can be useful in helping people see and understand the stress responses and compassion, and how the ways our brains are wired can get us into various difficulties (like fighting or withdrawing when we don't like something our partner has said or done, rather than staying present with compassion). Or as Gilbert sometimes calls this, "our tricky wiring," which often leads us away from our desired outcomes. Gilbert notes that our tricky wiring is "not your fault, but it is your responsibility" and emphasizes the importance of training our brains through mindfulness and compassion (Gilbert & Choden, 2015; see Chapter 13 to read about Gilbert's tricky brain).

Introducing the Three Components of Self-Compassion

My approach to integrating self-compassion training into couple therapy is based on my experience with couples in the CFC program, as well as my experience as a compassion trainer and a couple therapist. The CFC program integrates Gilbert's work with the MSC skills-training model to introduce self-compassion training in couple relationships. Researcher and co-developer of the MSC program, Kristin Neff operationalized the components of self-compassion: mindfulness, common humanity, and kindness (Germer & Neff, 2019). Notably, all must be present for it to be self-compassion. Let's take a closer look at how each of these three components can be utilized to help foster compassion in couples and other relationships.

Mindfulness

Mindfulness is a state of balanced awareness. Based in the present moment, it sees things as they are without adding on additional layers of judgment, reactivity, or other distress, and also without numbing ourselves or otherwise closing our vision. We cannot offer compassion without seeing and opening to distress—however, focusing only on the distress undermines our resilience and ability to be present with suffering. In working with relationship distress, mindfulness can be especially helpful in two ways: restoring safety and fostering wisdom.

Mindfulness Practices to Restore Safety. Mindfulness practices like soles of the feet, awareness of breath, and even mindful walking (especially in nature; Germer & Neff, 2019) can be helpful when we find ourselves overwhelmed. We can use mindfulness practices to come safely into the moment so that our physiology can recover. One way mindfulness can be useful with couples (or individuals) in the therapist's office is by inviting them to focus on an external object, such as a tree outside the window, and to describe, in detail, what they see. Placing their attention on a safe object outside of themselves allows their physiology to settle rather quickly. The therapist can help patients find the particular object of attention that feels safe for each patient, presenting it as a way to manage the stress response. The goal of using mindfulness in this way is not to get rid of one's feelings; opening to feelings is necessary in caring for ourselves and our partners. Rather, having a way to toggle back and forth between opening to our suffering and grounding in safety fosters gradual opening in a way that feels safer, and more approachable. And patients are better able to tend to that suffering.

Cultivating Wisdom: Mindfulness of Relational Patterns. When patients can begin to widen their perspective and more clearly comprehend what's happening, wisdom can emerge. From that nonreactive place, couples can become curious and explore—they start to ask what tends to trigger reactivity in us. What triggers reactivity in our partners? And what actions do we and our partners take when we get caught in that reactive place? What kind of relational pattern arises? Becoming curious about these things and holding them in the context of our human wiring is often the first step toward changing a downward relational spiral into an upward spiral.

As noted above, fostering awareness of relational patterns begins by introducing Gilbert's (2015) work on evolution and emotion regulation systems (see Chapter 2). The therapist can open up the topic by saying something like

> "I can see that you are both caught in a painful dynamic that has its roots in stress reactivity and our human wiring. I'd like to take a moment and share some information about how we are wired, how that can get in our way, and how we can find our way to being safely connected. Would that be okay with you?"

Most couples find that agreeable. The therapist can share a visual depiction of the systems (Gilbert & Choden, 2015), explaining them and pointing out how the order of the systems matters. Most importantly, therapists can also describe the types of behaviors we often exhibit when in each of these systems and how these behaviors can manifest in relationships. (See Becker, 2023, for a comprehensive exploration of this topic.)

The therapist can suggest that the threat/defense system is characterized by fight–flight–freeze, where fight turns into attacking or defending, flight turns into withdrawal or avoidance, and freeze turns into confusion or placating. As Gilbert (Gilbert & Choden, 2015) notes, we often recruit the drive system in an attempt to get out of the pain of the threat/defense system. Toward this end, we move into trying to fix the problem, control the situation, or fix our partners (which our partners experience as criticism). Neither the behaviors in the threat/defense system (attacking/defending, withdrawing/avoiding, and placating) nor those in the drive system (fixing, controlling, and criticizing) are likely to be helpful to our partners. Rather, these behaviors can make our partners feel less safe, activate their threat/defense systems, and foster a negative downward spiral.

The therapist can then note that when we open to the pain and each other and meet it with kindness, care system behaviors, such as noticing, allowing, holding, befriending, comforting, soothing, validating, and so on, can emerge. These care system behaviors foster safety for our partners, leading to increased authenticity and vulnerability, and ultimately increased intimacy. This is what we try to cultivate in our relationships, and when couples learn the skills of activating the care system, the whole landscape of the relationship shifts.

This psychoeducation helps them take a more accurate view of their patterns in a way that defuses the shame and blame so often present when looking at our unskillful behaviors. After explaining the systems and normalizing this by emphasizing that, this is how our human wiring for survival manifests—the therapist can ask each of them to name their go-to strategies. And then as therapists go along in couples work, they can interrupt negative relational patterns as they begin to arise and ask them which system they think they are caught in. Over time, they begin to understand each other's unskillful behaviors through the lens of these systems, rather than taking it personally. This de-escalates situations when they are held in the context of what Gilbert (Gilbert & Choden, 2015) refers to as our "tricky wiring." And it creates a pause that allows couples to break the reactivity of the threat/defense system and move toward the care system.

Following the psychoeducation on the affect regulation systems, therapists can help couples identify their strategies by offering them Practice P.1, "Exercise to Help Identify Relational Patterns," in the Appendix. The therapist can introduce the exercise by saying something to the effect of, "I'd like to offer you a way to identify your relational pattern. Would you be willing to try the exercise?" The therapist then offers the exercise as a guided reflection, or as a written exercise, depending on what the therapist deems most appropriate for the particular couple. Following the exercise, the therapist discusses the findings with the couple and encourages them to understand these patterns, unskillful as they may be, in the context of our human wiring and each partner's attempt to restore safety. Having done the exercise with couples in session, and identified and discussed the findings, the therapist can reference these patterns when they arise in situ with the couple. Couples are also invited to continue to notice which system they are in while relating to their partners and the effect it has on their partners.

Clinical Vignette: Mindfulness

Sam and Susie[1] were a good example of how this unfolds. I'd been seeing them in couple therapy for some time. One day, I got a text from Susie. She wanted to let me know that her biopsy was positive—she had cancer. I called her back right away and, as I acknowledged and felt the impact of the diagnosis on her, she mentioned she hadn't told Sam yet. A few days later, Sam and Susie were in my office for a session. Things were really difficult for them and Sam was upset that he wasn't the first person that Susie had called.

Susie was also upset. She explained that when Sam found out, he went into "fix-it mode." He called in all his connections to find the best treatment center for her. He got a copy of the pathology report and consulted with family and friends who were doctors about the type of cancer she had, the available treatments, and the prognosis. He let her know that her prognosis looked good. He was like a tornado of "helpfulness." Only Susie wasn't finding it helpful at all. Quite the opposite, she felt simultaneously bombarded and discarded. She felt like a broken toy that needed to be fixed. She wondered if he would discard her if it turned out she wasn't easy to fix. She needed some space to breathe and feel her feelings before deciding on her course of action. She was scared. What Susie needed first was for Sam to hold the very scary feelings with her. That way, she wouldn't be alone with them.

I could see a downward relational spiral was at play, so I interrupted them. With kindness and understanding, I pointed out to Sam that he had gone into fix-it mode. I wondered what was underneath that fix-it mode and what vulnerable feelings had been activated. To his credit, he was able to redirect toward his vulnerable feelings. He explained how scared he was of losing Susie, how she was the center of his life, and how, having recently lost a sibling, he didn't think he could bear another loss. As Sam landed more fully in his fear, Susie finally felt permission to talk about her fear. Her fear of dying, her fear of treatment, her fear of being too much for Sam, and how she feared he might discard her—it all came tumbling out. This time, instead of fixing Susie, Sam was able to be present with her. He comforted her as he looked into her eyes and reassured her that he wasn't leaving and he'd be there for her. I could see the effects on both of them. Their bodies softened and they leaned closer together as he held her hand. They shared some tears. It was still a difficult path ahead, but now they had each other. Sam softened when Susie explained that she had waited to tell him because she was afraid that he'd go into fix-it mode. Sam now knew what Susie needed. She needed him, his presence, his strength, his vulnerability, and his reassurance (adapted from Becker, 2023).

---

[1] All clinical vignettes have both names and details changed to protect anonymity.

When couples become more aware of these emotion regulation systems and see their patterns, it helps them to see more clearly and hold their distress more mindfully; one that opens to the distress, holds it in a larger context, and meets it with a warm presence. You can find a reflection I often offer couples to help them identify their relational patterns in Practice P.1, "Exercise to Help Identify Relational Patterns," in the Appendix.

Common Humanity

It's Our "Tricky Wiring." Common humanity, the second component of self-compassion as defined by Neff (Germer & Neff, 2019), refers to the universal aspect of suffering. This is an important aspect of cultivating compassion in couples as it helps couples see and understand how their relational behaviors are activated, how they lead to distress in their partner and their relationship, and to hold that discovery in the context of our "tricky wiring" and desire to restore safety. Couples feel less shame about the unskillful behaviors they sometimes exhibit. This increases the individual and collective capacity to tend to what is needed.

Just Like Me. One of the most important aspects of common humanity in couple therapy is what Thupten Jinpa (2015) refers to as "just like me." As couples hear their partners discover their relational patterns, there is an opportunity to see each other differently. Rather than taking their partner's behavior as a sign that they aren't loved, aren't important, or as a sign their partner thinks poorly of them, they can simply see it as a reflection of the system their partner is caught in. They realize that "just like me," my partner gets caught in their threat/defense and drive systems and is sometimes unskillful.

It's Not about Me. When one can see that their unskillful behavior is a reflection of the system they are caught in and not about how much they care about their partner, they begin to see their partner's unskillful behavior is about *the state their partner is in*, ***not*** a reflection on them, or how much their partner cares about them. It sometimes takes time for patients to recognize this, but when they do, it changes everything. Often, it leads to wanting to come closer and offer soothing and reassurance to their partner. I say "often," rather than always, because we do not want to tolerate harm. So, if the partner is doing something harmful, it is necessary to set limits and boundaries. Compassion doesn't tolerate harm. It skillfully sets limits and boundaries from a place of understanding the behavior as a reflection of the suffering the partner is in, rather than assuming it is a personal affront. So, how do we unpack this in therapy?

After helping partners uncover their own unskillful behaviors, couples are invited to reflect on whether that behavior was a reflection of how much they care about their partner. One way to invite this reflection is by using Practice P.2, "Exercise to Help Foster Common Humanity—Just Like Me," in the Appendix. The therapist can introduce the exercise by saying something like

> "Just as it was helpful to identify how your survival wiring can lead to unskillful behaviors with each other as we did in the prior exercise, it can also be helpful to reflect on what that behavior does and doesn't mean when it arises. Would you be willing to try another exercise with me?"

The exercise can be offered in the same session as the prior exercise, or in a later session. Again, the exercise can be offered as a guided reflection or as a written exercise and should be discussed with each other for maximum benefit. The entire exercise can be done in about 10 minutes and is usually more beneficial when done as a whole exercise, rather than just pulling out one question, but again, therapists can use their discretion as to which way works best with any particular couple. Having done the exercise and discovered that their partners' behavior is simply a reflection of their suffering—not a reflection of how much their partner loves them—the therapist can refer back to this learning by asking them to reflect similarly on situations that present in situ. When therapists intervene with this exercise, the negative downward spiral is interrupted, allowing for compassion for self and others to arise. This is often a profound shift in the treatment, untangling them from themselves and opening them to each other.

Clinical Illustration: Common Humanity

Jake and Stella were discussing a situation that happened the prior evening. Stella was upset because when she told Jake how angry she was that he let her down, he said he was going out and left her home alone with her feelings. Jake explained that he felt criticized by the way Stella was talking to him and he left to avoid saying something he would later regret, so he and the relationship wouldn't be further injured. Jake was able to say that he had been caught in the threat/defense system and withdrew. I asked Stella to name the system she was caught in. She could see she was also caught in the threat/defense system and was blaming in hopes that it would help correct the situation. I noted that even though both behaviors were an attempt to gain more safety, they had the opposite effect. Then I asked them to close their eyes and reflect on what was happening to them when they were caught in the threat/defense system and, even though they were upset with each other, whether they still loved their partner and wanted to be in a good relationship with them. Both were able to see that, though they'd been upset with their partner at that moment, it was only because their partner, and this relationship, was so important to them that they'd felt threatened in the first place. So I asked them to consider the possibility that their partner also loved them, and that's why their threat defense system was activated. Was it possible that their partner's behavior was more a reflection of the fear that they would lose that love than a reflection of whether they were loved? I could see each of them soften. As they opened their eyes and looked at each other again, they began to talk about how scared they each were and what they needed, and they were able to meet each other's fears with care and understanding.

Kindness

Comforting and Soothing in Difficult Times. The third component of self-compassion is kindness, treating oneself with care, understanding, and support, which also involves a willingness to take action in support of oneself. This is a good place to introduce a self-compassion practice, like Practice P.3, "Self-Compassion Break," in the Appendix. It's important when introducing this practice that neither partner is in their threat/defense system. It is also important to invite them to call to mind a situation that is causing them stress but doesn't involve their partner. Again, it is important to talk with couples about their experience of the practice. This helps them discover which part of the practice was most helpful: mindfulness, common humanity, or kindness through touch or words. Fostering awareness of what comforts and soothes them builds resilience and takes the pressure off of their partner, which often leads to their partner being more willing to turn toward them in difficult times. Once couples have the experience of comforting and soothing themselves, therapists can invite the use of the practice in moments when relational distress arises in situ.

It is surprising how little couples know about how to comfort and soothe each other. When talking about the care system, the therapist can invite a discussion about what comforts and soothes each of them. Some of us are soothed by a kind touch, some by reassuring words, some by having someone listen to them, and still others like company without talking, like taking a walk together. There are many paths to kindness. The problem is that most of us give our partner the thing we find comforting, rather than what they find comforting. Practice P.4, "Exercise to Foster Kindness," in the Appendix, can help couples find what is truly comforting to their partner. This exercise can be done as a guided reflection or a written exercise and therapists will find it most helpful to do the entire exercise with couples, rather than pulling out a single question. The power of the exercise comes from unpacking the learning with couples. Then, as the couple's therapy progresses, the therapist can remind the couple to consider what their partner would find comforting and soothing. The clinical illustration below illustrates the relief that can arise for individuals when they discover what their partner *actually* wants and needs.

Clinical Illustration: Kindness

I led Alex and Amrita in a compassionate listening exercise (see Becker, 2023, for the full exercise). In this exercise, partners take turns speaking and listening for 5 minutes. The speaker just listens, then has another 5 minutes to ask questions of the speaker for clarity. There is no discussion, just practice in speaking with compassion and listening with compassion. Once completed, I asked the couple how it went for them. Alex was bursting with excitement. "That's what she wants?!" he remarked, grinning from ear to ear. He then went on to explain that he always felt like he had to fix her problems for her. Discovering how much it meant to her that he'd just listened and cared about what she said was an enormous relief for him. Amrita was also smiling; it was a relief for her too. Alex was grateful that he finally knew what she wanted, he finally knew how to be successful in his relationship with her.

Strengthening the Foundation of Kindness. Finally, cultivating a practice of partner appreciation can help foster kindness and a safe connection. It helps to keep the appreciation about small things, like gratitude for their partner bringing them coffee in the morning. The formula therapists can use is "When you ___________, I feel ___________, thank you." For extra credit they can also name the positive quality in their partner that reflects. For example, "When you bring me coffee in the morning, I feel important to you and loved. Thank you. It shows your kind nature." Therapists can invite couples to take out their calendars and schedule partner appreciation times. For many couples, especially couples that are very reactive and in distress, we start each session with two notes each. It's amazing how a short practice like this can take them out of the reactivity of the threat/defense system and prime them for the care system. Sessions that begin this way have a different feel.

Conclusion

Helping couples foster the skills of compassion for themselves and each other through training in mindfulness, common humanity, and kindness can help couples move from relationship distress to resilience. When we learn to meet ourselves, our partners, and our relationships with care and understanding, our relationships become a shelter in the storm. In couple therapy, the therapist offers the couple what they want the partners to offer each other. Rather than "fixing" the couple, the therapist meets each partner and the relationship, just as they are, allowing themselves to be curious. With an attitude of understanding, acceptance, and warmth, the therapist uses their understanding of the factors and skills that lead to healthy relationships to help the couple find their unique way of embodying compassion in their relationship, emphasizing the importance of customizing practices to suit them.

The therapist takes an active stance, interrupts reactivity and downward relational spirals, offering a path toward the care system instead. The central question in self-compassion is "What do I need right now?" In guiding couples in compassion training the question is "What do you need right now?" followed by guiding the couple in finding practices that suit them. Offering couples psychoeducation and the skills of compassion through a focus on mindfulness, common humanity, and kindness helps couples drop their defensive strategies, see the good in each other and themselves, and relate to each other from a place of care and understanding, even when setting limits with each other. We and our partners don't need to be perfect to be loved. Nor is there a perfect path to cultivating compassion for every couple. When therapists develop their self-compassion practice and identify the patterns in their relationships with close others, the capacity to shepherd couples through the sometimes-rocky path from relational pain to resilience becomes readily available. Therapists can use the *Compassion for Couples* (Becker, 2023) book as a guide for couple skill training.

REFERENCES

Becker, M. (2023). *Compassion for couples: Building the skills of loving connection.* Guilford Press.

Bolt, O. C., Jones, F. W., Rudaz, M., Ledermann, T., & Irons, C. (2019). Self-compassion and compassion towards one's partner mediate the negative association between insecure attachment and relationship quality. *Journal of Relationships Research, 10*, e20, 1–9.

Geller, S. M. (2017). *A practical guide to cultivating therapeutic presence.* American Psychological Association.

Germer, C. K., & Neff, K. (2019). *Teaching the mindful self-compassion program.* Guilford Press.

Gilbert, P., & Choden, K. (2015). *Mindful compassion: Using the power of mindfulness and compassion to transform our lives.* Constable & Robinson.

Jinpa, T. (2015). *Fearless heart: How the courage to be compassionate can transform our lives.* Hudson Street Press.

Lathren, C., Rao, S., Park, J., & Bluth, K. (2021). Self-compassion and current close interpersonal relationships: A scoping literature review. *Mindfulness, 12*(5), 1078–1093.

Miller, K., & Kelly, A. (2020). Is self-compassion contagious? An examination of whether hearing a display of self-compassion impacts self-compassion in the listener. *Canadian Journal of Behavioral Science, 52*(2), 159–170.

Neff, K., & Beretvas, N. (2012). The role of self-compassion in romantic relationships. *Self and Identity, 12*(1), 78–98.

Neff, K., & Pommier, E. (2013). The relationship between self-compassion and other-focused concern among college undergraduates, community adults, and practicing meditators. *Self and Identity, 12*(2), 160–176.

Shaver, P. R., Mikulincer, M., Sahdra, B., & Gross, J. (2016). Attachment security as a foundation for kindness toward self and others. In K. W. Brown & M. R. Leary (Eds.), *The Oxford handbook of hypo-egoic phenomena* (pp. 223–242). Oxford Academic.

Welch, A. C. (2023). *Compassion for couples: An initial evaluation of an online self-compassion training for couples*. Doctoral dissertation, Florida State University. ProQuest Dissertations and Theses Global.

Yarnell, L., & Neff, K. (2013). Self-compassion, interpersonal conflict resolutions, and well-being. *Self and Identity, 12*(2), 146–159.

18

Self-Compassion and Teens

Lisa Shetler
Lorraine M. Hobbs

Adolescence is a tender and unique period of life. As such, teaching teens self-compassion requires sensitivity, nonjudgment, acceptance, and most importantly, embodied presence. This chapter discusses how to integrate self-compassion training into a therapeutic context to help teens build resources and skills to face challenges and promote self-care.

How Self-Compassion Helps Teens

It is widely accepted that adolescence begins with puberty and ends around ages 24–25, with some noting that adolescence now begins as early as ages 10–11. Specific changes in personal, social, and neurophysiological development differentiate this stage from other phases of development. Consequently, this differentiation in maturity and emotional health may influence a teen's ability or willingness to embrace self-compassion.

Kristin Neff (2011), a pioneering researcher in this field, conceptualized self-compassion as having three distinct components: (1) self-kindness versus self-criticism, (2) mindfulness versus overidentification, and (3) common humanity versus isolation. A closer look at these three components reveals the potential for self-compassion to guide teens to cultivate and integrate a healthier state of well-being.

Self-Kindness versus Self-Criticism

Adolescence is a time of reconstruction when teens are taking steps toward independent living and shifting their attachment from their parents to a peer group. They typically struggle with issues of confidence, social comparison, and fitting in. Their self-worth, often based on their self-esteem, fluctuates based on performance and can leave teens feeling "not good enough." Self-compassion and self-kindness can help stabilize the emotional ups and downs of adolescence, especially as teens struggle with discovering who they are and finding their voice versus identifying with the voice of the inner bully.

Mindfulness versus Overidentification

Jon Kabat-Zinn (2013) defines this second component, mindfulness, as "cultivated by paying close attention to your moment-to-moment experience while, as best you can, not getting caught up in your ideas and opinions, likes and dislikes" (p. 21), which can be particularly beneficial for teens who struggle with anxiety, attention deficit, or other neurological disorders. Mindfulness can train attention, interrupt overidentification, and increase awareness of the inner chatter or storyline that often perpetuates suffering. Furthermore, mindfulness can also improve interoceptive body awareness, leading to better cognitive and emotional functioning, a healthier perspective on life, and the skills to recover from emotional turmoil.

Common Humanity versus Isolation

Adolescence is a time of uncertainty and isolation, making the third component, common humanity, particularly relevant to this stage of life. It is a time when many teens experience disconnection, often exacerbated by digitalization and social media. In this very tumultuous time, teens need to know they are not alone, that other teens face similar challenges, and that suffering is part of life. Common humanity can help foster a deeper connection to self, others, and humanity, and can help bridge the gap created by a world that marginalizes individuals and groups that don't fit the norm.

Working in the Window of Adolescent Development

The Reconstruction Process

During this developmental period, the brain begins pruning away the things it no longer needs and forming new connections as it learns the skills needed for adulthood (Siegel, 2015). The teenage brain is under major reconstruction, a bit like a house undergoing renovation. Imagine a room that was fit out and decorated just right for a young child, that is now undergoing major change to suit the style and needs of a young adult. In time, the completed project will be impressive and have the latest technology and all kinds of new furniture and features. However, during the renovation phase, the room is a mess, nothing works as it should, and it's difficult to imagine the result. Parents might similarly describe teens: as a bit of a mess, inconsistent, and difficult to see how they are going to become functional adults! Keeping these ideas of reconstruction and renovation in mind, we can begin to appreciate the immense effort required for growth and maturation through the teenage years. Teens are simultaneously capable and dependent, holding on to some things from the past while trying to make way for the new. All the while they're comparing themselves to those around them and wondering whether they are "good enough." It can be a challenging time for both teens and those around them.

Once the renovation and construction process concludes, we hope that the finished product (the young adult) is more cohesive and better equipped for the demands of adult life. Part of this process involves young people engaging in social comparison with their "real-life" peers and with the global, social space of "influencers," mass media, and cultural norms and expectations. Throughout the process, teens are questioning what makes them acceptable and worthy of connection and belonging, and what is likely to lead to their exclusion or failure as human beings. As parents of teens and those working with teens well know, figuring this out often involves teens engaging in a lot of experimentation. It's as if young people are trying things on for size to see what fits. This is all part of the process of individuation and integration.

Many things can support young people through their teenage years with more ease. Not the least of which is a robust support network (Qi et al., 2020), with as many people as you can gather to offer their time, wisdom, skills, presence, and care to the teen. With a good foundation and a good team around them, many teens will have a relatively smooth renovation experience. Unfortunately, for a wide range of reasons, many teens will not. Setbacks and being ill equipped to handle them can give rise to maladaptive ways of coping, relationship difficulties, and mental illness, which can permeate the entire building project with far-reaching effects both in the moment and in the years to come.

Teaching teens self-compassion is more than adding a tool to their toolkit. It is about empowering them with a complete operating system with which they can manage difficulties as they arise in ways that are self-supporting and foster greater connections to others.

Case Vignette

The following case vignette[1] demonstrates the importance of meeting a teen where they are and taking a flexible approach to introducing self-compassion into therapy.

> When I (Lisa) greeted Kyra in the waiting room for the first time, she had all of her defenses up. Arms folded, eyes fixed on the floor, adamant that she didn't need to see me and wasn't going to talk. "No worries," I said, "you don't have to talk." She met my gaze, puzzled. She was attending therapy after all. Her mother, her teachers, and her school counselors had all told her she needed to go and *speak* to someone about her mood and behavior. Kyra had experienced sexual abuse as a child. Her parents were separated, she was frequently in trouble at school, friendships were turbulent, and it was clear that she was suffering from extremely high levels of anxiety. While the need for therapy to address her past trauma was evident, Kyra was underresourced to begin such work. She was unaware of her internal experience and miscued her needs for comfort, reassurance, and acceptance. She had a fierce inner critic that bullied her relentlessly about her appearance, resulting in hours each day being spent on looking "perfect."
>
> As Kyra was not one to "meditate" in the traditional sense, we explored mindful awareness in creative ways: drawing, listening to music, and using the sense of touch to find textures and objects that felt soothing before focusing more on building awareness of thoughts, feelings, and body sensations. We began building a compassionate voice through the use of an imagined compassionate figure—in this case, a celebrity whom Kyra adored and felt would offer her wisdom and comfort. Sessions were spent considering the function of her inner critic and the behaviors that resulted from it bossing her around. We involved Kyra's mother in sessions focused on understanding the protective role her inner critic was playing and how her mother could provide both validation of this while modeling a kinder self-assessment. Communication back to Kyra's school involved sharing insights into the needs that underpinned her behaviors and agreeing to accommodations that helped Kyra feel safer and more supported at school. While the trauma work in therapy was still tough, the foundation of mindfulness and self-compassion increased Kyra's confidence in her ability to cope in the face of pain and more effectively identify, communicate, and meet her needs.
>
> Now very comfortable in therapy, Kyra comes into the room without makeup on, kicks off her shoes, lies on my couch with her feet up, and speaks

[1]The case vignettes presented in this chapter are intended to serve as illustrative examples derived from a variety of cases encountered in clinical practice. These vignettes are crafted to represent typical situations faced when working with teens. To ensure the utmost protection of client confidentiality, all identifying information and personal details have been deliberately altered or fictionalized. Any resemblance to real individuals, living or deceased, is purely coincidental.

openly about the various ups and downs of teenage life. Periodically she'll ask me to do "one of those kindness meditation things" because they help her feel calm and remind her that she's awesome, just as she is.

Mindfulness through Music

Building a teen's capacity for mindful awareness is an integral component of building toward greater interoceptive awareness and self-compassion. As psychotherapists, you can use this music practice to introduce teens to mindfulness and establish greater trust and rapport in the therapeutic relationship.

Exercise 1: Mindfulness through Music[2]

- Invite the client to choose a song that they feel connected to in some way.
- Listen to the song together (perhaps multiple times) and invite awareness of various components: the lyrics, the melody, the beat, individual instruments, and then the song as a whole again.
- Experiment with listening to different versions of the song if possible (e.g., instrumental, remix, acoustic) or print the lyrics to invite awareness of how this impacts the client's experience.
- Inquire about what feelings and sensations arise while the client is listening to the song/reading the lyrics.

Holding Space for Teens

In your role as a therapist, you have the opportunity to help onboard a new operating system that your young clients can carry with them into adulthood. Through your gentle manner, embodied presence, and compassion; your skillful holding of space and thoughtful responding; and your skill in guiding inquiry, you create the conditions needed for a young person to experience a loving connected presence and ultimately cultivate loving-kindness toward themselves.

As therapists, you know the importance of creating a safe space for your clients in which they feel held, heard, and seen. Boundaries are also needed to provide safety and containment at times. This firm but kind approach, along with a good dose of humor, fosters a therapeutic relationship that allows teens to drop their defenses and become more authentic, present, and curious, without fear of judgment or invalidation. While this

[2]See Practice T.1, "Mindfulness through Music," in the Appendix for expanded guidance on leading young clients in this practice.

may all sound fairly standard in regard to creating trust and safety with a client in therapy, it can sometimes be challenging to maintain equanimity when working with teens.

Teenagers can be prickly. They walk around with their walls up and social masks on. They push boundaries, speak their mind, and can lack perspective and experience. In the life of an adolescent, some things change quickly, and other things change painfully slowly. Teens are caught in between the total dependence of childhood, where adults hold a lot of control and are responsible for meeting their needs, and the natural drive for independence. This shift can be both exciting and terrifying and will almost certainly involve some degree of conflict with the key adults in their world. As therapists, you need to balance holding the teen as both capable and responsible for helping themselves and acknowledging that they still need considerable guidance and support.

Case Vignette

The following case vignette is an example illustrating how well self-compassion can be integrated into psychotherapy and can support teen clients in cultivating skills for self-care.

> Now 23 and preparing to move into their own home, I (Lisa) first met Riley when they were 16 years old. Riley had seen many therapists before me and "none of them helped." There was a long list of concerns: severe self-harm, multiple past suicide attempts, past trauma, unstable home life, substance abuse, struggling at school, and most recently, the emergence of a serious eating disorder. By 18, the language of borderline personality disorder was being written on Riley's hospital discharge summaries.
>
> In the early days of seeing Riley, I hadn't yet encountered self-compassion teachings for myself, let alone begun incorporating it into my work. I followed the treatment protocols for dialectical behavior therapy, cognitive-behavioral therapy, acceptance and commitment therapy, and schema therapy—I threw it all at the problem list only to remain feeling frustrated at the lack of progress. Riley remained stuck in a cycle of dysfunction. Just as they would reach a level of relative stability, things would fall into crisis all over again.
>
> After my training in mindful self-compassion and later mindful self-compassion for teens, Riley was one of the first clients I began using the teachings with. For the first time, we started to gain real traction. They stayed out of the hospital, the self-harm was reduced, and they were eating. Over time, Riley's self-talk began to shift, and there was a sense of care for themselves and hope for their future. The language of self-compassion wove itself so easefully among the other therapies we had used and soon became the cornerstone of our work together. It also sustained me as a therapist. In difficult sessions, hearing graphic stories, and sitting with the uncertainty of Riley's safety,

> I found myself taking just one mindful breath, applying kindness for myself and my client, coming back to the present moment and softening, time and time again. Riley reflected one day, "I used to only hear bad voices in my head, then I started hearing your voice—being kind to me, and now I hear my own voice, my own compassionate voice."

A Compassionate Friend

Teens may find it difficult initially to imagine offering themselves kindness. Using a practice such as the one below to invite them to imagine a wise or kind figure that can offer them support is a gentler way of uncovering their own kind inner voice. They may begin by imagining the therapist offering them kindness, as in the case example above, or choose any other figure that feels relevant to them.

Exercise 2: A Compassionate Friend[3]

- Begin by inviting the client to sit or lie down in a position that is comfortable to them.
- Suggest that the client call to mind a time recently in which they felt stressed or upset.
- Now invite the client to summon a wise and kind figure to come and support them through this difficult time.
- Have the client take a moment to imagine what this figure might say or do to bring them comfort. Ask what kind and compassionate words this figure has just for the client.
- Ask the client to notice what it feels like to hear these words from someone who cares for them deeply. Suggest that this kind voice is already within them.
- After the practice, you may invite young clients to journal about or draw their wise and kind figure and the words they found comforting.

Why Do Teens Resist Self-Compassion?

There are many reasons that self-compassion can feel uncomfortable for teens. Resistance is often an indicator of how disempowered and vulnerable teens feel. While learning self-compassion may sound like a good idea to the adults around them, for many teens, it may increase their sense of

[3]Find an expanded version of this guidance in Practice T.2, "Modified 'Compassionate Friend' Practice" in the Appendix.

vulnerability and exposure, feelings of being overwhelmed, or fears of being judged. Remember, teens don't generally arrive on your doorstep voluntarily. They are typically referred to you by parents, school counselors, or doctors because they are struggling in some way, and at least one adult in their lives is paying attention and believes they need help. Avoidance or resistance has likely been a valuable coping strategy that may have provided protection and safety for a teen, and it is unwise to attempt to rob them of this at the outset of therapy. As discussed above, it is essential to first establish psychological safety and trust before beginning to help soften the edges of resistance in a teen and invite discovery of their capacity to turn toward their emotional pain.

Below is a list of behaviors that may indicate resistance in a teen:

- Irritation or anger at what they are being asked to do
- Becoming disruptive
- Shutting down, withdrawing, becoming silent
- Changing the topic
- Blaming others
- Moving into thinking mode
- Rumination or overthinking
- Restlessness and agitation
- Indifference
- Insolence
- Making jokes
- Tightening of the chest, restricted breathing
- A sensation of numbness
- Feeling outside of the body, dissociation

When there is evidence of resistance in the room, therapists can invite awareness of what they are observing, give language to the client's experience, invite reflection on how resistance has served the client well in the past, and gently provide an opportunity to utilize self-compassion as a tool for moving forward.

Meeting Resistance with Self-Compassion

The following are phrases that you can utilize in meeting clients' resistance with compassion and curiosity: "I hear you. I believe you. Thank you for letting me know that you don't want to talk about this right now. I'm not here to make you do anything that you don't want to do"; or our personal favorite, "I can see how this resistance has helped to protect you in the past and I appreciate that it's showing up now to keep you safe in the only way you know how." These are the phrases we frequently use with teens. When resistance shows up, it's telling you something and it's meeting a need for the young person. As a psychotherapist, maintaining your practice becomes integral to your ability to model curiosity, acceptance, patience, and kindness, while allowing the teen to maintain a sense of safety and control. To push against resistance or plow through it, would only rupture the trust and safety of the therapeutic relationship. Instead, we invite the teen to get to know it. We build their capacity for mindful awareness so that they can better notice and communicate about what is arising in their moment-to-moment experience and how the resistance is serving them. Ultimately, we hope to create a greater sense of choice between using an old defense mechanism and the possibility of a new way of responding to their fears, pain, and suffering. At times, due to developmental or environmental circumstances, teens may not be ready or able to completely let go of the safety systems that they have in place. We can still plant seeds of self-compassion through our presence and acceptance of them, meeting them where they are, and inviting them to consider new ways of responding to their experiences.

Case Vignette

The following case vignette shows another way of softening and adapting a self-compassion practice to make it more accessible to a teen with trauma.

> When I (Lisa) arrived at work, everyone was talking about the accident. A child had died. Toby, just 13 years old, was there when it happened. A referral was rushed through to me by well-meaning adults who were certain Toby would need psychological support. He, of course, did. But when I first met him, Toby was jovial, smiling, and keen to tell me about the online game he was into at the moment. By the end of the initial consultation, with no mention of the incident, I gingerly asked whether he knew why he had been referred to me. He stared at me and said, "Not really." I double-checked my notes to ensure that I was seeing the right kid. "I was told you experienced something really traumatic. You haven't been back to school. You're having nightmares about the incident." I could see his body stiffen at my mention of it. "I want you to know that we're not going to talk about that today. In fact, I'm never going to ask you to tell me what happened unless you want to," I said. He relaxed.
>
> In time, we agreed to address the incident. His mom had let me know that he was feeling immense guilt that his friend had died and not him. We had done some work on mindfulness, relaxation, and grounding. Toby had aphantasia, so in place of visualizations, we used music, tactile fidgets, and storyboards to help us. When I asked Toby to think about what happened, he told me firmly that he couldn't remember anything. I told him I believed him. We took some time to learn together about his amazing brain and all the ways that it was protecting him from feeling and experiencing things that were really distressing for him.
>
> In subsequent sessions, Toby began sharing fragments of what happened. We sat together in the awfulness of it. Simply noticing and naming what was present and grounding as needed. Initially, the guilt was too strong to allow for any sort of direct self-compassion practice, but over time I could feel the resistance softening. Toby acknowledged that punishing himself wouldn't change

what had happened. Using the language of "kindness" felt too strong, but "comfort" became more accessible to him as he considered what he would want his friend to receive if the situation were reversed. Learning to cradle one hand within another and rest them gently in his lap, this supportive gesture opened the door to deeper acceptance and comfort of his pain.

Holding Your Own Hand (Modified Soothing Touch)

Teens are not always ready for the array of soothing gestures offered through self-compassion. Therefore, modifying a soothing touch as a simple "holding-your-hand" gesture can be a relief and often is more successful with teens who are experiencing resistance. Such modifications help make the practice more accessible while still providing physical comfort and activating the caring system within the brain.

Exercise 3: Holding Your Own Hand (Modified Soothing Touch)[4]

- Begin by sitting comfortably anywhere you would like.
- Experiment with ways that you can "hold your own hand," perhaps with fingers interlocked, one hand resting on top of another, or whatever feels okay for you.
- Try a few different ways, and then stay with the one that you like best.
- Notice what it's like to support yourself in this way.

Inquiry: A Path to Self-Exploration

Christopher Germer (2009), co-developer of the mindful self-compassion program, describes inquiry as an intimate exchange between a teacher and student that evolves organically over time. This implies that teachers are embodied and fully present in this exchange—that they cultivate an attitude of curiosity, nonjudgment (mindfulness), and warmth (loving-kindness) in order to guide the inquiry process with a teen who may be resistant and vulnerable (see Chapter 10 for more about the inquiry process in psychotherapy).

Inquiry in self-compassion is designed to help teens identify less with the problem or story and build skills in self-care, self-acceptance, and self-kindness. It is present-moment oriented and relies on interoceptive body

[4]See Practice Q, "Holding Your Own Hand Practice (A Modified Soothing Touch)," in the Appendix for the expanded practice.

awareness: the ability to investigate the more subtle layers of emotion and sensation in the body, the purpose of which is to build skills in emotional regulation and resilience (Hobbs & Tamura, 2022). This process of inquiry is rooted in a gentle awareness of the experience and the experiencer. The questions are not "why" questions, as they are in psychotherapy, but questions of "what and how" that are intended to inspire perspective taking and curiosity into what is arising at this moment, not the causes and conditions of a teen's suffering.

The following questions are good examples of inquiry-based questions that are useful in working with teens: "So, how was that?"; "What happened in this exercise? What did you notice or learn?"; and "Is there anything else you noticed, such as a particular physical sensation or perhaps a strong feeling?" These questions support an exploration of what is unfolding in their inner landscape and help to connect a teen to their personal experience so they can begin to identify what they may need in the moment.

It can sometimes be difficult to assess what a teen might need when they withdraw, shut down, or become silent. Silence may be concealing suffering or may indicate that more time is needed to process their current experience. Most teens are uncomfortable if they are in the spotlight for too long. As such, it is wise not to linger in inquiry for too long and to be attuned to your young clients' cues of when to lean in and when to back off.

Compassion for the System

One of the key considerations when working with adolescent clients is the management of multiple relationships, including the teen and all key stakeholders in their life, such as caseworkers, teachers, health professionals, coaches, and others. Often, these investors can have different priorities about what is most urgent or important. At its best, this extended network enhances the available resources and can help to scaffold and support positive change in teens' lives. At its worst, it may be a contributing source of their dysfunction and distress, perpetuating their suffering and hindering their ability to make use of what is offered in therapy.

When you begin working with a teen, time is well spent developing an eco map, considering which relationships are supportive, which areas of their life they are struggling with the most, and determining the things within their control and those that are not. You can then negotiate together who else may need to be physically present during therapy appointments in order to make meaningful changes in their world and whether those people can do what we're asking of them.

Case Vignette

The following vignette shows how self-compassion can be integrated into family therapy and the benefits of showing compassion for the system and yourself in the course of supporting a teen.

> One of my (Lisa) most heartbreaking self-compassion interventions was with a 13-year-old girl with separated parents. She was desperate for a connection with her father. During one of many family therapy sessions involving the teen, her mother, father, and stepmother, this young girl bravely and tearfully told her parents that she was depressed and suicidal, unable to continue living in the hostility between her mom and dad.
>
> The invitation was for her parents to increase kindness and compassion toward each other and their daughter. The father flatly refused. My heart began racing, a mix of panic and anger. "I'm telling you that your daughter is desperate for a relationship with you and would rather die than keep living like this, and you're telling me that you refuse to show her warmth and kindness?," I said, pressing my own feet into the floor to ground myself. Her father sat across from me with arms folded across his chest. He looked me square in the eyes and said, "I'm not doing it." I took one mindful breath, drawing on my own self-compassion training and personal practice to assess my internal reaction and options for responding. This man was suffering too, but he was not asking for my help. I stood up, opened the door, thanked him for his time, and calmly excused him and his new wife from the therapy room.
>
> In the sessions that followed, my young client processed the grief of this lost relationship, the rejection, and the lack of care. Self-compassion was the only antidote to this young girl's suffering. She rose valiantly to the challenge of learning to meet her own needs, care for her own broken heart, and lean into relationships that offered comfort and shelter. We frequently revisited the practice of loving-kindness phrases to help her identify what she needed most. We spoke often of common humanity to remind her that she was a human, deserving of love and care just like everyone else. In time, she was able to do the thing that her father could not. She was able to generate forgiveness and kindness toward this person who had rejected her. She was also able to make use of self-compassion to meet her own needs while continuing to live in an underresourced system. Yes, teens can be challenging to work with at times, but their flexibility and capacity for change is truly remarkable.

Thankfully, many families are both willing and capable of learning and growing alongside their teens. Supporting multiple parts of the system around a teen to learn and integrate self-compassion into their lives is likely to lead to better outcomes for the teen. Indeed, if a teen is resistant or not ready to engage in self-compassion-focused therapy, look to the broader system and consider inviting parents, carers, or extended family to engage in self-compassion training. If the family is in a high state of chaos and unable to attend therapy regularly, consider working with the school, sports club, or other community spaces that influence the young person's world. The intention is to try and resource the system around the teen, through psychoeducation and consultation so that wherever they turn with their distress, they are met with a compassionate response. In addition to individual therapy, there is utility in offering teens the opportunity to attend a self-compassion-focused group program to provide extra exposure to the content, so they may truly experience common humanity through connection with other young people who are struggling too.

Risks and Considerations

There are no firm contraindications for using self-compassion with teens—however, consideration of the factors below is prudent to minimize the risk of overwhelm or rejection of the approach. For teens with existing mental illness, the advice here is to assess and treat as normal, using all of your clinical training and expertise, utilizing all of the tools in your therapist toolkit, and drawing heavily from your own personal practice of self-compassion. Before asking clients to come into contact with their pain and suffering, we want to ensure a level of stability in their mental health along with an established understanding and use of mindfulness in daily life. Self-compassion alone cannot take the place of good clinical treatment, risk assessment, and safety planning.

There are a range of mental health conditions that commonly emerge in adolescence. Of particular note are eating-, body-, and gender-related concerns. While the application of self-compassion is highly relevant for these clients, the intense focus on the body as a focal point of awareness, the notion of soothing touch, and even the language of acceptance can be extremely activating due to an often entrenched inner-critical voice, experiences of shame, and potential of trauma stored in the body (Laricchiuta et al., 2023). An individualized approach is needed that caters to a teen's high need for control, along with modification of the language and focal points of common practices, such as body scans and soothing gestures, to make them more accessible. Inviting curiosity about the teen's experience and experimenting with what words or gestures feel comfortable to them, along with ways in which they already practice self-care, is as much about engaging them in the practice of self-compassion as any formal meditation.

Difficulties can arise with teens who overidentify with their illness or symptoms, or where there is secondary gain either for them as an individual or within their family system, to remain in distress or display distress in a certain way. Some teens may tell you that they find self-compassion to be an invalidation of the legitimacy of their struggle. They may be skeptical and opposed to learning that the path to wellness involves accepting and befriending their experiences, especially when they believe strongly that their pain is intolerable and expect the therapist to collude with their perceived need to be rid of it. As a clinician, you may need to spend additional time orienting teens to the mindset of "acceptance," establishing that this doesn't mean passive resignation of how things are and ensuring that they truly understand the balance between actively creating change where they can in their lives and in the world *and* softly holding and comforting themselves when pain is present.

Similarly, for clients who are prone to suicidality, therapists need to be mindful of continuing to monitor risk, as they may perceive acceptance of suffering as confirmation that they will never be rid of their pathology. Suicidal teens may be unable, as a result of their neurodevelopmental limitations, to imagine having a different relationship to their negative thoughts and feelings and may be unwilling to live with their distress. Ongoing risk assessment and safety planning remain important as you work with young people to build a sense of hope for their future and skills in meeting their pain in new ways.

Conclusion

Self-compassion is arguably one of the most valuable skills we can offer teens who are growing up in a challenging and constantly changing world. Teens are prone to feel things more intensely and don't yet have reliable healthy internal resources available to them to cope. This combination can fuel a myriad of mental health difficulties, all of which will benefit from increased awareness, kindness, and a sense of belonging.

As you as a therapist move forward in bringing self-compassion into your clinical practice with teens, we emphasize the importance of cultivating and continuing your own personal practice in self-compassion. This foundation ensures that you're teaching from a place of embodied presence and also supports and sustains you in this sometimes challenging work.

As teens move toward individuation and independent living, the skills of self-compassion can be a lifelong resource that will support healthy relationships, good decision making, and the ability to respond in skillful ways to the challenges they will face as adults. Teens need to know that the promise of self-compassion is in recognizing their suffering and responding with kindness, tenderness, and warmth, not to make themselves feel better but because they *are* suffering.

REFERENCES

Germer, C. K. (2009). *The mindful path to self-compassion: Freeing yourself from destructive thoughts and emotions.* Guilford Press.

Hobbs, L., & Tamura, N. (2022). *Teaching self-compassion to teens.* Guilford Press.

Kabat-Zinn, J. (2013). *Full catastrophe living.* Bantam Dell.

Laricchiuta, D., Panuccio, A., Picerni, E., Biondo, D., Genovesi, B., & Petrosini, L. (2023). The body keeps the score: The neurobiological profile of traumatized adolescents. *Neuroscience and Biobehavioral Reviews, 145,* 105033.

Neff, K. (2011). *Self-compassion: The proven power of being kind to yourself.* Morrow.

Qi, M., Zhou, S.-J., Guo, Z.-C., Zhang, L.-G., Min, H.-J., Li, X.-M., & Chen, J.-X. (2020). The effect of social support on mental health in Chinese adolescents during the outbreak of COVID-19. *Journal of Adolescent Health, 67*(4), 514–518.

Siegel, D. J. (2015). *Brainstorm: The power and purpose of the teenage brain.* Tarcher/Penguin.

19

Mindfulness and Self-Compassion for Chronic Pain

Ronald D. Siegel

It's easy to see why the urge to escape pain is one of our most basic instincts. Having an inclination to avoid sharp stones, painful falls, and toxic foods obviously helped our ancestors to survive and pass on their DNA. But as it turns out, this same impulse often traps modern humans in chronic cycles of pain, fear, avoidance, and more pain.

Fortunately, mindfulness and self-compassion can help free us from these cycles. Numerous studies suggest that mindfulness and self-compassion practices indeed help to mitigate the fear and avoidance that lock people into chronic pain and disability. Mindfulness practice has been shown to bring about modest decreases in pain and pain avoidance (Hilton et al., 2017; Pardos-Gascón et al., 2021), while several studies suggest that higher levels of self-compassion are associated with less pain-related anxiety, pain catastrophizing, depression, and disability, as well as greater pain acceptance and success in valued activities (Lanzaro et al., 2021; Torrijos-Zarcero et al., 2021).

Unfortunately, however, mindfulness and compassion practices are often not enough on their own. They typically don't by themselves break people out of chronic pain cycles, allowing them to lead full and rich lives (Sharpe et al., 2024). But when embedded in a comprehensive approach to rehabilitation, they can actually do this. To understand how, this chapter explores the dynamics of chronic pain cycles and ways that mindfulness and self-compassion practices can help interrupt them.

Chronic Pain Cycles

When we humans experience physical pain, we naturally assume that it's due to an injury, illness, or structural abnormality. After all, when we cut or bruise ourselves, the relationship between tissue damage and pain is unmistakable. While most acute pain indeed signals such conditions, countless patients suffer from chronic pain (lasting for several months or longer), which can have little or no relationship to damaged or diseased structures. Instead, they are trapped in cycles in which fear and attempts to avoid pain play central roles.

All mammals share an ancient, sophisticated, fight–flight–freeze emergency response system. When we're threatened, our sympathetic nervous system and hypothalamic–pituitary–adrenal axis are activated, resulting in increased adrenaline in the bloodstream and countless other physiological changes. Respiration, heart rate, body temperature, and muscle tension all increase—the better to flee from danger or fight an enemy.

Imagine, for example, that a bunny grazing in a field notices a fox. It freezes, hoping not to be noticed, while becoming vigilant and physiologically aroused in preparation to run (rabbits aren't big fighters). If the fox wanders off, the rabbit's arousal decreases and its physiology returns to baseline.

But what if the rabbit had a highly evolved cerebral cortex like ours, allowing for complex anticipatory thought? Once the fox left, the rabbit might think, "Will it return?," "Will it find my family?"—not to mention whether it can save up enough carrots for retirement. Such thoughts would continue to activate its fight-or-flight system, which would remain stuck "on."

From Fear to Pain

There are two major ways that this sort of ongoing fear contributes to chronic pain. The first involves muscle tension. Take a moment to act terrified. (Go ahead, ham it up, as though you were in a drama class.) You'll probably notice that your skeletal muscles contract. And tight muscles can be painful—whether it's the aching in our neck and shoulders after a stressful day, or the pain when a calf muscle spasms. If we then become frightened of the pain, our muscles tighten further, creating a vicious cycle. A wide variety of chronic neck, back, jaw, foot, shoulder, knee, pelvic, and chest pain is maintained this way.

Fear also amplifies the subjective experience of pain. In a classic experiment, subjects' hands are placed in ice water. If they're told that the experiment will only last a minute, their pain ratings at 30 seconds are relatively low. If told, however, that they'll need to keep their hands in the ice water for 10 minutes (a more frightening prospect), pain ratings at 30 seconds are much higher.

Countless studies confirm that factors such as pain catastrophizing (Martinez-Calderon et al., 2019), pain avoidance (Meulders, 2019), and conditioned pain anticipation (Meulders, 2020) play central roles in maintaining and amplifying chronic pain.

What about Underlying Medical Conditions?

But what about other causes of pain, such as tumors, infections, or structural damage? This presents a diagnostic challenge. Consider the possible causes of a loud chord from an electric guitar. The chord might be loud because the guitarist is strumming the strings forcefully, or it might be loud because the amplifier is turned up. For many common chronic pain disorders, there's little correlation between what can be observed through medical imaging and the degree to which a person experiences pain. The amplifier (which is strongly affected by our thoughts, feelings, and behavior) is the main problem. But for some individuals, there's actually a strong signal coming from peripheral tissue disturbance. It's therefore often helpful to be agnostic with our patients: "We can't know with certainty the proportion of your pain that's due to psychological and behavioral factors, but they're likely playing a role, and we can work together to reduce them."

Chronic Back Pain as an Example

We can readily see how pain is maintained and amplified in a typical *chronic back pain cycle* (Siegel et al., 2002). The cycle begins with a fundamental misunderstanding. Most patients and, until recently, most health care professionals, have naturally assumed that persistent back pain must be due to damage to the disks or other structures of the spine. Most research findings, however, question this assumption. They point to a lack of correlation between the condition of the spine as revealed by imaging and the presence of pain (Kasch et al., 2022). While structural abnormalities can sometimes be the cause of chronic back pain, in many instances, they are merely coincidental to it. In other cases, they play a role, but the pain is greatly amplified by fear and avoidance.

The chronic back pain cycle can begin with an injury from an accident or overuse or can seem to appear out of the blue, without a clear physical precipitant. Once the pain has persisted longer than expected or reached high levels of intensity, fear becomes a factor. Virtually everyone knows someone with a frightening story of chronic back pain—the prevalence of magnetic resonance imaging, with its ability to reveal variations in spinal structure in great detail, contributes to fear by presenting patients with frightening images of a decaying spine.

This fear can have several problematic effects. Many people abandon physical activities that previously helped to reduce stress, keep their muscles strong and flexible, and provide meaningful engagement in life. Concerns about disability then lead to anxiety, frustration, and anger, all of which further activate the fight-or-flight system. This arousal in turn contributes to muscle tightness, worsening the pain, at the same time that the muscles are deprived of the normal movement that previously helped them relax. Fear, as mentioned earlier, also amplifies the pain sensations coming from tight muscles. A cycle of pain–fear–disability–tension–pain becomes established.

Once a person becomes worried about chronic muscular–skeletal pain, they naturally try to figure out which movements or positions seem to make it better or worse. Every time they engage in an activity they think is damaging, they become more anxious and tense. Increased pain follows, reinforcing the belief that a given action is hazardous. This conditioned reaction, termed *kinesiophobia* (fear of movement), has long been known to be a better predictor of back pain chronicity and disability than medical diagnosis (Bordeleau et al., 2022; Leeuw et al., 2007; Luque-Suarez et al., 2019).

In the same way we try to avoid physical pain, most of us use a variety of strategies to push out of awareness painful thoughts, feelings, images, desires, and memories. But these efforts are usually only partially effective. As one of my clients aptly put it, "When we bury feelings, we bury them alive." Disavowed mental contents are easily reawakened, and when they get close to our awareness, we experience anxiety.

Our propensity to feel anxious when unwanted mental content is aroused is proportional to how much of our experience we've split off or disavowed. Trauma survivors in particular often have many memories, thoughts, and feelings that their minds work to keep out of awareness. And the anxiety they cause, like the fear of movement, can constrict muscles and amplify pain sensations.

The Recovery Cycle

Recovery from chronic pain cycles begins by interrupting them. For most muscular–skeletal pain, this involves a combination of (1) *cognitive restructuring*, (2) *resuming full physical activity*, and (3) *working with negative emotions* in order to address pain-related fear, fear of movement, and fear of unwanted affects (see Siegel et al., 2002, for step-by-step details).

Before beginning a rehabilitation program, patients need a thorough physical examination to rule out potentially serious medical causes of their pain. These disorders, which include tumors, infections, injuries, and unusual structural abnormalities, have long been known to cause only a small percentage of chronic back pain cases (Atlas & Deyo, 2001). For some other types of chronic pain such medical causes are more frequently significant, while for others they play a similarly small role. For all, a medical evaluation is needed to avoid overlooking a treatable medical disorder, to facilitate cognitive restructuring, and to grant trustworthy permission to resume activity when appropriate.

Because many medical providers still don't fully understand the role of psychological and behavioral processes in chronic pain syndromes, they can inadvertently make things worse by offering patients frightening diagnoses—many of which describe in Latin normal changes associated with aging that are not necessarily causing pain. It can therefore be helpful to have patients inquire whether their provider has "evidence that, were I to engage in normal life activities, I'd irreparably damage my body." Since there are now considerable data, particularly in the case of neck and back pain, that it's usually safe to exercise vigorously in the presence of chronic pain (Rainville et al., 2004), many providers respond to this question with permission to move normally.

Mindfulness and Self-Compassion in the Recovery Cycle

Since fear, catastrophic thinking, the avoidance of activity that flows from it, and disavowed difficult emotions play such a central role in chronic pain cycles; mindfulness and self-compassion practices, combined with other strategies, can be very helpful in interrupting them.

Mindfulness for Cognitive Restructuring

The capacity to see thoughts as thoughts, rather than representations of reality, is one of the powerful benefits of mindfulness practice. This metacognitive awareness can support the shift in perspective that's necessary to interrupt chronic pain cycles. It's important to start with psychoeducation about the stress-response system and the role of fear in tensing muscles, disrupting normal body functioning, and amplifying pain sensations. Mindfulness practices can then help patients see these effects in action, noticing how often fearful pain-related thoughts arise (sometimes every few seconds) and how much tension is generated in the body in response (usually a lot). They can help patients observe the interplay among pain, fear, and behavior, illuminating the role that thoughts and emotions play in their suffering.

Case Vignette

Juanita had been suffering from back pain for years. Despite the fact that doctors never found anything more than a mild disk bulge, she was sure that she had a "bad back" and was in constant danger of reinjuring herself. She avoided sitting for more than a few minutes, carrying heavy objects, twisting or bending—convinced that her body couldn't tolerate the stress this put on her spine.

After being introduced to mindfulness during therapy, Juanita took to it—but only lying down. It became much more difficult when she tried practicing in a chair. Her attention constantly went to her lower back, monitoring it for pain. She wanted to get up as soon as she experienced a twinge.

Sticking with the practice, Juanita eventually noticed that her urge to get up was coming more from fear of the pain getting worse than from the intensity of the pain itself. She also saw how her mind would "budget" her chair time, thinking that if she already hurt after 5 minutes, she'd never be able to sit for 20.

Seeing streams of fearful thoughts arise, followed by anxiety, increased muscle tension, and more pain helped Juanita open to the idea that her mind and behavior might be playing a role in her problem. It also helped her see that she didn't need to act immediately on every urge to alleviate discomfort.

Mindfulness can also increase cognitive flexibility. For most patients, it's useful to explain how fear and avoidance maintain and amplify pain. If relevant to their particular diagnosis, it's also helpful to share research studies questioning the connection between pain and tissue damage, and if they're medically cleared, why expanding activity, even if it's painful, will likely aid recovery.

Mindfulness practices can then be used to observe the arising and passing of fearful thoughts. Patients may notice how their minds are full of frightening ideas picked up by doctors, friends, and others. These observations can help them consider that their assumptions about structural damage or disease might be socially conditioned thoughts, not necessarily objective conclusions about reality.

Like Juanita, most people struggling with chronic pain can also be invited to try an exercise such as Practice R.1, "Mindfulness of Pain-Related Thoughts and Feelings," in the Appendix to explore the role of fear and worry in their condition.

Mindfulness and Self-Compassion for Resuming Activity

The second step of the recovery process, resuming normal physical activity if medically permitted, serves many functions. It is an exposure-and-response-prevention intervention for kinesiophobia and fears of disability. Instead of avoiding activity, we work to open to, and befriend, the pain and fear that arises while we pursue it. This provides physical exercise for muscles that have become short and weak and helps reduce psychological stress. Resuming activity helps us begin enjoying our lives again by connecting with others and redirecting our attention from preoccupation with pain and its alleviation to more meaningful pursuits.

When we resume relinquished activities, our pain usually increases initially. This is both because tight, weak muscles are painful to use and because anxiety increases when we do something we fear. Mindfulness practice can help patients move through this difficult step.

Pain Does Not Equal Suffering

There is robust literature, dating back to Melzack and Wall's (1965) famous gate-control theory of pain, which can be expressed in a simple formula: pain × resistance = suffering. It points to the fact that the psychological suffering associated with pain is amplified dramatically by our aversion responses to pain sensations. While one needs to be quite adept at mindfulness practice to not suffer in the presence of extreme pain, even a little practice can help us suffer less from moderate pain.

Learning how to separate aversion responses from pain sensations themselves can go a long way toward increasing pain tolerance. This increased tolerance can allow us to resume normal activities, even if they're painful, thus supporting the active rehabilitation that helps interrupt chronic pain cycles. See Practice R.2, "Separating Pain from Aversion," in the Appendix for a mindfulness and self-compassion practice that can help us see aversion responses as separate from pain sensations, increasing tolerance for discomfort.

Working with pain in this way can help us to tolerate greater levels of discomfort, thereby supporting a much wider range of activity. Also, by bringing attention to the present moment, the anticipatory anxiety that is at the heart of most chronic pain cycles is reduced, lowering muscle tension and reducing the perceived intensity of pain.

Working with Urges to Escape Pain

A major obstacle to reengaging in life activities is the compulsion most of us feel to get rid of the pain. Very often, patients will squirrel up the courage to try a previously relinquished activity, only to feel an uptick in pain, accompanied by an aversion response, and then a strong urge to stop the activity. While for some medical conditions it may make sense to take a rest or back off when pain increases, in many circumstances, the pain is not actually signaling damage to the body, and this avoidance only feeds into fear–pain–avoidance cycles. Waiting for an activity to be pain-free may involve waiting forever.

Mindfulness and self-compassion practices can be used to work directly with counterproductive urges to escape pain. See Practice R.3, "Compassionate Urge Surfing for Pain," in the Appendix, for an exercise constructed to work with pain associated with sitting, yet it can be modified for any activity associated with discomfort.

In addition to learning to surf urges to escape pain with exercises such as this one, many people need regular reminders that uninhibited movement is not dangerous (assuming that this is the case for their condition). Also, to help extinguish conditioned associations between particular activities and pain, it helps to engage in the activity several times weekly for a few weeks, using mindfulness and self-compassion practices to work with any aversion responses that arise. Most people notice fluctuations in pain levels during this period, despite consistency in activity. This helps us realize that the activity itself is safe, further supporting a return to a full life.

Mindfulness and Compassion for Self-Soothing

Living with chronic pain is hard. And when we have no clear options for relief, we often experience fear, frustration, and anger that further tense muscles and amplify pain sensations.

A critical factor in how long this emotional distress persists is our capacity to self-soothe. Developmental trauma survivors and people with problematic attachment histories often have great difficulty self-soothing, since they missed out on caregivers to help them modulate their arousal with a loving, caring presence. They also have reason to think that the world is unsafe, which makes pain more threatening, and they often imagine it will last forever. Without memories of "it's okay, sweetheart" in which to take refuge, distress about pain tends to persist.

While not panaceas, mindfulness and self-compassion practices can help here too. By repeatedly returning attention to the present moment, mindfulness practices provide a refuge from the future-oriented catastrophizing that plays a central role in pain and disability. They also provide a comforting, structured activity that doesn't feed into the spiral of aversion responses, increased pain, and disability. Particularly if learned in the context of a supportive therapeutic relationship, and perhaps offered for home practice with an audio recording of the therapist's voice, mindfulness practices can also connect patients to a sense of safe, soothing social connection. A focused attention practice can help to stabilize the mind, adding to a sense of safety.

Self-compassion practices can also help provide the soothing that people in chronic pain need. Self-kindness can serve as an antidote to the self-critical narratives that often come with the territory: "I never should have shoveled the snow"; "I should have gone to the doctor sooner"; or "I shouldn't have listened to that surgeon—I had a bad feeling about them."

Connecting to common humanity can also help. Considering all the people in the world right now who are also in pain, while daunting, can give us a sense that we're not all alone in our suffering. And conjuring up images of caring figures comforting us can add to a sense of safe social connection that helps our nervous system to calm down.

It can be helpful to explore with patients, whether they've experienced self-criticism, isolation, or self-preoccupation associated with their chronic pain, and suggest self-compassion exercises explicitly to counter these difficulties.

Mindfulness and Self-Compassion for Difficult Emotions

For many people, learning that their pain is not primarily due to structural damage (when this is the case), seeing for themselves how chronic pain cycles operate, approaching their pain with mindfulness and self-compassion, and reengaging in normal life activities goes a long way to free them from the disorder. For others, however, a return to normal activity and a shift in attitude toward the physical pain is not enough. These are often people for whom difficult emotions beyond concerns about pain are contributing to persistent fear and muscle tension.

Case Vignette

Everyone thought that Carl was a really nice guy—but he hadn't always been. As a boy, he was a real troublemaker, regularly getting into fights. As an older teen, Carl turned his life around and became an exemplary young man. And now as an adult, he rarely argued and was almost always well mannered. He was often anxious—but not angry. Not surprisingly, Carl was very faithful in following my suggestions in therapy. He recognized how frightened he had been about his pain, and dutifully resumed activity.

Carl was frustrated, though, that his pain persisted. As it became clear that he had difficulty recognizing and expressing anger, I encouraged him to pay attention to feelings of annoyance. At first, he drew a blank. But then, as he started practicing mindfulness, the aggression became more apparent. He noticed that when angry thoughts arose, he tried to talk himself out of them. As his therapy and mindfulness practice continued, he was increasingly able to acknowledge his anger. But this brought up a lot of shame. Carl recalled how difficult he was with his parents, teachers, and siblings. So, I introduced self-compassion practice. At first, he thought of it as making excuses but eventually came to see how harsh his inner critic was and how isolated he felt when thinking about his past bad behavior. Bit by bit, he began to get it that everyone feels anger at times—it's only human. As he became more at home with his aggression, his anxiety lessened, and he began to feel less pain.

When we're unable to acknowledge or tolerate a thought or feeling, our fight-or-flight system reacts to the threat of it emerging much as it reacts to external dangers. As the stress physiologists say, "We respond to the tiger within with a system designed to respond to the tiger out there." Since life experiences continuously trigger unwanted cognitions and affects, our fight-or-flight system can be on overdrive. This overdrive can contribute to the muscle tension and pain-signal amplification that maintains chronic pain cycles.

Mindfulness practice can help bring previously unnoticed thoughts, feelings, and memories into awareness, and help us tolerate them. Seeing these as impermanent, arising, and passing makes them easier to bear. Self-compassion practice supports this process by cultivating an inner atmosphere of love and acceptance, allowing us to embrace our full range of emotions more deeply, and it gives us the confidence that we can soothe ourselves when difficult feelings arise. Together, these practices allow us to relax our defenses more, opening more fully to whatever arises in our awareness.

Conclusion

Chronic pain is a complex problem fueled by remarkably varied psychological and physical processes. Fortunately, by understanding its typical dynamics while exploring each individual sufferer's unique mix of psychological and physical drivers, the cycles that maintain chronic pain can often be interrupted. Mindfulness and self-compassion practices can facilitate this work by helping individuals increase cognitive flexibility, tolerate the pain and fear that often accompany a return to normal activity, and work effectively with the negative emotions that can maintain the condition, all with warmth and kindness. These practices can also support recovery by helping us learn to relinquish control, embrace impermanence, accept our mortality, and become less self-preoccupied.

For a surprising number of people with whom I've worked, mindfulness and self-compassion practices, when integrated into a comprehensive approach to rehabilitation, have helped free them from chronic pain cycles entirely. Others have used them to temper the forces that maintain and amplify pain that persists because of underlying medical conditions. And they can help almost all of us move in the direction of leading fuller, more engaged lives despite the challenges of being embodied mammals.

REFERENCES

Atlas, S. J., & Deyo, R. A. (2001). Evaluating and managing acute low back pain in the primary care setting. *Journal of General Internal Medicine, 16*(2), 120–131.

Bordeleau, M., Vincenot, M., Lefevre, S., Duport, A., Seggio, L., Breton, T., et al. (2022). Treatments for kinesiophobia in people with chronic pain: A scoping review. *Frontiers in Behavioral Neuroscience, 16*. www.frontiersin.org/articles/10.3389/fnbeh.2022.933483.

Hilton, L., Hempel, S., Ewing, B. A., Apaydin, E., Xenakis, L., Newberry, S., et al. (2017). Mindfulness meditation for chronic pain: Systematic review and meta-analysis. *Annals of Behavioral Medicine, 51*(2), 199–213.

Kasch, R., Truthmann, J., Hancock, M. J., Maher, C. G., Otto, M., Nell, C., et al. (2022). Association of lumbar MRI findings with current and future back pain in a population-based cohort study. *Spine, 47*(3), 201–211.

Lanzaro, C., Carvalho, S. A., Lapa, T. A., Valentim, A., & Gago, B. (2021). A systematic review of self-compassion in chronic pain: From correlation to efficacy. *Spanish Journal of Psychology, 24*, e26.

Leeuw, M., Houben, R. M. A., Severeijns, R., Picavet, H. S. J., Schouten, E. G. W., & Vlaeyen, J. W. S. (2007). Pain-related fear in low back pain: A prospective study in the general population. *European Journal of Pain, 11*(3), 256–266.

Luque-Suarez, A., Martinez-Calderon, J., & Falla, D. (2019). Role of kinesiophobia on pain, disability and quality of life in people suffering from chronic musculoskeletal pain: A systematic review. *British Journal of Sports Medicine, 53*(9), 554–559.

Martinez-Calderon, J., Jensen, M. P., Morales-Asencio, J. M., & Luque-Suarez, A. (2019). Pain catastrophizing and function in individuals with chronic musculoskeletal pain. *Clinical Journal of Pain, 35*(3), 279–293.

Melzack, R., & Wall, P. D. (1965). Pain mechanisms: A new theory. *Science, 150*(3699), 971–979.

Meulders, A. (2019). From fear of movement-related pain and avoidance to chronic pain disability: A state-of-the-art review. *Current Opinion in Behavioral Sciences, 26*, 130–136.

Meulders, A. (2020). Fear in the context of pain: Lessons learned from 100 years of fear conditioning research. *Behaviour Research and Therapy, 131*, 103635.

Pardos-Gascón, E. M., Narambuena, L., Leal-Costa, C., & van-der Hofstadt-Román, C. J. (2021). Differential efficacy between cognitive-behavioral therapy and mindfulness-based therapies for chronic pain: Systematic review. *International Journal of Clinical and Health Psychology, 21*(1), 100197.

Rainville, J., Hartigan, C., Martinez, E., Limke, J., Jouve, C., & Finno, M. (2004). Exercise as a treatment for chronic low back pain. *Spine Journal, 4*(1), 106–115.

Sharpe, L., Richmond, B., Menzies, R. E., Forrest, D., Crombez, G., & Colagiuri, B. (2024). A synthesis of meta-analyses of mindfulness-based interventions in pain. *Pain, 165*(1), 18–28.

Siegel, R. D., Urdang, M., & Johnson, D. D. R. (2002). *Back sense: A revolutionary approach to halting the cycle of chronic back pain*. Harmony/Rodale.

Torrijos-Zarcero, M., Mediavilla, R., Rodríguez-Vega, B., Del Río-Diéguez, M., López-Álvarez, I., Rocamora-González, C., & Palao-Tarrero, Á. (2021). Mindful self-compassion program for chronic pain patients: A randomized controlled trial. *European Journal of Pain, 25*(4), 930–944.

20

Integrating Self-Compassion into Acceptance and Commitment Therapy and Other Third-Wave Cognitive-Behavioral Therapies

Benjamin Weinstein

There have been significant shifts in the theoretical foundations and clinical delivery of cognitive-behavioral therapies (CBTs) in the last 25 years. These changes are reflected in the emergence of the "third wave" of CBTs, which emphasize mindful awareness, psychological flexibility, and value-guided behavior in context. In the last decade or so, there has been burgeoning attention to self-compassion as shown in an enormous surge of scholarly, clinical, and popular interest. The data are growing by leaps and bounds every year, pointing toward self-compassion as an important element in treatment and personal growth (Neff, 2023). As Neff summarizes in her recent review:

> Self-compassion is not just a good idea, it is something one can do . . . because it is a powerful way to alleviate suffering that is accessible to anyone at any moment. It can be learned and practiced, and it is not rocket science. (p. 211)

Clinicians with different allegiances around the globe are incorporating self-compassion interventions into counseling and therapy because they work both for us and for our clients.

Focusing on acceptance and commitment therapy (ACT), which has a well-specified clinical model, this chapter shows how self-compassion converges and fits with ACT's experiential nature and core clinical model in such a way as to facilitate comprehensive and seamless integration. This also applies to third-wave CBTs using mindfulness, acceptance, and value-guided action. A full treatment of the issues is beyond the scope of a brief clinically focused chapter. This chapter begins with a brief overview of conceptual convergence and moves to ACT-consistent clinical applications of self-compassion practices, including concepts, practices, and metaphors that smooth and empower the integration of self-compassion into ACT and other CBTs.

Self-Compassion Fosters Psychological Flexibility

Emphasizing the flexible, transdiagnostic, and transtheoretical utility of self-compassion, Finlay-Jones (2023) refers to self-compassion as a "house with many doors" (p. 435). Indeed, self-compassion as a concept and clinical toolkit embodies psychological flexibility since it doesn't require adherence to any theoretical or clinical model.

Although caring is emphasized as an essential component in the ACT therapeutic relationship, compassion or self-compassion were not explicit elements in the original ACT model (Hayes et al., 2011). ACT's originators now acknowledge the importance of the construct for impactful ACT work. Steven Hayes (2014) has written, "At the level of psychological process, it turns out that compassion is integral to psychological flexibility. Indeed, it is arguably essential" (p. xvi).

Various authors (Germer, 2023; Germer & Neff, 2019; Gilbert, 2009, 2010, 2019) have highlighted how compassion and self-compassion are based on complex, evolved, neurobiological systems. For example, self-compassion practices directly soothe sympathetic nervous system arousal and stimulate parasympathetic calming (Germer, 2023). Gilbert (2009, 2019) hypothesizes that neurological soothing/caregiving and reward-seeking motivational systems underlie the different facets of the experiences and responses we label as compassion and kindness. Thus, self-compassion has an embodied and commonly shared reality: Any person can directly experience self-kindness and learn how to direct this resource to themselves when they need it.

Understanding the evolved, physiological, grounded, and shared nature of self-compassion is key to understanding self-compassion's role in psychological flexibility. Reflexive and automatic experiential avoidance of aversive, internal experiences is a central feature of the ACT model. Thus, behavior is less flexible and adaptable when we're in pain. When we're aware and can soothe our pains, we're more able to direct our behavior effectively. As ACT prefers using metaphors over other forms of psychoeducation (which increase the risk of getting tangled up in intellectual, analytical discussions), here is a metaphor I use with clients that captures the nature of self-compassion, the *muscle metaphor*:

> "Compassion and self-compassion are natural resources that are inherent to being human. Self-compassion isn't a concept or a theory—it's like a muscle. Every one of us already has the capacity for self-compassion and kindness in the same way that each of us already has a full set of muscles in our body. So, you already have this kindness muscle. Depending on your history and experiences the muscle may be well developed, underdeveloped, or not developed at all. If the muscle is underdeveloped or undeveloped, simply beginning to use that muscle will spark and engage the process of development. Even if you never used it, you already have this muscle and the nature of the muscle is to grow, little by little, when stimulated, just like any muscle."

Mapping Self-Compassion onto the Psychological Flexibility Model

ACT (Hayes et al., 2011) is designed as a process-based, experiential behavioral therapy that posits psychological and behavioral rigidity, driven by fusion and experiential avoidance, as the root causes of human suffering in general and maladaptive behavior in particular. ACT's overall clinical goal is fostering and empowering psychological flexibility in the service of engaged, valued living. Psychological flexibility is operationally defined by six psychological processes that are hypothesized to influence flexibility or rigidity. These six processes comprise the ACT clinical model for case formulation and intervention: flexible attention to the present moment, acceptance, defusion, values, committed action, and self-as-context (Harris, 2019).

ACT emphasizes the importance of a caring and connected therapeutic relationship (Hayes et al., 2011). ACT clinicians recognize that they are being influenced by the same processes in the psychological flexibility model as the client, which Hayes and colleagues refer to as "We are all in this stew together" (p. 151). From the perspective of self-compassion, this is a recognition of common humanity that deeply connects the therapist and client. ACT encourages "radical respect" for the client's direct experience. Thus, ACT explicitly values a connected, compassionate relationship.

The psychological flexibility model outlines the six processes currently regarded as crucial for fostering engaged living without getting tangled up in one's mind (see Figure 20.1). Situated in a hexagon, this model forms a map that ACT therapists can use to guide themselves. The model is divided into

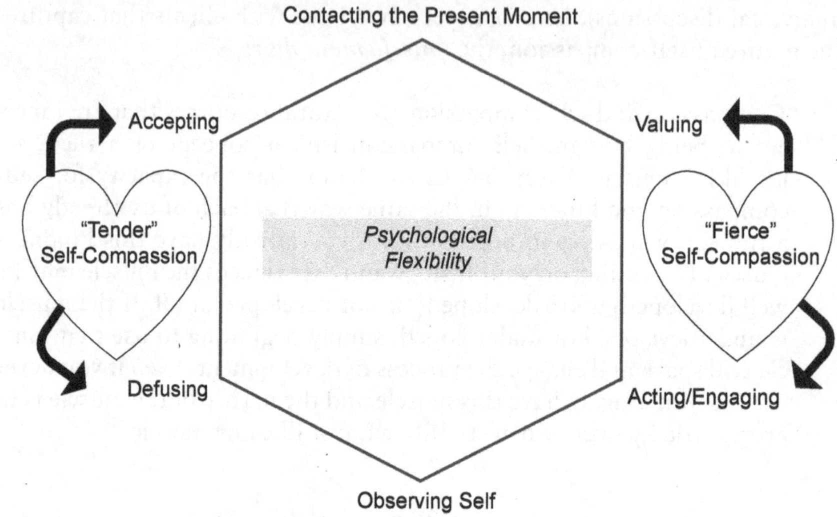

ACT Model:	Mindfulness and Acceptance Processes		Commitment and Behavioral Activation Processes
Integrating Self-Compassion:	"Tender" Self-Compassion Techniques and Practices		"Fierce" Self-Compassion Techniques and Processes

FIGURE 20.1. How self-compassion interventions and practices "map" onto the ACT model of psychological flexibility.

two, overlapping sides. The left side of the model comprises the processes that foster mindfulness and acceptance (contacting the present moment, acceptance, defusion, and observing self). In contrast, the right side of the model comprises the processes that foster and support commitment and behavior change (contacting the present moment, valuing, engaging/acting, and observing self). Therapists working from an ACT orientation attempt to move back and forth flexibly within the model in the service of the client's values and goals.

Through in-session direct observation and dialogue, the therapist observes where the client/therapeutic moment is on the map and offers an ACT-consistent response targeting that process in the service of the client's goals and values. When the client then moves into another part of the map, the ACT therapist observes this with mindful awareness and flexibly moves together with the client, shifting to a different technique/response that suits the evolving present moment.

It turns out that self-compassion converges with and naturally fits within an ACT framework. There are three powerful illustrations of this:

First, ACT clinical work and self-compassion practices are grounded in very similar models of emotion. A core tenet of ACT is that experiential avoidance is one of the normal human psychological processes that creates and perpetuates suffering and dysfunction. Our efforts to avoid, resist, and escape from our feelings drive lasting unhappiness, not the feelings themselves. Therefore, ACT emphasizes the willingness to "show up" for painful emotions over controlling or avoiding them. This is the same rationale that is provided for self-compassion practice. In the mindful self-compassion (MSC) program, participants are taught "What you resist will persist and what you can feel, you can heal" (Germer & Neff, 2019). The spirit of both ACT and self-compassion is oriented to acceptance and opening for painful affects that are a natural, inevitable part of human life.

Second, at a clinical level, ACT and self-compassion are both experiential, not conceptual. During ACT therapy, the clients need to directly experience the processes within sessions so this experience can be generalized outside of the sessions. ACT furthermore privileges the client's direct experience of workability. Based on radical respect, the client is the person most able to judge whether their actions and choices are working to produce the life that matters to them. Likewise, self-compassion, as noted above, is a shared, biologically grounded reality built into our human brains and nervous systems and is best learned by clients not as an abstract concept but as a tangible, embodied skill set that can be practiced in a variety of ways and directly experienced. Thus, both in ACT and self-compassion, the client has the authority to guide themselves based on their own direct experience as the therapist creates the environment that facilitates direct experience.

Third, self-compassion can be mapped comprehensively onto the psychological flexibility model—that is, self-compassion skills span the full scope of the psychological flexibility model from mindfulness/acceptance processes on the left side of the hexagon over to the commitment/behavioral engagement processes on the right side of the hexagon. It's a common misconception about compassion that compassion and self-compassion refer exclusively to soothing, gentle, and soft elements of kindness. Kindness is not always gentle and soft. Germer and Neff (2019; Neff, 2021) highlight the crucial distinction between tender/yin and fierce/yang self-compassion. It is the former that most people associate with self-compassion, the sense of warmly comforting, soothing, and consoling. And yet, self-compassion also comprises a fierce/yang side, which can protect, provide, and motivate. Fierce self-compassion harnesses the inner resource of self-compassion to actively engage through encouraging and motivating action in specific contexts. Because of this misconception, many cognitive-behavioral and behaviorally oriented therapists have not appreciated how vital and empowering self-compassion can be across the full spectrum of cognitive and behavioral interventions. Figure 20.1 shows how tender self-compassion naturally aligns and fits with the left-side processes of the psychological flexibility model (acceptance and defusion as responses to painful, aversive affects and cognitions) and fierce self-compassion aligns with the right side of the model (valuing and committed action).

Thus, there is a compelling convergence between ACT clinical work and self-compassion. The following sections amplify how self-compassion maps beautifully onto the psychological flexibility model. There are numerous self-compassion techniques, and this brief chapter presents only a few.

Tender Self-Compassion Supports Mindfulness, Acceptance, and Defusion: From Co-Regulation to Self-Regulation

On the left side of the psychological flexibility model (see Figure 20.1), the therapist is working with their own and the client's responses to painful private experiences, such as shame, anger, numbness, discomfort, and so on, and fused mental content. It's a persistent challenge in psychotherapy to help a diverse range of clients learn to tolerate and accept painful private experiences so they can engage with what matters in their lives. Like ACT, self-compassion also begins by contacting the present moment and this naturally supports moving left on the model to opening up for present-moment experience. Being aware of pain directly in the present moment is a precondition for self-compassion to also arise. It's a necessary but not sufficient precondition since the client also needs the intention to be kinder to themselves when in pain.

Approaching the client compassionately in an emotionally safe and connected therapeutic relationship helps the client contact and regulate the experience. Cultivating client self-compassion in psychotherapy operates in part through the establishment of a connected, secure base within the therapeutic relationship that allows the therapist's embodied compassion to be conveyed to the client. Depending on their attachment histories and how they experience attachment, clients vary in their need for co-regulation.

These experiences foster the client's capacity for self-compassion and gradually increase the client's capacity to regulate themselves inside and outside of sessions. In cases where the client doesn't develop the requisite internal intention to be kinder to themselves, the experience and skills may not generalize outside of sessions. Self-compassion tends to act as an accelerant to ACT work by speeding up the movement from co-regulation to self-regulation. As a form of behavioral therapy, CBT therapists in general and ACT therapists in particular value this kind of intervention.

Two practical skills of tender self-compassion can easily be adapted for psychotherapy, which many clients find impactful. These are compassionate touch (see Practice G, "Soothing or Supportive Touch," in the Appendix) and the self-compassion break (see Practice A, "Self-Compassion Break," in the Appendix"; Germer & Neff, 2019). They are both concrete, behavioral exercises the client directly experiences for themselves. Both skills help regulate central nervous system activation and painful emotions. When we practice any self-compassion skill, we invite the client to reflect on whatever has connected for them experientially and to think about how to apply that in their daily experience. The spirit of both ACT and tender self-compassion is to empower flexibility and creativity in how the client applies these skills to make their lives more workable.

The client is thus empowered, both with the therapist and on their own, to adapt their practice to fit their own experience. I describe this simple empowerment to a client using the *recipe metaphor*:

> "When you learn a recipe from a cookbook, the first few times, you tend to stick with the cookbook version. As you cook the recipe for yourself more and more, you don't have to follow the cookbook recipe. You make it the way that tastes delicious to you. You might add more of one ingredient and even drop ingredients altogether as you like. You let your experience guide you. Practicing self-compassion is the same way—when you practice, you don't have to do it according to the book or how I guide you in session. There's no one else to please. It's not about doing it 'correctly.' As you use it, you notice what connects for you and focus on that, practicing in the way that works best for you."

Case Vignette: Integrating Tender Self-Compassion Practices

Bilyana is a 41-year-old working single mother who presents for therapy after her 6-year-old child was diagnosed with cancer during the COVID-19 pandemic and her workplace has been unsupportive. She presents for therapy feeling overwhelmed and relates her history of insecure attachment and unsatisfying relationships, saying, "I myself alone am not enough." Bilyana is hardworking and analytical, with inflexible standards and is disconnected from herself and the present moment. In the early stage of treatment, she prefers mindfulness interventions that increase awareness. Despite getting great relief and support from the therapist's connection and compassion, the self-compassion skills we practice together in session don't connect well for her. Later in therapy, Bilyana discovers that her partner has been having an affair, filling her with despair and anger. We practice the self-compassion break together again in session and for the first time, she describes feeling connected deeply with herself and her pain and being able to speak lovingly to herself in a way that feels authentic. Bilyana begins to practice the self-compassion break regularly on her own while standing up for herself more, little by little. She says that while she's still in pain, her practice is helping her to believe in her own resources and help her face the future.

While some clients respond rapidly to self-compassion practices, Bilyana is an example of a client for whom it takes more time and practice in the context of a connected, safe therapeutic relationship to develop her resource of self-compassion. This is common with clients who experience forms of insecure attachment.

Beginning to Work in Session with "What Do I Need?"

There is a broad range of tender self-compassion skills and practices that therapists can offer to the client to help support being present, opening up, and noticing thinking. For example, the MSC training course alone offers more than two dozen guided meditations and other skills for daily life and compassion-focused therapy (CFT; Gilbert, 2010) offers many more. Beyond specific techniques, it's possible to cultivate client self-compassion within the therapeutic dialogue using a simple set of questions:

1. Present-moment question: "What's happening right now? What are you feeling?"
2. Self-compassion question: "When you're feeling this way, what do you need?"
3. Alternate self-compassion question: "If you had a dear friend feeling this same way, what would you say or do to support and encourage them?" or "What do you wish someone would say or do for you right now?"

As other chapters in this book also explore the question "When I'm feeling this way, what do I need?," the question captures the essence of practicing self-compassion. This question guides people to become an ally implicitly and explicitly for themselves. As embodied in the practice of the self-compassion break, "What do I need?" begins with a pause and shifts attention to the present moment. For many clients, this is a significant shift from the constriction of efforts to escape/avoid/control their experience with an associated narrow attentional focus produced by intense negative affect.

When having a discussion with the client about these questions, it's important to focus on the client's directly lived experience and not get tangled up in different kinds of analytical discussions. For example, do not get into a discussion about what a need is or isn't. In the context of self-compassion, asking, "What do I need right now?" is the functional equivalent of asking, "What will help me to live this moment?" or being asked, "How can I help?" While the responses frequently fit within existing paradigms like coping skills or emotion regulation, posing the question in this way empowers the client to pause, check in with themselves, and crucially, begin to (1) experience themselves as an active agent engaging with their own lives and (2) with a kind and supportive intention directed at themselves. From an ACT perspective, posing the question can sometimes help clients defuse from struggling with painful thoughts and feelings. When encouraging the client to engage with the question and explore whatever it means for them, the focus is on the process, not the answer, since there is no "correct" answer and the only person who can know what they need is the client themselves.

Two important distinctions can help therapists work fluidly and pragmatically with "What do I need?" First, there is a distinction between a need and what meets that need for the client in the specific context. Many of the needs clients have are universal needs like belonging, safety, connection, courage, and so on. While universal needs might not vary, how a client might satisfy those needs can vary enormously. So, ACT clinical work in this vein can focus more on what practice or action helps this client meet that need for themselves in a specific context (i.e., at a specific moment and place). For example, when a client is longing for connection and at that moment no one else is available to connect with, what will help the client to meet that need for themselves, even just a little bit?

This brings us to the second distinction, which is to recognize that meeting needs partially is frequently sufficient. Needs are not simply met or unmet. Many clients derive relief from internal pressure by adopting this frame of meeting their own needs "just a little—even just a drop" to enable them to move toward what matters.

So, in ACT "What do I need when I feel this way?" can become "What do I need when I feel this way to help me live in the way that matters to me here and now?" Therapists and clients can easily become fused with the concept of needs; the "What do I need?" discussion benefits from having a flexible, light, and playful flavor with a pragmatic focus grounded in a specific moment in the client's life.

Case Vignette: "What Do I Need?" as a Clinical Tool Driving Dialogue

Mara is a divorcee in her late 50s who presents with symptoms of burnout because her life has fallen apart during the COVID-19 pandemic. She lost her long-term job in a humiliating way and took another job that didn't go well and she left after only a year. In the last year, she has wandered while feeling unsettled, and in her initial session, she says, "I'm at sea . . . I'm not really anywhere." Mara is self-critical, particularly about her lack of focus and her emotions. She observes that "I tend to suppress and not be aware of my emotions." At the same time, attempting to think about her future triggers intense fear and hopelessness, which she's been suppressing. When introduced to her, she initially finds the question "What do I need?" befuddling and is at a loss to respond. At first, she opts for behavioral coping, finding that going for long walks seems to help soothe and comfort her. With more in-session practice and as we work with backdraft, other impulses gradually surface, including an internal, felt sense of "Maybe I shouldn't be so hard on myself. . . ." Mara is invited to notice how this experience feels in her body and to contrast that experience with how criticizing herself feels. Guiding her attention to her felt, direct experience has traction and throughout about a dozen sessions practicing other skills, her lifelong self-criticism diminishes significantly as does her emotional distress, allowing her to explore a new direction for her life.

"What Do I Need?" Is a Bridge from Pain to Action

ACT is fundamentally a behavioral therapy, built on a functional–contextual model. It includes interventions that foster engaged action, supporting clients to engage with and move toward what matters to them. "What do I need?" can easily function as a clinical bridge between the sides of the model (Figure 20.1). It helps guide the in-session process from mindfulness-acceptance processes toward commitment and behavioral activation processes.

Imagine a client who feels intensely anxious in the session at the thought of breaking up with their partner. Suppressing and controlling these feelings has led the client to remain in a dysfunctional relationship. An ACT therapist might guide the client into opening up using a variety of ACT exercises to be with, allow, and kindly make space for the experience. At some point in the dialogue, the therapist can inquire, "When you feel this way, what do you need to help soothe and comfort you?" At that moment, a subtle shift has already occurred. Even the smallest effort of meeting emotional pain with self-compassion already has a bit of fierce self-compassion built into it, starting with the active intention to do something to alleviate one's own suffering. The client is shifting from simply being with their experience kindly to actively engaging with ways of taking care of that experience. This is a crucial shift. When the client takes steps to identify what they need, aligned with their values, and then give themselves whatever that is, this is already a form of committed action. In the example of Bilyana above, gradually developing her ability to observe and soothe her feelings of inadequacy and distress eventually empowered her to also stand up for herself. This is how fierce self-compassion, in the form of an intention to provide for one's own needs, flows naturally over into committed action. So, Russ Harris's (2006, p. 8) pithy summary of ACT as "Embrace your demons and follow your heart" when combined with self-compassion becomes "What do I need so I can embrace my demons and truly follow my heart, even just a little, here and now?"

Fierce Self-Compassion Tools Supporting Commitment and Behavior Change

On the right side of the model (Figure 20.1), ACT empowers valued living through valuing and engaged action. ACT therapists use the metaphors of "standing up" and "standing for something" to convey the quality of valuing and committed action. This metaphor also captures the spirit of fierce self-compassion that can be harnessed to support valuing and engaged action.

Neff (2021) further divides the functions of fierce self-compassion into protecting, motivating, and providing. At some level, all expressions of fierce self-compassion represent standing up for oneself in some form. This framework can be a helpful launching point for exploring the range of possible ways that clients can be there for themselves as a friend and ally.

ACT therapists and other therapists integrating ACT are familiar with how valuing can give rise to experiential avoidance and fusion. Getting in contact with what matters tends to bring up pain in clinical populations; in ACT parlance, what truly matters to us is where most of our emotional pain lives. This makes self-compassion and common humanity vital ingredients in accelerating the client's ability to connect with what matters to them while honoring their personal, human history of experiences that make it painful for them to do so. Therapists support this engagement by placing this experience firmly in the context of common humanity, and the reality of having an evolved brain, nervous system, and body.

Case Vignette: From Tender to Fierce

Jenny, single and in her mid-30s, presents for therapy seeking help to manage her emotions and cope with stress. Jenny's career involves living and working in high-stress environments delivering humanitarian programs and moving every 3–4 years to a new assignment. Jenny struggled with obsessive–compulsive disorder as a teenager but is currently free of compulsions. She tends to suppress her emotions and seek approval. She's frequently triggered by work or social interactions and experiences intense feelings of shame and inadequacy. Starting early in therapy we cultivate her awareness to recognize and name what's happening while practicing compassionate touch and the self-compassion break together. Jenny is surprised and pleased to find that these practices soothe her. Although her own practice is halting and inconsistent, she continues to practice as she moves on to her next assignment. Jenny is gradually more and more able to soothe herself and is less frequently triggered, which she finds empowering. This empowers her to work on fierce self-compassion guided by an image of being a mama bear both comforting and protecting the little girl inside of her. She gradually becomes less reactive and significantly more able to set and hold emotional boundaries with coworkers. Interactions that used to cause her intense worry, doubts, and shame no longer bother her, and she describes herself as "leaning into life."

A Kind Coach for Committed Action

Moving toward committed action sometimes becomes a stumbling block in therapy. Self-compassion empowers a motivational shift from self-criticism to self-encouragement that supports committed action. Most people tend to motivate themselves with various forms of self-criticism. Fierce self-compassion offers a powerful alternative to this universal routine. We invite clients to support, encourage, and motivate themselves with kindness, in the same way that a kind, caring coach would. This allows us to help clients connect with valued directions in a way that feels supportive rather than critical. It's helpful to guide a simple in-session practice called "Kind Coach," which can be practiced as a guided visualization or as a written reflection (see Practice S.1, "Kind Coach," in the Appendix for instructions).

Bringing Tender and Fierce Fully Together: The Four *N*'s of "What Do I Need?"

The full clinical utility of "What do I need?" can be harnessed for ACT clinical work using the four *N*'s worksheet I developed for working with clients (see Figure 20.2). It is a simple, intuitive framework that's easy for ACT therapists and clients to apply. The client is invited to use four *N*'s that help orient to the present moment with self-compassion and engaged, value-guided action.

Figure 20.2 shows the steps in brief and can be shared as a handout with clients. It can be used in a variety of ways. First, it can be used as a framework to gradually introduce basic concepts of self-compassion to clients in a simple, intuitive model that fosters effective behavioral coping. I usually start with the first two *N*'s and then move forward at a pace suitable for the client. Second, the four *N*'s model helps clients who are already familiar with tender and fierce self-compassion practices begin to sort through (1) which form of self-compassion they need in a given moment/context and (2) what that might look like as a form of action. Third, because it takes time for most clients to develop a clear sense of what their authentic needs are in different contexts, it's a useful tool for fostering in-session dialogues that help the client explore and experiment with what their needs are and what might help meet their needs. And finally, it helps to overcome clients' rigid standards and perfectionism by focusing only on the next small step in context.

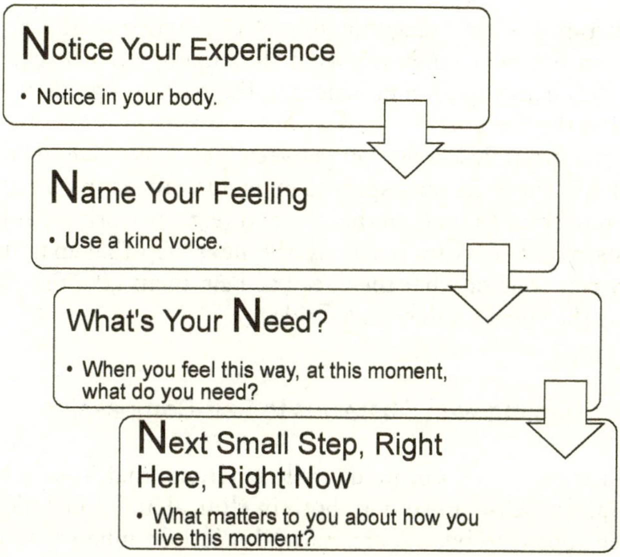

FIGURE 20.2. The four *N*'s of "What do I need?"

1. *Notice:* Notice the experience in the present moment with an emphasis on embodied noticing. Notice what you're experiencing right now: feelings, sensations, memories, thoughts, images, and so on. This can be supported by asking one of the questions above: "What am I feeling right now?"
2. *Name:* Name what you're experiencing using a kind tone of voice. It's possible to name the experience by speaking to yourself the same way you'd speak to a friend feeling the same way.
3. *Need:* Stop and ask yourself, "When I'm feeling this way, in this moment, what do I need right now?" This helps to develop your ability to be there for yourself when you're in pain. For beginners, this takes some time, energy, and practice to figure out. Is the kind of self-compassion that you need right now more tender or maybe fiercer?
4. *Next step:* The next step depends on you and what matters to you. Based on where you are right now, what small step helps you to move toward what matters to you? There are many different possibilities: this might be comforting and soothing yourself, taking a break, shifting your attention, finding a way to cope, giving yourself permission to be how you are at the moment, saying no, setting a boundary, standing up for yourself, or so many different things.

The therapist must engage flexibly in this dialogue and privilege the client's experience as a guide for what they might need. It can be useful to refer to the client's lived experiences in the past as a guide to what they might need in the present.

There is a dynamic interaction between Step 3, Need, and Step 4, Next Step. What a client needs in a specific moment/context frequently depends on what's important to them in that context (e.g., at work vs. at home). So, some clients might need to articulate the next step that matters to them before they can contact what they need to help them take that step. It can help to raise the client's values as a guide.

Dealing with Obstacles to Self-Compassion

There are a set of common, predictable reactions that arise when people begin to practice self-compassion, both in clinical and nonclinical populations. These appear to be, in part, natural reactions inherent in the underlying evolved systems regulating compassion and self-compassion. In CFT, these are referred to as the fears of compassion and collectively as fears, blocks, and resistances. There is evidence that clients in therapy may have more fears of compassion and self-compassion than the general population (Kirby, 2019) so therapists can expect these responses and prepare to recognize and respond with openness and compassion.

In the MSC program, these experiences are collectively called "backdraft," which refers to distress or discomfort arising when the client practices self-compassion. The course teaches that "love reveals everything unlike itself" (Germer & Neff, 2019, p. 109), such that when clients try to proactively love themselves using self-compassion, it will reveal "the conditions under which we felt unloved in the past" (Germer & Neff, 2019, p. 109). This fits well with the ACT views that every human being is carrying their learning history with them wherever they are.

Clinically, working with fears/doubts about self-compassion and backdraft are important milestones, not obstacles, in the development of self-compassion. From both an ACT perspective and the perspective of self-compassion practice, the experience of backdraft shouldn't be seen as a problem; it's avoiding/controlling backdraft that perpetuates the cycle. Describing the range of possible ways to work with fears of compassion and backdraft is beyond the scope of this chapter. See Practice S.2, "Suggestions for Working with Fears of Compassion and Backdraft in ACT," in the Appendix for suggestions on how to work with backdraft in an ACT-consistent fashion.

Some ACT clinicians may fear that self-compassion can become a form of experiential avoidance. This is a fear that's similar to the common fears and doubts described above. Rather than supporting avoidance, authentic self-compassion tends to surface old pains so they can be soothed while fostering workable engagement with what matters.

Conclusion

Self-compassion converges and fits comprehensively with the ACT clinical model and can be seamlessly integrated into ACT and other third-wave CBTs. The raison d'être of ACT is making space for painful, aversive private experiences while sustaining behavioral engagement with what matters. ACT fosters flexibility and creativity in the service of vitality and valued, workable living. When woven into ACT work, self-compassion accelerates the process of helping clients to acknowledge, make space for, and even embrace painful, fused private experiences while engaging with what matters to them. Self-compassion is a skill set, not just a concept; it is a living, embodied reality. It can be experienced and practiced by anyone in their daily life, and as Neff (2023) tartly noted above, "it is not rocket science" (p. 211). Self-compassion practices can enhance ACT clinical work across the whole ACT model, potentially making it more present, alive, and connected for the client and the therapist. ACT and self-compassion deeply empower the client's flexibility and self-directed engagement with their life.

REFERENCES

Finlay-Jones, A. (2023). A house with many doors—Toward a more nuanced self-compassion intervention science. In A. Finlay-Jones, K. Bluth, & K. Neff (Eds.), *Handbook of self-compassion* (pp. 433–454). Springer International.

Germer, C. (2023). Self-compassion in psychotherapy: Clinical integration, evidence base, and mechanisms of change. In A. Finlay-Jones, K. Bluth, & K. Neff (Eds.), *Handbook of self-compassion* (pp. 379–415). Springer International.

Germer, C., & Neff, K. (2019). *Teaching the mindful self-compassion program: A guide for professionals.* Guilford Press.

Gilbert, P. (2009). Introducing compassion-focused therapy. *Advances in Psychiatric Treatment, 15*(3), 199.

Gilbert, P. (2010). An introduction to compassion focused therapy in cognitive behavior therapy. *International Journal of Cognitive Therapy, 3*(2), 97–112.

Gilbert, P. (2019). Psychotherapy for the 21st century: An integrative, evolutionary, contextual, biopsychosocial approach. *Psychology and Psychotherapy: Theory, Research and Practice, 92*(2), 164–189.

Harris, R. F. (2006). Embracing your demons: An overview of acceptance and commitment therapy. *Psychotherapy in Australia, 12*, 70.

Harris, R. (2009). *ACT made simple: An easy-to-read primer on acceptance and commitment therapy*. New Harbinger.

Hayes, S. (2014). Building a cooperative, caring, and productive relationship: ACT and CFT as a test case. In D. Tirch, B. Schoendorff, & L. Silberstein (Eds.), *The ACT practitioner's guide to the science of compassion: Tools for fostering psychological flexibility* (pp. xv–xviii). New Harbinger.

Hayes, S., Strosahl, K., & Wilson, K. (2011). *Acceptance and commitment therapy: The process and practice of mindful change*. Guilford Press.

Kirby, J. N. (2019). The "flow" of compassion: A meta-analysis of the fears of compassion scales and psychological functioning. *Clinical Psychology Review, 70*, 26–39.

Neff, K. (2021). *Fierce self-compassion: How women can harness kindness to speak up, claim their power, and thrive*. Penguin.

Neff, K. D. (2023). Self-compassion: Theory, method, research, and intervention. *Annual Review of Psychology, 74*, 193–218.

Concluding Reflections

Integrating Self-Compassion into Psychotherapy

Shari Geller
Galia Tyano Ronen

While we began this book with a strong vision of supporting therapists to incorporate self-compassion in psychotherapy, we learned from these masterful authors new ways of doing so. Our shared experience of developing various trainings and teaching therapists how to incorporate self-compassion into psychotherapy has taught us about how valuable this approach and way of being is, yet developing ways to teach this to therapists is a phenomenal task.

The authors contributed their expertise and wisdom, deepening this vision and teaching us much more about the many nuances of taking a self-compassionate approach in therapy. We are inspired by the model of Christopher Germer (Chapter 1) to view self-compassion as implemented through three vehicles: compassionate therapeutic presence, relationship, and interventions. We use this model to reflect here on some of what we learned in this writing and editing journey. Yet before we do, we want to share more about the nuanced yet powerful theoretical basis for self-compassion in psychotherapy.

Foundations of Self-Compassion in Psychotherapy: A Theoretical Framework

As has been reiterated in this book, self-compassion is a way to care for our suffering in the way we would care for someone we truly love. Many authors utilized Kristin Neff's (2011) definition of self-compassion, which has three components: (1) mindfulness (being aware of our experience before we can bring compassion to it), (2) common humanity (knowing we are not alone in our human experience of suffering), and (3) self-kindness (bringing warmth, soothing, and care to our human pain and suffering). Both mindfulness and self-compassion are powerful ways to approach our experience and therefore help to cultivate present-moment and kind awareness so that we can meet our pain directly and bring transformation to our experience. This is equally beneficial to clients (to hold their pain and suffering with compassion) and to therapists (to meet our own experience of pain and the resonance of pain with clients with kindness so we can be more present and available).

Buddhist and humanistic perspectives recognize that at the core of who we are there is a deep potential for wisdom, growth, and wholeness. Mindfulness practice helps us release a sense of identity, needs, hunger for attention, longing, greed, and desire, which allows our innate wisdom to be illuminated. Self-compassion supports us in approaching pain and difficulties with warmth and kindness. Trusting in this natural wisdom and wholeness (Buddhist) and actualizing tendency toward growth (humanistic) allows us as therapists to meet the barriers to human experience, deep pain, and suffering with compassion, and trust in that transformation. In psychotherapy, we change emotions with other emotions. Bringing compassion to emotional pain (i.e., sadness or anger) helps transform it.

It is also powerful to change our perspective of self as separate, as our Western tradition has taught us, and shift to seeing self in relationship. Humanistic therapy based on Carl Rogers has taught us this fundamental wisdom—we grow and evolve in relationship with others. More recently neuroscience challenges the notion of self as separate and this is directly relevant with compassion. Weisbaum and colleagus (Chapter 3) offer a paradigm shift in this way. The authors share how seeing the self as separate and encased in a physical body is a top-down construction, "informed by our subjective lived experience of having a physical body." This narrative is a barrier to both inner and outer compassion. Instead, they offer the view, which we adopt in this reflection, of having three levels of compassion: (1) inner compassion (our inner world), (2) intercompassion (our interpersonal relationships with others and nature), and (3) intracompassion (our integrated relationship that combines these to a holistic perspective of me (inner) plus we (inter) as MWe (intraconnected).

Being intraconnected, we regulate through relationships. We impact one another from a neurophysiological perspective, according to Porges's polyvagal theory as highlighted by the first author (Geller; Chapter 6). We are bidirectionally attuned with one another. We have a ventral vagal system that includes a social engagement system. Being in contact with a grounded, present, and compassionate therapist allows clients to feel safe, felt, and seen, so they can explore their pain and trauma in the safety of the therapeutic relationship. So, whether we see ourselves as existing as separate, or we see ourselves as directly interconnected with others, this self and other distinction and relationship is imperative to understanding how our compassion as therapists can directly impact clients' self-compassion.

Evolution of Compassion

It further guides our understanding of compassion when we learn from Gilbert (Chapter 2) how compassion and self-compassion are based on complex neurobiological systems that have evolved in mammals. Compassion from this lens is viewed as an evolved mechanism in humans rooted in the development of self-awareness. As self-aware humans, we encounter challenges such as fears, blocks, and resistance. Self-compassion helps us meet those challenges and work through them with wisdom, courage, and commitment. We help clients develop a secure base within themselves, as self-compassion helps us reparent ourselves by approaching our challenges and difficult emotional experiences with kindness and the willingness to help.

Compassion and self-compassion become natural responses to suffering. With practice and within a compassionate relationship, we can develop an awareness of suffering and find ways to reduce suffering on three levels: physical (care and sustenance of the body and physical needs), relational (caring for relationships by both feeling others' experience and taking action to care about them), and psychological (caring for our emotional and psychological suffering and being mindful of how these express themselves to others).

Self-Compassion as a Vehicle for Growth: Mechanisms of Change

The mechanisms of change when viewing self-compassion through the lens of psychotherapy are multifaceted. Particularly, they target reducing experiential avoidance and enhancing emotion regulation, acceptance, and presence. Research supports these mechanisms as well as the reduction in cognitive rumination and the increase in positive coping and resilience that can help clients to thrive. Below, we highlight essential themes that reflect how self-compassion helps in psychotherapy.

Emotion Regulation

Self-compassion helps clients develop emotion regulation skills, which is at the heart of how it can help in a therapeutic context. Bernabé and Díaz

(Chapter 5), Germer (Chapter 1), and others highlight how this occurs in part through reducing fear and soothing the sympathetic nervous system. When secondary reactions to emotions (such as shutdown, aversion, judgment, or overwhelm) are reduced, clients can feel safer accessing their initial primary natural emotion responses, which helps them feel more regulated and able to express and work through these primary emotional states. By meeting experiences with a compassionate therapist and a self-compassionate mindset and approach, as Shapiro and colleagues (Chapter 7) describe, regulation becomes more possible.

Reducing Shame

We understand shame as prevalent in clients, especially those with depression, trauma, and addictions. Germer (Chapter 11) describes how self-compassion is a resource and an antidote for clients' shame. Given that shame is both hidden and pervasive in many disorders and at the heart of the experience of trauma for many clients, it is powerful to learn how self-compassion exposes clients to shame, reduces their self-criticism, and offers an opportunity for transformation. The emphasis across chapters includes directing self-compassion toward underlying emotions and not just the issues (i.e., shame or grief underlying depression or addiction or trauma).

Wishart (Chapter 12) sees reducing shame as a central mechanism within addiction frameworks. Shame often goes unnoticed, yet therapists working with self-compassion can reduce clients' shame as both an underlying and responsive factor to addictions. As shame underlies depression, Gilbert (Chapter 13) demonstrates from a compassion-focused therapy approach how the mind can help activate the body (through imagery or exercises, such as compassionate letter writing) and how the body can support the mind (i.e., via compassionate care with diet, exercise, posture, and breathing techniques).

Self-compassion is also a helpful approach for therapists who experience shame or self-doubt that gets in the way of offering a therapeutic and compassionate presence to clients. In Chapter 6, the first author (Geller) describes how internal barriers to being fully present with clients, such as self-doubt, shame, or self-criticism, can be quieted with a stance of self-compassion. It can help soften the critical voice that can be activated and distract the therapist from staying in the unknown and unfolding of the moment. It also provides therapists with ways to recognize and access with compassion the deeper experiences that have contributed to self-doubt. Offering compassion to our own vulnerabilities, we strengthen our ability to be compassionate with clients, and in turn, strengthen the relational bond with them.

Breaking the Cycle of Self-Criticism

Relatedly, the self-critical cycle perpetuating shame can be interrupted with a self-compassionate approach. These mechanisms were highlighted in working with people suffering from trauma and eating disorders, with teens, and with people with borderline personality disorder (BPD) where self-loathing as a result of trauma is ever present. Stiglmayr (Chapter 14) recommends using a self-compassionate approach early in treatment with clients with BPD and describes how self-compassion is the missing ingredient when working with this population. We learn that loving-kindness and self-compassion lowers self-criticism and improves self-kindness and acceptance in clients with BPD.

Anxiety is seen by Roemer and colleagues (Chapter 15) as partially related to having a problematic and critical relationship with our internal experience, which may lead to avoidance, isolation, and disengagement in meaningful relationships. Self-compassion practice helps counter the self-criticism that is part of our difficult relationship internally, allows clients to see experience as transient, therefore reducing avoidance, and reengaging in meaningful relationships. It can also reduce internalized racism.

Exposure

Interesting to us as editors was how many authors described exposure principles as core to the mechanism of change with self-compassion. Exposure to difficult emotions is core to change from a behavioral perspective generally, and self-compassion helps expose clients to their painful emotions with a pace and approach that is kind and warm. Like being with a dear friend who is suffering, we help clients befriend their own difficult emotions with kindness.

Using self-compassion practices such as those offered throughout this book, with a present therapist and in a safe and supportive therapeutic relationship, can help clients increase tolerance to difficult underlying emotions and have the resources to work through them.

Non-Avoidance

Relatedly, non-avoidance may also elucidate how self-compassion works in therapy. We know that the avoidance of traumatic memories and difficult emotions is the hallmark of those who suffer from posttraumatic stress disorder and anxiety, which increases related pain and anxiety. The acceptance of and working through traumatic memories and difficult emotions is more possible within a compassionate therapeutic relationship and by utilizing self-compassion practices.

Self-Soothing

A key mechanism within a self-compassionate therapeutic framework is the ability to self-soothe through a kind and caring touch, intentions, gestures, or words, toward one's own pain and suffering. It can deactivate the threat response and enhance safeness, demonstrated in part physiologically through the reduction of cortisol levels. Stiglmayr (Chapter 14) affirms this in clients with BPD who have suffered complex trauma, as their ability to self-soothe in difficult moments dramatically increased after engaging in self-compassion.

Chronic pain, as shared by Siegel (Chapter 19), can enhance fear, anger, and frustration, which further exacerbates the pain cycle. The capacity to self-soothe reduces this emotional distress. Self-compassion teaches clients, such as those who did not necessarily have a model of caregiving that helps modulate distress through care and touch, to self-soothe. This helps reduce emotional reactions to physical and traumatic pain, which further reduces the actual pain itself.

Therapists also benefit from self-soothing, as when they sit with the deep pain and suffering of clients, their own resonance of pain (and possibly their own triggers of pain) can be elicited. This can allow therapists to prepare for presence prior to session as well as work with their vicarious pain elicited in therapy (not to mention their personal pain and struggles). This also offers a model from which clients can benefit when they see our hands on our own hearts as we sit with and feel our clients' pain and can invite them to do the same. Both of us teach therapists in our chapters and our professional lives to offer self-compassion as a way to be with the difficult resonance of pain that shows up inside of us, and to remove the barriers to presence in the therapy encounter, as well as to care for ourselves amid this deep and important work we do as therapists. This is a powerful offering, as psychotherapy training often does not focus on helping therapists work with their own experience and pain in the therapy dyad.

Self-Compassion as a Resource in Multicultural Counseling

In our therapeutic work, we find enormous importance in bringing more sensitivity and compassion to the nuances and challenges of cross-cultural psychotherapy. Spears and Ochester (Chapter 4) help us be more socioculturally self-aware and work through the barriers to that, such as shame, self-judgment, and self-isolation. We must stay curious and have the tools to work through the shame and judgment that might occur when we meet our marginalized clients. It is important to stay open as we try to understand clients with challenges related to privilege and power and our own possible contribution that may cause alliance ruptures. By bringing self-compassion to both the development of cross-cultural competence and the challenges that can occur in a therapist–client dyad, we have an important resource to meet our clients and work through ruptures that are complicated by differences in identity, power, and privilege.

Self-Compassion as Transdiagnostic and Transtheoretical

Both of us come from different theoretical backgrounds, using different models and working with a broad range of clients. Yet the beauty of incorporating self-compassion into psychotherapy is that it can be a transtheoretical and transdiagnostic model. It can enhance changes through the embodiment of compassion with therapeutic presence and a deepening therapeutic relationship that is both interconnected and separate.

This perspective inherent in this book teaches us that therapists' presence within compassionate therapeutic relationships is the groundwork for self-compassion in psychotherapy. Therapeutic presence and relationships are each common factors in psychotherapy in their own right, but together and when combined with interventions incorporating self-compassion practices, clients can experience a reduction in symptoms of rumination and experiential avoidance, so they can approach their pain and experience in session with greater ease.

Self-compassion in this way can serve as an anchor in a stormy sea, so we do not just shut down or further the harm. Pain is inherent and consistent across theories and diagnoses. It is a part of being human. Knowing how to approach pain can enhance the perspective and approach we come from. It is beneficial for clients and therapists alike. It can also serve us to see our intertwining nature with others; when we know we are not separate, then the compassion we bring to ourselves and our clients is inextricably linked and felt. This view provides us with a model of self-compassion in psychotherapy that we began this journey with and have a deeper understanding from the wisdom of the authors in this book.

A Model of Self-Compassion in Psychotherapy

A model of self-compassion put forth by Germer (Chapter 1) allows us to highlight the three main avenues from which self-compassion has an impact: compassionate therapeutic presence, therapeutic relationships, and interventions.

Therapeutic (Compassionate) Presence

The essential quality of being present with ourselves and our clients in the therapy encounter is the basis for a strong alliance and effective therapy. This includes being grounded, immersed in clients' experience, spacious, and compassionate. It also involves being receptively attuned to clients' experience, attuned with our own experience in the moment, and in contact with each other and the relationship between us.

My (Geller, 2017) work and training on therapeutic presence and self-compassion has helped to discover that presence and compassion/self-compassion work in synergy with each other. Compassion is an essential part of the model of presence, yet it is also a practice that helps to cultivate presence. We also understand as therapists the challenges of being so intimately in contact with clients and their suffering. Having a self-compassionate practice, as highlighted by multiple authors in this book, helps us to be with the pain of others while holding ourselves.

In our chapters (6 and 8), we elucidate the powerful role of inner compassion to work through the barriers to presence, such as shame, self-doubt, overwhelm, and shutdown, as well as outer compassion to be with clients' trauma and pain in a way that can help transform it in the safety of the therapeutic relationship.

Therapists' presence was highlighted by many authors, illuminating this essential stance in a self-compassion-based therapy. For example, Hickman (Chapter 10) encourages having this openhearted presence as we bring curiosity to our clients' experience of self-compassion practice. Mastering the skill of inquiry is essential as we put aside interpretations and instead ask questions about clients' practice of self-compassion with a not-knowing curious approach—being present to the unfolding of clients' experience. This helps foster the resource of clients' self-compassion. Spears and Ochester (Chapter 4) share the value of having cultural humility, which includes presence to the unknown and openness to understanding clients' sociocultural experience, rather than making assumptions about their background.

Many authors shared the importance of adapting traditional self-compassion practices to the client's personal style, issues, and needs. This includes the flexible ability of the therapist to adapt the practice to the client based on the experience in the moment. This demands a cultivated compassionate presence, so these adaptations result from therapists' attunement to clients' moment-to-moment experience in session. As Wishart (Chapter 12) notes, offering the right amount of practice and number of exercises—not too structured and not too minimal—comes from therapists' presence and ability to read the moment.

Therapists' presence and compassion not only create safety for clients but also offer a model for clients to be with their own experience and with others. In her work with couples, Becker (Chapter 17) emphasizes that therapists' embodied presence and compassion with the couple and both partners offers a model for how couples can be present and compassionate for each other, which helps to glimpse new ways of relating with each other.

Similarly, embodied presence is at the heart of working with teens, as Shetler and Hobbs (Chapter 18) emphasize. It creates the conditions for a teen to experience a present and compassionate other and internalize those qualities within. Given this tender and unique period of life, therapists' nonjudgment and acceptance allows them to sensitively read the client's experience as well as be nonreactive and understanding to the challenging and sometimes prickly and defensive way teens can relate. Cultivating an embodied state of presence then is one of the three foundations of how self-compassion can be felt and expressed in the therapeutic encounter.

The Therapeutic and Compassionate Relationship

The second vehicle for compassion is the therapeutic relationship. As clients feel and experience the embodied presence and compassion of their therapist, they feel safe and held, and then in turn the therapeutic relationship strengthens. In time, this received compassion helps the client to internalize and turn compassion toward themselves. From a neuroscience perspective, therapists' and clients' nervous systems are in constant communication, so feeling that compassion and presence from therapists acts as a buffer and co-regulator for clients. The intraconnected aspect of self, MWe, means that feeling compassion for the client is felt in this intraconnection, and the relationship deepens in response.

Gilbert (Chapters 2 and 13) shares how the therapeutic relationship infused with compassion acts like an attachment relationship providing both a secure base and a haven for clients. Roemer and colleagues (Chapter 15) highlight how the therapeutic relationship is core for helping clients cultivate self-compassion, as it allows them to disentangle from anxious responses and engage meaningfully in their lives. Biasetti (Chapter 16) affirms how self-compassion is established first and foremost in the therapeutic relationship in the recovery process for clients with eating disorders. Through modeling compassion, offering validation, and being compassionate, clients begin to invite a new way of approaching their own experience.

Many approaches, such as in discussions of therapeutic presence by the first author (Geller; Chapter 6) and of acceptance and commitment therapy by Weinstein (Chapter 20), emphasize the importance of a caring, connecting, and compassionate therapeutic relationship. The therapeutic relationship is the instrument for change, helping clients be in contact and regulate their experience—and then moving them to internalize the compassion they receive.

Learning self-compassion through the therapeutic relationship, modeled and felt via therapists' presence, complemented with home practices with the therapist's voice, can help clients connect to a safe, soothing social connection. As well, offering self-compassion practices to the client, and being present to suffering while practicing together in session, deepens the therapeutic relationship.

Self-Compassion-Based Interventions

The third way self-compassion is developed for clients in psychotherapy is through interventions, practices, and compassionate questioning. Self-compassion is a learnable skill that can be experienced relationally and practiced internally.

Adaptation of Practices

While this book provides several different practices throughout the chapters and in the Appendix, in psychotherapy, it is important to be present and flexible and adapt practices for clients based on their style and moment-to-moment experience and needs. When applying therapeutic interventions, we want to avoid, as Gilbert (Chapter 13) points out, manualizing forms of practice where "one size fits all." Interventions need to be adapted and tailored to the particular challenges and style of the client. This is possible when therapists also have a personal self-compassion practice to draw from.

Also, we encourage therapists to employ creative uses of mindful and self-compassion practices when adapting to different clients. For example, Shetler and Hobbs (Chapter 18) describe creative ways to enhance mindfulness and self-compassion with teens, such as through arts, music, and holding your own hand. They also emphasize an individualized approach to cater to a teen's high need for control, along with modification of the language and focal points of common self-compassion practices to make them more accessible.

For clients with challenging emotions or behaviors, such as teens or those with trauma or BPD, authors suggested visualizing a compassionate other or receiving and internalizing compassion from the therapist as a more reasonable and effective way of generating self-compassion. In working with trauma, Pollak (Chapter 9) encourages therapists to offer clients opportunities to slow down, practice with eyes open, not start with the breath, and bring choice to their engagement with practice. This reduces the backdraft or overwhelming emotions that can occur when approaching experience and traumatic memories with self-compassion. As Wishart (Chapter 12) emphasizes, individuals who have experienced neglect and trauma in their attachment and care histories can experience distressing memories being reactivated when they begin compassion training. Starting with psychoeducation can be a helpful way of working with compassion more gently.

Psychoeducation

Something that struck us was the pervasive use of psychoeducation across different authors. In working with people with BPD, through dialogue and compassionate questioning, therapists can start with theory, which is essential, as going straight into a practice can be triggering and evoke backdraft and further pain and shutdown in people who have suffered great pain. Psychoeducation to understand how anxiety increases through shutting down emotions can generate self-compassion. In working with eating disorders, offering a self-compassionate reframe can help clients see their experiences more kindly. Becker (Chapter 17) offers therapists a way to introduce self-compassion skills to couples by first helping them to understand the way human brains are wired to respond to stress. Offering psychoeducation and compassion-based skills can help couples lower defenses and see the good in each other and themselves. In working with pain, Siegel (Chapter 19) guides therapists to start with psychoeducation about the stress-response cycle and how tensing muscles amplifies chronic pain, as the groundwork for working more directly with practices. Weinstein (Chapter 20) provides a set of questions to cultivate self-compassion within the therapeutic dialogue. Offering self-compassion in dialogue with clients can be incorporated across different theoretical approaches.

It's All in the Tone

We learn through our own self-compassion practice that it is about how we talk to ourselves more than what we say. When offering self-compassion practices to clients, it can be helpful for therapists to not get too caught up in the specific words of the practice we are suggesting to clients in a practice. The words are less important in what clients are saying to themselves than the tone. Gilbert (Chapter 13) points out his shock when he saw that offering self-compassion was not helpful for clients with depression and that the reason lay in how cold the tone was.

Self-Compassion Does Not Replace Treatment as Usual

The contributors to this volume generally shared that self-compassion, while transtheoretical and transdiagnostic, does not replace therapy as usual and instead can complement and expedite the therapeutic process. As clients are with a present therapist, in a compassionate therapeutic alliance, and learning self-compassion interventions, they can more easily be with their pain so that they can work through it. Stiglmayr (Chapter 14) describes ways that self-compassion can be integrated into dialectical behavior therapy to enhance this approach. And Weinstein (Chapter 20) highlights how self-compassion can accelerate the acceptance and commitment therapy work of moving clients from co-regulation to self-regulation.

Instead of an alternative therapeutic approach, self-compassion can be viewed as a complement to treatment. For example, Siegel (Chapter 19) emphasizes that mindfulness and compassion practices are not enough in working with pain and do not break the pain cycle on their own. However, when embedded in a comprehensive rehabilitation program, they do help to break this cycle and have eliminated pain for some clients. With teens, Shetler and Hobbs (Chapter 18) advise therapists to assess and treat as they normally would, using therapists' clinical training while also drawing from their personal practice of self-compassion.

The Importance of Personal Practices for the Therapist

Both of us have had a regular practice of mindfulness and inner and outer compassion for many years. We believe that it is essential for us as therapists to have a personal self-compassion practice to enhance our therapeutic presence and embody presence and compassion for clients, as well as take care of ourselves. It is a pervasive and validating belief shared in this book that therapists need a personal self-compassion practice to both care for themselves and balance the intensive emotional work they do with clients.

As well, offering self-compassion to clients from this embodied place of presence and compassion brings an authentic offering of practices with more personal experience to draw from. It also allows us to pause in difficult moments within a therapeutic moment that is emotionally challenging, to offer ourselves a moment of self-compassion. Our personal practice of self-compassion also helps model for clients self-compassion and provides the grounds for offering compassion and validation to clients, which can then help them cultivate their own experience of self-compassion and compassion.

The second author (Tyano Ronen; Chapter 8) describes the underlying fruits of practice and guidelines and suggestions for therapists to develop and maintain a personal practice. Chapter 8 also presents the therapist and client as a mini-*sangha*—through practicing together in session, both benefit and the relationship deepens.

A *sangha* is a community practicing together in order to bring about and maintain a compassionate awareness. The essence of a *sangha* is awareness, understanding, acceptance, harmony, and love. A beautiful walking path may be part of a *sangha*, but a good cushion can be also. We can make many things into supportive elements of our *sangha*. If we do not have a supportive *sangha*, we may not be getting the kind of support we need for our practice, that we need to nourish our desire to cultivate compassion and wisdom in ourselves. Sometimes, we call it a beginner's mind, beautiful and strong. In a healthy *sangha*, there is encouragement for our beginner's mind. So, the *sangha* is the soil and we are the seed. No matter how beautiful or how vigorous our seed is, if the soil does not provide us with vitality, our seed might die. When we allow ourselves to be in a *sangha* the way a drop of water allows itself to be in a river, the energy of the *sangha* can penetrate into us, to transform and heal.

Many authors shared this need for therapists to have a personal practice. And we add the benefit of doing so in *sangha*, in relationship with others. Both taking care of ourselves and optimally teaching clients self-compassion need to emerge from an embodied place of understanding.

Implications for Psychotherapy Training and Supervision

We propose that psychotherapy training include self-compassion across therapeutic approaches. This includes training therapists to cultivate therapeutic presence, develop and sustain therapeutic compassion relationships, and learn various self-compassion-based interventions. This would include helping therapists to ground themselves first in their own personal practice and then learn to attune to clients and their moment-to-moment experience in session. They can then offer self-compassion interventions that are attuned to clients' styles, needs, and experiences in the moment.

In programs that have already started incorporating this approach, therapists in training are sharing that they find it very nourishing and preventive of burnout. When applying self-care, and practicing mindfulness and self-compassion, it is serving as a protective factor for therapists.

Self-Compassion-Based Supervision

Self-compassion as a foundation in supervision can be used to transform painful experiences and gain insights during a supervision session, hence influencing the session with the client. The practice of self-compassion can help a person (therapist, client, supervisee) process unresolved and painful issues that interfere with therapists' presence in session, creating a safe and caring bond with themselves.

In self-compassionate supervision, we are attentive to the challenging events that therapists may experience with their clients. The supervisor helps the therapist to be aware of the pain and transform it by bringing a kind and caring attitude to themselves. This helps them return to the psychotherapy process with their client in a new, present, and compassionate way. The supervisee learns to recognize the painful and unprocessed experiences in themselves (such as despair, uselessness, tiredness, emptiness, etc.) and other painful experiences connected to their psychotherapy work and relate to themselves with care and self-compassion.

The supervisor serves as a caring witness to their painful experiences and re-creates a supportive kind bond with themselves. It enables emotional and physiological regulation of the supervisee's experience that is more flexible, open, and reconnected to the client. It influences the way the supervisee feels about themselves, the clients, their relationships, and the challenges brought to supervision. It changes the supervisee's way of being at a supervision session and consequently in the subsequent psychotherapy session. It creates a ripple effect, as the supervisors, therapists, clients, and all their relationships are wrapped in a compassionate envelope, enabling eventually the creation of a more compassionate world.

Final Words: Contributing to a Compassionate World

Feeling our intraconnectedness and being part of this web of human life led us to feel a sense of caring and responsibility toward all sentient beings. Our vocation as therapists stems from a sensitivity to the suffering of beings and the deep intention to alleviate suffering. We each took our own creative path, searching for the ways and means to do so, and found the practice of self-compassion a powerful way of life, mindset, and practice for ourselves as therapists, supervisors, and our clients. The possibility we have to take care of ourselves, as well as caring for others in various ways, is a huge resource that is shared in this volume. Through this care, and the many moments of compassion felt and taught to our clients, we can contribute to a myriad of relationships and a larger global world that is infused with compassion.

When we practice mindfulness, inner and outer compassion, walking, and working, we create a more compassionate society, inspiring confidence and compassion all around us. This could be one way to avoid letting despair overwhelm us. It might also help our environment to not lose hope, living our daily life in such a way that demonstrates that a compassionate future is possible.

The presence of a *sangha* that practices together (supervisor–psychotherapist–client and into the world) is a wonderful opportunity to allow for the collective energy of compassion. We systemically profit from that collective energy, implementing compassion and self-compassion in health care systems and organizations—for example, therapists in an agency practicing self-compassion together. Although we can rely on the energy of mindfulness and compassion that is generated by our personal practice, sometimes it is not enough. Yet, if we know how to use that energy in order to benefit from the collective energy of the whole, we will have a powerful source of energy for our therapeutic practice and our personal and collective transformation and healing.

When we understand that inner wholeness, inter- and intraconnected relationships, and compassion are evolved states in mammals, we can widen and deepen our awareness of them, bringing compassion to ourselves and others, creating a ripple effect of kindness and caring, and hopefully reducing suffering in our global world.

REFERENCE

Geller, S. M. (2017). *A guide to cultivating therapeutic presence.* American Psychological Association.

APPENDIX

Practices and Exercises

The practices in this appendix are accompaniments to the chapters and are referred to in the chapters. Many of these practices have audios that accompany them that can be enjoyed or shared as guided audio meditations. You can find these audios, which have been recorded either by the authors or by other self-compassion teachers, at *www.guilford.com/tyano-ronen-materials*. You can read the written scripts below or play the relevant audios as guided meditations with clients, but we encourage you to practice first with yourself. We hope these written practices and audios support your journey to being a self-compassion-based psychotherapist.

PRACTICE A

Self-Compassion Break

(Germer & Neff, 2019)

Christopher Germer (Chapter 1)

- To start, please think of a situation in your life that is difficult, that is causing you stress right now, such as a health problem, a problem in an important relationship, or perhaps a work problem. Please choose a specific problem in the mild to moderate range, not a big problem. (*Pause*)

Mindfulness

- Now allow yourself to drop into the situation and recall how it felt at the time or even notice how you feel right now. Notice how distress feels in your body. (*Pause*)
- And see if you can discover where in your body you feel the sensation of stress the most. (*Pause*)
- Allowing your experience to be just as it is, perhaps making just a little *more room than usual* for the experience of stress or discomfort in your body. (*Pause*)
- And if you like, try labeling the experience for yourself in a gentle and kind way—"This is uncomfortable," "This hurts," "This is stressful"—validating your experience as you might for a good friend. (*Pause*)

Common Humanity

- As you do this, know that what you are experiencing right now is *part of the human experience.*
- You are not alone. Others might feel just as you do, or did, in the same situation.
- Stress is part of being human; it's part of our common humanity.

(continued)

Self-Kindness

- Now let's see if you can respond to distress in a new way. Perhaps by giving yourself some kindness simply *because* you're having a moment of discomfort.
- If you like, perhaps *placing a hand* on the part of your body that feels the most stress. (*Pause*) Just feeling the sense of compassionate touch, and if you like, sending kindness through your fingers into that part of your body that is holding stress for you, or gently massaging that part of your body. (*Pause*)
- And consider for a moment what you would most like to hear in a moment like this—perhaps words of comfort or support. For example, "I'm here for you," "I love you," "You are a good person." What might those words be for you? (*Pause*)
- Allowing yourself to repeat these words for yourself, over and over, in your own mind, in your own way. (*Pause*)
- Taking a few more moments to offer yourself kindness in a way that feels just right for you, savoring compassionate touch or offering yourself words of kindness, just *because* you feel distress, not trying to change it or make it go away. (*Pause*)
- And when you're ready, beginning to release the practice, letting the practice settle. (*Pause*) Allowing yourself to feel just as you do right now, letting the practice be just as it was, and allowing yourself, if only for this moment, to be just as you are.
- And when you're ready, slowly open your eyes.

PRACTICE B

Giving and Receiving Compassion

(Germer & Neff, 2019)

Christopher Germer (Chapter 1)

Savoring the Breath

- Begin by turning your attention inward and feel the physical sensation of your body breathing in and breathing out.
- If you like, allowing yourself to be internally rocked and caressed by the rhythm of your breathing.

Warming Up Awareness

- Then, focus your attention on your *in-breath* only—letting yourself savor the sensation of breathing in, one breath after another, perhaps noticing how the in-breath energizes your body.
- As you breathe in, if you wish, breathing *kindness* and *compassion* in for yourself—feeling the quality of kindness and compassion as you breathe in.
- Breathing in for yourself as often as you need to. Then, when you're ready, shifting your focus to your *out-breath*—feeling your body breathing out. Feel the ease and relaxation of the body exhaling.
- And as you breathe out, sending the ease and well-being to your client.
- If you wish, also sending *kindness* and *compassion* with each out-breath, one breath after another.

"In for Me, Out for You"

- Finally, focus on the sensation of breathing *both* in and out, savoring the sensation of breathing in and the sensation of breathing out. Allowing the in-breath to always be for yourself.
- If you like, sending *kindness* and *compassion* along with your breathing.

(continued)

PRACTICE B *(page 2 of 2)*

- Find just the right balance. Give yourself permission to breathe in for yourself as often as you need, one breath after another, and when your cup is full, begin breathing out for others.
- Let go of any unnecessary effort, allowing this meditation to be as easy as the body breathing itself.

PRACTICE C

Compassion Practice Sequences to Aid Cultivating Compassion Brain, Body, and Mind States

Paul Gilbert (Chapter 2 and Chapter 13)

This practice is offered as a full practice, which comprises four shorter practices within it. It can be followed in full, or you can focus on just one aspect if you prefer a shorter practice. The corresponding audio reflects the option to listen to the full practice or to listen to the smaller practices on their own (C.1, C.2, C.3, C.4).

Compassion Practice Sequences to Aid Cultivating Compassion Brain, Body, and Mind States

I'm delighted to offer you some recordings and exercises. Compassion-focused therapy is what we call a biopsychosocial approach, which means that we try to develop practices that will influence our bodies, our minds, and our social behaviors.

So what I'm going to do in these practices, I'm going to put a whole series of practices together for you, and when you listen to the sequence, you can then play it again and stop at any point where you want to spend time just engaging in a specific practice.

C.1. Grounding and Breathing

So we're going to begin with the body. So first we sit comfortably in the chair and we lift the shoulders up and back so they're sitting in line with the hips.

Now this will open your chest, but it will also open your diaphragm and it will create a small inward curve in your back. So that's the first part of the exercise is practicing posture, which lifts your diaphragm and gives you a small curve

(continued)

---

in your back, your lower back. This now allows us to breathe in a way, which will stimulate your vagus nerve and balance your autonomic nervous system.

So I'm going to invite you to do what we call a five and five. Now there are many breathing patterns that you can use, that you can discover on the internet, which facilitates your vagus nerve. This one is going to invite breathing in for 5 seconds, holding for around 2 seconds, breathing out for 5 seconds, and resting for 2. In some breathing practices, you can spend longer on the outbreath because the outbreath is the breath that has a particular impact on the vagus nerve.

So let's do this together then.

So breathing in, two, three, out, two, three, in, two, three, four, out, two, three, four, in, two, three, four, five. Out, two, three, four, five.

So that is our basic rhythm. As you're breathing to that rhythm, try and feel the air going down into the diaphragm. So your diaphragm is doing the work of the breath to feel your diaphragm rising and falling. And you can even imagine the breath going down to the base of your spine. So you want no movement in your shoulders. Your shoulders should be stable and you're just in all the breathing with your diaphragm. So I'm going to leave you for 1 minute for you to practice that, but you can stop the recording at any time and spend more time on this part of the posture and breathing exercise. (*Pause*)

Now that you've got a sense of the pattern, just allow yourself to feel into the rhythm of your body, and as you're breathing in and out in this way, noticing your body settling down, let your body settle into the chair. So your shoulders are up and back, you're sitting upright, you have that curve in your back, just allow the chair to take your weight. So we call this grounding, sitting like a mountain with your feet flat on the floor, grounded.

C.2. Voice Tone

The exercise is about how we use our voice tones in our minds. Now, when we have various thoughts, sometimes anxious thoughts or angry thoughts, they take on the emotional tone of the thoughts. But here we're going to practice deliberately creating friendly, compassionate tones. So on the out-breath, I'm going to invite you simply to say hello to yourself and you can compare and contrast what it's like when you say hello in a neutral way, or when you make a real effort to create a sense of friendliness.

(continued)

So my name is "[therapist's name]." So on the out-breath, I will be saying, "Hello, [therapist's name]," and notice how the voice moves up slightly in a welcome.

So there's a joyous and a friendliness in the voice tone. So I'm going to give you a minute just to practice on the out-breath saying hello to yourself in a friendly way and try and feel into that voice tone so that you can feel the friendship that you want to offer in that voice tone.

Now whenever you are having various thoughts that are trying to be helpful to you, always remember to create that friendly impassionate voice tone. So, if you use mantras such as "May I be happy" or "May I be well," always use that voice tone.

C.3. Facial Expression

So now we're going to focus on our facial expressions and we're also going to do an imagery task. So we are sitting there in the chair, our shoulders are up and back, and we've got a curve pointing toward lifting the diaphragm. We're going at about four breaths per minute.

We've created a curve, a friendly voice tone in our minds with a compassionate texture.

Now create a friendly facial expression as if you are greeting somebody who you really like, a real friend of yours. And notice what happens when you do that. If, for example, you go from a neutral face, which is probably what you have at the moment, and then deliberately try to create a friendly voice. You're not going to be able to do that. Make a friendly face and focus on the feeling of friendliness that you're trying to convey. Imagine that you're looking at your friend, you can see their eyes, you can see them smiling back at you. Focus on that sense of friendliness.

Now focus on the fact that if your friend was struggling a little bit with something, had a little life problem, nothing too major—because this is a practice, imagine how much you want to be helpful to your friend, how much you want to be there for them, how much you would like them to turn to you for help. So this is priming your compassion motivation, noticing what it's like that you really want to be there for them, you really want to help them, and how much joy you would get if you could help them and they came through that life to a goodie because you helped them, right?

So just focus on that wish. As you sit with your friendly face and your friendly voice, just really focusing on that real wish to be helpful: "May I be helpful."

(continued)

The more we practice imagining and stimulating these areas of the brain over time, those areas of the brain, which are linked to our motivation to be helpful and our pleasure of being able to be helpful, will become strengthened.

Now we're going to change the imagery slightly. Sometimes people have a little bit more difficulty with this one. But just hang in there and keep going. Because now I'm going to invite you to imagine that rather than your friend you are imagining, you see an image of yourself. Okay, now that's maybe an image of you that's maybe a little anxious or worried about something.

Once again, stick with your breathing at about four breaths per minute, a bright posture, friendly voice. Friendly facial expression, now focusing on the wish to be helpful to this part of you.

Don't get pulled into the distress of the part you're looking at, stay with the part that's wanting to be helpful, that's wanting to reach out and be helpful to the part of you that's maybe struggling a bit. Maybe some ideas come into your mind of what you would like to say to that part that's struggling a little bit.

So now you have been trying out your compassionate self and your compassionate motivation just a little bit, just to touch it. In your next practices, you can begin to focus on the qualities you would like with this part of you that's sitting there now, like a mountain, with compassion and motivation, and how you would like to see this part of you grow. So keep your friendly smile and think what would you like to develop as the compassionate self.

Maybe more patience, maybe more tenderness, maybe more toughness, maybe more assertiveness. You can choose whatever you want. Just focus on this idea of growing, cultivating, developing, and feeding this part of you. This part of you that wants to be helpful, that wants to be supportive, that wants to see others flourish from what you do, and that includes yourself, of course. Sometimes it can help if we choose one quality and then over a week, we practice that one quality, so the quality could be taking time out, relaxing more or becoming more patient or being more friendly.

You can choose anything, really, that you feel will help you on your journey to developing and growing your compassionate self.

C.4. Tricky Mind

We will now bring to mind the reality of being human.

This is basic wisdom, and your compassionate mind has wisdom and courage, and the wisdom is all living things. It has been built by DNA. Everything that

(continued)

exists, that is alive, has all been built by genes. And no living thing chose its design.

And that includes you and me. We didn't choose to have two arms and two legs. We didn't choose to have to breathe every few seconds, otherwise we keeled over. We didn't choose to have to eat. We didn't choose how to keep fit. We didn't choose that some of the foods we can put a lot of weight on.

We didn't choose any of that. There is so much about being a human that we never chose and we never chose to have the brain that we've got. We didn't choose to be the gender that we are.

We didn't choose to be the ethnicity that we are, and we didn't choose the day or the place of our birth. We didn't choose anything. What we discovered is that we are a consciousness existing in a body that's been built by nature. And that nature is designed to survive and reproduce.

And therefore, our brains have been built in such a way that we can have some fantastic qualities, but also some very dark ones. It's easy for the human brain to fall into anxiety, depression, or rage. Inside of us is the capacity of wonderful compassion, but the most terrifying vengeance. But we didn't design any of it. It's all being built for us.

And so, the compassion journey is to become mindful of a mind that is being built for us, to become conscious that we exist as a consciousness in a body with the brain that is being built for us.

In order for us to pursue compassion, we will work out as best we can how it works. So for the next minute or so just spend time in a friendly way saying hello to your body and to your brain because it's being designed for you. Not by you, as if you're designing any of it, but that you will try as best you can to get to understand it so that you can work it in a way that it's not harmful to you or to others, because brains can be very tricky. And so this brings us to the end of our practice together.

End of Full Practice

Together where we looked at how to help the body support the mind, our posture, opening up the diaphragm, engaging in soothing rhythm breathing, grounding in the body, using the voice to convey friendliness and compassion, using the face to convey and stimulate friendliness and compassion in our brain, focusing on priming compassion motivation by bringing a friend to mind that we really want to help, and then doing the same with ourselves. Then bringing in the wisdom that we've all just found ourselves here, trying

(continued)

to make the best sense that we can with a brain and a body that's being built for us, not by us. And that's quite a challenge. So I wish you well on your practices and of course, there are many other practices for you to explore in compassion-focused therapy and indeed other compassion therapies and mindfulness approaches.

So I wish you well. "May you be well," "May you be happy," and "May you develop the wisdom and courage to guide you through the rest of your life."

PRACTICE D

Compassionate Practices

Elli Weisbaum, Shelby L. Alsup, and Daniel J. Siegel (Chapter 3)

Practice D.1. Forgiveness

This meditation expands on the "Kind Awareness" portion of the "Wheel of Awareness" practice. The focus here is on offering forgiveness for whatever pain or harm someone else may have caused you in the past and then asking yourself for forgiveness for something you may have done to cause pain or harm to someone else. Forgiveness is not stating that what happened was right or good; forgiveness, as my colleague and friend Jack Kornfield has suggested, is giving up all hope for a better past. As you take this time to feel forgiveness toward another and offer forgiveness to yourself, you can repeat the following phrases quietly in your mind or even say them softly aloud:

First, take a breath and say:

"May all living beings be happy . . . May all living beings be as healthy as they can . . . May all living beings be safe . . .
May all living beings flourish and thrive."

Second, taking a deeper breath say to the person you are extending forgiveness to:

"May you be happy . . .
And live with meaning, connection, and equanimity . . . And a playful, grateful, and joyful heart.
May you be as healthy as you can . . .
And have a body that gives me energy and flexibility . . . strength and stability.
May you be safe . . .
And protected from all sorts of inner and outer harm.
And may you flourish and thrive . . .
And live with ease of well-being."

(continued)

These compassionate practices are used with permission from Daniel J. Siegel, MD, and are adapted from his book *Becoming Aware: A 21-Day Mindfulness Program for Reducing Anxiety and Cultivating Calm.*

Last, allow yourself to forgive yourself for something you have done or said that caused another person pain:

"May I be happy . . .

And live with meaning, connection, and equanimity . . . And a playful, grateful, and joyful heart.

May I be as healthy as I can . . .

And have a body that gives me energy and flexibility . . . strength and stability.

May I be safe . . .

And protected from all sorts of inner and outer harm.

And may I flourish and thrive . . .

And live with the ease of well-being."

Practice D.2. Connecting to the Collective MWe

Our self is not only what exists in the inner life of the body—the "I" of who we are. We are also part of an interconnected whole, part of a relational "we." But how can we integrate this differentiated bodily me or I with a relational us or we? Integration is the honoring of differences and then their compassionate, respectful linkage. If we integrate "me" and "we," we come up with an integrated identity, one that we can name with a new term: *MWe*. Extending on the "Wheel of Awareness" practice, here is an additional short meditation—you might try for 5 or 10 minutes—that will focus your awareness on the collective MWe.

Find a comfortable place to sit or lie and focus your breath. Now let your visual focus of attention scan over your body—the source of your inner identity as an I or me. Now let your visual attention widen to take in the world around you—other people who might be nearby, the room, or the natural world you might be in. Now let your mind take in the images of all the people you know, and now all human beings, to our whole human family. Expanding this lens of identity, letting your relational belonging broaden, see if you can sense your being a part of all of nature—you belong to all people and the planet. Your inner identity is me, your relational identity is we, and together your integrated identity is Me plus We equals MWe.

Now that you've used your mind's lens to move from a close-up focus to a wide-angle view on identity, you can take this inner and relational self inside and offer positive wishes of kind intention to MWe. Repeat the following phrases aloud or say them silently in your mind as you continue to breathe deeply:

(continued)

"May MWe be happy . . .

And live with meaning, connection, and equanimity . . . And a playful, grateful, and joyful heart.

May MWe be as healthy as MWe can . . .

And have bodies that gives energy and flexibility . . . strength and stability.

May MWe be safe . . .

And protected from all sorts of inner and outer harm.

And may MWe flourish and thrive . . . And live with the ease of well-being."

Reflection

How did it feel to widen your identity lens and focus on the collective MWe of an integrated identity and broadened belonging? Did any particular faces of individuals you know, or know of, come into your mind? Did your heart move toward any communities in particular either, that you are a part of or know only from reading about them or seeing images on television? What did MWe feel like to you?

PRACTICE E

Working with Challenges of Cross-Cultural Psychotherapy with Self-Compassion

Sydney Spears and Tracy Ochester (Chapter 4)

Practice E.1. My Inner Container of Self-Kindness Exploration

This invitational practice involves finding an empty physical container of personal choice, which can symbolically represent one's sociocultural self and body. The prompts are invitations to mindfully pay attention to external sensory information and practice self-kindness. Since relational oppressive dynamics can be replicated within cross-cultural dyads, this practice was created by Sydney Spears (Chapter 4) as an exploration for the therapist to compassionately join (with the client's permission) and participate in exploring the practice with client as an anti-oppressive, relational ally in real time.

Script for the Practice

If you would like, you are welcome to take a moment and find a piece of paper, pen, or pencil and find a simple, empty container of any size, shape, or condition in your space for this self-kindness activity. This empty container of your own choice could possibly be a self-kindness container—if that is something you are open to experiencing. Your container of choice could be an old box, bowl, cup, glass, plastic cup, or something else [pause to allow time for client to select paper, pen, and container].

I am wondering if it might be okay with you if I participate in this exploration too. Please let me know how you really feel about this and no worries at all if you would prefer to explore this practice on your own. [*Note:* If a client agrees to therapist participation, say, "I have selected a container for myself—Are you interested in viewing my self-compassionate container?"] You are welcome to share or not to share your experience of this container exploration at any time.

When you are ready you might begin to notice some details about your self-kindness container. Perhaps the colors, design, shape, size—if it is accessible to you, feel free to run your fingers around different parts of the container

(continued)

to possibly feel the texture. (*Pause*) I will do the same thing and participate with you.

If you would like, call to your mind or maybe write down what details you noticed about your container. (*Pause*) What might be one detail of your container that you liked or felt neutral about? [*Note:* Therapists can choose to share their response.]

Now you might take a few moments and recall the main things we talked about during our session connection today. (*Pause*)

Now feel free to take a moment to think about one simple message or phrase that is positive, supportive, or uplifting to you—even if you do not believe it right now. What positive phrases or mini-messages might make you feel seen, understood, and truly valued? (*Repeat question and pause*)

Perhaps you would like to claim an uplifting, supportive, kind phrase or message from an ancestor, a cultural community, a personal cultural value or belief, particular person, spiritual or religious figure, an animal if it could talk, or from nature. What about a line from your favorite song, there may be a quote that you like, or the title of a book or movie that you like. (*Pause*)

You are welcome to write these kind words or phrases down on a piece of paper perhaps two or three times if you would like to do so. (*Pause*) Now, if you want to, place your words or message in your possible self-kindness container and maybe say the words to yourself a few times. (*Longer pause*) Then, [*Note:* Therapists can share their message with the client and describe what was personally experienced.] invite the client to write down their responses, hold responses in their awareness, or verbally share the following if they are open. What was it like to find your own container and your kind mini-message? Would you be open to adding more kind words or messages you like in your container during your next session or perhaps this coming week—no worries if you are not open to this. Is there anything else you might want to share about this activity?

Practice E.2. Self-Compassion Practice for My Social and Cultural Identities

The intention of this relational practice is to support client–therapist self-kindness, cultural appreciation, compassion, and sense of empowerment toward any of their sociocultural marginalized, disowned, or minimized identities rather than self-criticism and shame. As an alternative to a meditative practice experience, this script can also be shared as a client–therapist reflective relational discussion or a complete written activity.

(continued)

Script for the Practice

Take a moment to pause—and rest into this moment. Maybe take a few breaths if that is accessible for you. Breath is an expression of your aliveness—and your humanness. Feel free to allow the muscles of your body to release any tension that might be there. Just rest into this moment of time by settling in and maybe letting go of striving, proving, or doing. You are welcome to bring to mind two cultural parts of you.

Your social and cultural identity parts might be named as your gender, ethnicity, race, body features, sexual orientation, age, appearance, ancestors, personality, abilities, values, roles, family, community, language, celebrations, customs, stories, traditions, art, music, beliefs, activities, or other ways of being in the world. What two cultural parts come to mind that you tend to like—even a little bit? (*Pause*) What do you really like about these social and cultural parts? (*Pause*) What feelings or thoughts did you experience (if any) when focusing on these social or cultural parts? (*Pause*)

If your own likable cultural parts could talk, what messages might they send to you that are supportive, protective, or motivating? Maybe messages that you need to remember right now. (*Repeat, then pause*)

Your social and cultural identities are valuable parts that live within you—they are good enough and always worthy wherever you are.

Now, if you would like, call to mind one social or cultural identity you tend to struggle with at times. (*Pause*) What words might describe your identity struggle—such as *difficult, discrimination, hurt, not true, injustice*, or something else? (*Pause*)

You were not born with these thoughts about your identity of struggle. So, how did you learn about your difficult identity? Where did that information come from? (*Pause*)

If your own likable cultural parts could talk, what messages might they send to you that are true, motivating, and empowering about your identity of struggle? (*Pause*)

As you end this practice, feel free to write down any other important messages you may want to remember as a kind and empowering cultural resource for yourself.

PRACTICE F

Soften, Calm, Allow

José Ramón Yela Bernabé and Antonio Crego Díaz (Chapter 5)

Practice F.1. Labeling Emotions (Germer & Neff, 2019)

As you relive this situation, notice if any emotions arise within you. And if so, see if a label for an emotion comes up, a name. For example:

- Anger
- Sadness
- Grief
- Confusion
- Fear
- Longing
- Despair

If you are having many emotions, see if you have a name for the strongest emotion associated with the situation.

Now repeat the name of the emotion to yourself in a gentle, understanding voice, as if you were validating for a friend what they were feeling: "That's longing," "That's grief."

Practice F.2. Pause for Self-Compassion (Germer & Neff, 2019)

Find a comfortable position, sitting or lying down, close your eyes, and take three relaxing breaths.

Place your hand on your heart, or another soothing place, for a few moments to remind yourself that you are in the room and that you, too, are worthy of kindness.

Let yourself recall a mild to moderately difficult situation that you are in right now, perhaps a health problem, stress in a relationship, or a loved one in pain.

(continued)

Do not choose a very difficult problem or a trivial problem—choose a problem that can generate a little stress in your body when you think of it.

Visualize the situation. Who is involved? What's happening?

Practice F.3. Soften-Soothe-Allow (Germer & Neff, 2019)

Now soften into the location in your body where you feel the difficult emotion. Let the muscles soften, let them relax, as if in warm water. Soften . . . soften . . . soften . . . Remember that we're not trying to change the feeling—we're just holding it tenderly.

If you wish, just soften a little around the edges.

Now soothe yourself because of this difficult situation.

If you wish, place your hand over the part of your body that feels uncomfortable and just feel the gentle touch of your hand. Perhaps imagine warmth and kindness flowing through your hand into your body. Maybe even thinking of your body as if it were the body of a beloved child.

And are there some comforting words that you might need to hear? If so, imagine you had a friend who was struggling in the same way. What would you say to your friend? ("I'm so sorry you feel this way," "I care deeply about you.") Can you offer yourself a similar message? ("Oh, it's so hard to feel this," "May I be kind to myself.")

If you need to, feel free to open your eyes whenever you wish or let go of the exercise and just feel your breath.

Finally, allow the discomfort to be there. Make room for it, releasing the need to make it go away.

Allow yourself to be just as you are, just like this, if only for this moment.

If you wish, you can repeat the cycle with your emotion, going a bit deeper each time, sticking with the sensation if it moves in your body or even morphs into a different emotion. Soften . . . soothe . . . allow. Soften . . . soothe . . . allow.

Now let go of the practice and focus on your body as a whole. Allow yourself to feel whatever you feel, to be exactly as you are in this moment.

(continued)

Practice F.4. Discovering Core Values (Germer & Neff, 2019)

Now expand your awareness to your body as a whole.

Recall the difficult situation again and scan your body for where you feel it most easily. In your mind's eye, sweep your body from head to toe, stopping where you can sense a little tension or discomfort.

Just feel what is "feelable" in your body right now. Nothing more.

Now if you can, choose a single location in your body where the feeling expresses itself most strongly, perhaps as a point of muscle tension, a hollow feeling, or even a heartache.

In your mind, incline gently toward that spot. Allow your awareness to fully inhabit the physical sensation of the emotion in your body.

PRACTICE G

Soothing or Supportive Touch

(Germer & Neff, 2019)

Shari Geller (Chapter 6) and Galia Tyano Ronen (Chapter 8)

This practice can help clients find a way to physically comfort, soothe, or support themselves by using a somatic, through physical touch. Soothing touch refers to the tender side of self-compassion and supportive touch refers to fierce compassion. Both are forms of caring. A simple body gesture like putting a hand over the heart can influence how we think and feel; it has been shown to reduce the stress hormone cortisol.

Some clients might be resistant, or even unable, to do this. In these situations, we might invite clients to share how they comfort themselves already with touch. The focus of this practice is finding a physical way to comfort and support oneself, such as holding a pillow, rubbing a smooth stone, or stroking a pet.

Instructions

Therapists may invite clients to stretch, saying that touch is a key signal of compassion for all mammals; this is why physical touch is a powerful gateway to self-compassion.

Invite the client through the following gestures to discover where the experience of touch is genuinely soothing or supportive.

Invite the client to close their eyes, partially or fully, to connect with their inner experience.

Some options that can be offered:

- Palms gently pressed against one another.
- One hand cupped in the other.
- One hand over the heart.
- Two hands over the heart.

(continued)

- Cupping one hand over a fist over the heart.
- One hand over the heart.
- Gently stroking one's chest, back and forth, or in small circles.
- One hand over the heart and one on the belly/abdomen.
- Two hands on the belly/abdomen.
- One hand on a cheek.
- Cradling one's face in the hands.
- Crossing one's arms and giving a gentle hug.
- Stroking one's arms.
- Gently rocking or swaying one's body.
- Cupping the hands in one's lap.

Now invite the client to explore soothing or supportive touch on their own for another minute. Then it is possible to use it whenever they feel the need to soothe themselves.

PRACTICE H

Embodied Presence Practice: Core Body Centering

(adapted from Geller, 2017)
Shari Geller (Chapter 6)

This presence practice is focused on centering and embodying a sense of presence. Learning to center can occur through three dimensions of the body: length, width, and depth. Accessing presence through the body involves aligning ourselves internally through the following steps:

1. *Length:* Firmly plant both feet on the ground, becoming aware of your posture, and aligning your body with gravity so that you feel effortlessly supported. Place feet slightly apart, knees unlocked, and pelvis rocked forward slightly to straighten the spine. Sense the bottoms of your feet, where the soles rest firmly against the ground. Allow your gaze to be soft, maintaining awareness with your peripheral vision. Imagine that the top of your head is connected to the sky as if it were held by a string. Allow your attention to drop to the center of gravity in your body, 2 inches below your navel.
2. *Width:* Gently rock your weight from right to left until you come into stillness with both feet fully on the ground. Find the neutral balanced position in the center of the width of your body. A helpful image is to imagine walking in a room, knowing that you fully belong, and feeling an expansion in your chest that gives you a sense of taking up space.
3. *Depth:* Allow your awareness to be with the front and back of your body. Gently rock back and forth, from heel and toe, until you come into stillness with all four corners of the feet on the ground. Allow yourself to be supported by both the front and back of your body, allowing your belly to soften and open—sensing the center of your body, that point or area that aligns you from top to bottom, side to side, and front to back.
4. *Breathe:* Now rest in the experience of centeredness and grounding while taking a few full breaths.

Regular practice of this embodied presence exercise can help develop a greater ability to shift and return to an internally centered place before the session. Therapists can also use this practice in session to recenter when their attention moves away from the moment or emotions become overwhelming. In session, therapists can simply bring awareness to the feet as they make contact with the ground to help anchor awareness when it has wandered.

PRACTICE I

Self-Compassion in Practice

Shauna Shapiro, Shayda Roohparvar, and Jill Lillie (Chapter 7)

We invite you to call to mind a current challenge you are facing with a client or within a therapeutic context. Perhaps you are feeling overwhelmed, or perhaps you made a mistake that you are ruminating on. Choose one struggle that you want to work with.

Mindfulness

Please write down the situation as clearly and objectively as possible. Notice how you feel as you write about it. See if you can mindfully acknowledge your emotions and become aware of any accompanying body sensations (e.g., tightness in my throat, fear in my chest). Also, be aware of how you may be judging yourself for what happened. Write down anything you notice.

Kindness

Write down some kind statements that you could make to yourself in the face of this situation—for example, "This is painful. I am here with you"; "You are really worried about your client. This is scary for you"; "It's okay to make mistakes, I am learning"; or simply, "I care about you." As you write these kind statements, you may want to pause and put your hand on your heart as a gesture of self-care. When we place a hand on our heart it releases oxytocin, the hormone of safety and connection.

Common Humanity

Remind yourself how natural it is for hard times to arise, and for you to feel scared, frustrated, or sad. Reflect on all the other people in the world who might be in a very similar situation right now. Write down your reflections—for example, "It is natural to feel confused. Many therapists struggle with knowing what to do." As you connect in your mind and heart with others in

(continued)

your same situation, try sending them and yourself compassion and kindness. For example, "I care about my client. I feel scared about his safety. I imagine many therapists are scared about their clients right now. I am sending compassion to myself and all therapists."

Once you have completed writing, take a moment to set down your pen and paper, close your eyes, and allow the teachings of this practice to settle in. Inviting in a few deeper breaths in and out and let yourself absorb the nourishment and wisdom of this practice. Trust that the seeds you are planting will continue to grow. The key is practice. What you practice grows stronger.

PRACTICE J

Cultivating the Practice of Self-Compassion

Galia Tyano Ronen (Chapter 8)

Practice J.1. Sitting Compassion Meditation Practice

- I invite you to sit comfortably, letting your shoulders be relaxed.
- Letting your chest be open and the belly soft.
- Putting your feet on the ground.
- Feeling the ground underneath you, your sitting bones in contact with the chair or the cushion. Your hands resting in your lap.
- Breathing in a smooth relaxed way.
- Resting in open awareness.
- Relax your mind and remain present.
- Don't try to focus on anything in particular or control your mind, yet do not get lost in thoughts either.
- Breathing, being present.
- Leave all the senses open.
- Leave all of the senses' doors open, without trying to block any aspect of the experience.
- If it is difficult to remain present, bring your awareness to the breath.
- Simply know that you are breathing.
- Breathe gently, letting the breath come to you.
- Soft breath.
- It caresses you from the inside in a soothing way.
- If you notice one part of the breath, such as the belly rising and falling, or the feeling of air entering your nostrils, allow this but do not keep your mind fixed on any one sensation or feeling. You could use the sounds that come to your ears as guides.
- Still letting everything coming through your senses be present in your experience now.

(continued)

- From time to time, relax your mind into a state of alert presence and bring it back to the breath if you find yourself getting distracted.
- You might consider listening to the sounds around us.
- Relax your mind, open to anything around us and inside us.
- I invite you to put a hand over your heart, feeling the warmth and the soft touch, the support of your hand, acknowledging your presence in an appreciative way.
- Letting go and resting once again in open soft awareness. Open soft awareness.

Practice J.2. The Practice of Self-Compassion with Equanimity (Neff & Germer, 2018)

This exercise is intended for use in actual caregiving situations. It is a way of being compassionate with ourselves while maintaining a connection to others. It combines the "Giving and Receiving Compassion" meditation with phrases that cultivate equanimity. Equanimity is balanced awareness in the midst of pleasant or unpleasant emotions.

Please find a comfortable position and take a few deep breaths to settle into your body and into the present moment. You might like to put your hand over your heart, or wherever it is comforting and soothing, as a reminder to bring affectionate awareness to your experience and to yourself.

Bring to mind someone you are caring for who is exhausting you or frustrating you—someone whom you care about who is suffering. Visualize the person and the caregiving situation clearly in your mind and feel the struggle in your own body.

Now please listen carefully to these words, letting them gently roll through your mind:

"Everyone is on his or her own life journey.
I am not the cause of this person's suffering,
nor is it entirely within my power to make it go away,
even if I wish I could.
Moments like this are difficult to bear,
yet I may still try to help if I can."

Aware of the stress you are carrying in your body, inhaling fully and deeply, drawing compassion inside your body, and filling every cell of your body with

(continued)

compassion. Letting yourself be soothed by inhaling deeply, and by giving yourself the compassion you need. As you exhale, sending out compassion to the person who is associated with your discomfort, or to others in general.

Continue breathing compassion in and out, allowing your body to gradually find a natural breathing rhythm—letting your body breathe itself. "One for me, one for you." "In for me, out for you."

Occasionally scanning your inner landscape for any distress and responding by inhaling compassion for yourself and exhaling compassion for others.

If you find that anyone needs extra compassion, directing your breath in that direction.

Noticing how your body is caressed from the inside as you breathe.

Letting yourself float on an ocean of compassion—a limitless ocean that embraces all suffering.

And listening to these words once again:

"Everyone is on their own life journey.
I am not the cause of this person's suffering,
nor is it entirely within my power to make it go away,
even if I wish I could
Moments like this are difficult to bear,
yet I may still try to help if I can."

Now letting go of the practice and allowing yourself to be exactly as you are in this moment.

Gently open your eyes.

Practice J.3. Meditation in Action

Each morning, set the intention to be mindful throughout the day and to be gentle with yourself. You might add to any of these suggestions a gentle touch, putting a hand over your heart and feeling the supportive touch. Bringing warmth and appreciation to yourself.

- Remind yourself of this intention as often as you can.
- Pick moments to remind yourself throughout the day, such as during breaks, at mealtimes, or when you get up to do something.

(continued)

PRACTICE J *(page 4 of 4)*

- Place reminders, such as sticky notes or stickers, around your home and office in places where you will see them frequently.
- When you remember this intention, relax your mind into a state of alert presence, or bring awareness to the breath or sound.
- Avoid trying to control your mind or block certain experiences from occurring.
- Embrace whatever manifests, even difficult thoughts, painful feelings, and situations that you normally try to avoid.

PRACTICE K

Self-Compassion

Susan M. Pollak (Chapter 9)

Practice K.1. Awareness of Sounds Practice

- Start by sitting, standing, or lying down, finding a relaxed and comfortable posture. Eyes can be open or gently closed. As you settle, see if you can get in touch with your essential dignity.
- Let yourself be present in the room. Feel your feet on the floor, or the chair you are sitting on. Allow yourself to listen to the sounds around you. There is no need to name them or judge them, just listen. Let yourself rest and relax.
- Listen with your entire being. Become aware of sounds in front of you, behind you, above you, below you. Let them come to you. Just notice. There is nothing you need to do.
- Let them arise and pass away. No need to hold on to them. If your mind wanders, don't worry. Just return to the sounds in the moment.
- Return to your essential dignity and if it feels right, your innate kindness as you close the practice.

Practice K.2. Self-Compassion Life Saver Practice

This simple three-part practice is an accessible way to introduce self-compassion and some of its benefits into trauma therapy.

- Think of a situation that is causing you some discomfort. Choose something that is mild to moderate but does not cause a huge problem.
- Bring in a moment of *mindful awareness*. Perhaps saying, "This is a moment of difficulty, this hurts." Try to add a "soothing touch" as well. A hand on the heart or a hand on the heart and belly can increase comfort and agency.

(continued)

Adapted from Pollak, Pedulla, and Siegel, *Sitting Together* (2014, p. 206).

- See if you can expand your awareness of what we call *common humanity.* Try saying, "I'm not alone. Many people have experienced this."
- Bring in some *kindness* if you can. Try, "May I be kind to myself." If that isn't good, try "May I aspire to be kind to myself." Some survivors like to add humor, such as "May I learn to be kind to myself in this lifetime."

Practice K.3. Anchoring Safely in the Body Practice

- Stand comfortably, keeping your eyes open, with the feet hip distance apart. Arms can be in front of you, behind you, or at your sides. Feel your feet connected to the ground. Let them anchor you.
- Become aware of any sensation you notice in the toes, the soles of the feet, and the heels. You can shift your weight between your feet to feel the sensations more clearly.
- Start walking, remaining relaxed and alert. Feel your feet touching the ground. Silently note to yourself, "The earth is holding me. The earth is supporting me."
- Bring attention to the movement, the flow, of walking.
- Let yourself be present. You might want to say to yourself, "In this moment, I am here, I am safe." Some patients like to say, "Peace with every step," or "Kindness with every step."
- Become aware of the light, the colors, the sounds, and smells around you.
- If you become overwhelmed or get hijacked by a memory or thought, this is part of the process. Bring your awareness to the feet touching the ground, bringing kindness to the earth and yourself.
- When you are ready to stop, return to your feet touching the ground. Feel the earth holding you and supporting you. Feel the air around you. The sky above you. If you like, you can send gratitude and compassion to the earth.
- If at any point it feels overwhelming, it is fine to stop and rest.

Practice K.4. Loving-Kindness and Compassion for Yourself

The following phrases of loving-kindness and compassion can help clinicians in this challenging but rewarding work. If you are feeling overwhelmed or you notice that you are out of your zone of tolerance, try some of these phrases:

- "May I learn to care for and nurture myself so I can attend to the needs of others with generosity, balance, kindness, and presence."
- "May I let go of expectations of healing or curing others."

(continued)

- "May I see my client with a freshness of mind and an openness of heart."
- "May I see the goodness, intelligence, and vulnerability in this person."
- "While I care about your pain and suffering, I can't make choices for you or control your life."
- "May I accept the limitations of others with warmth and compassion, and may I accept my own limits with the same kindness."
- "May I let this moment be as it is, not as I want it to be."
- "May I look after myself with ease; may I look after others with ease."

PRACTICE L

Self-Compassion Break for Shame

Christopher Germer (Chapter 11)

This practice is based on the three components of self-compassion and can be practiced in part of in full whenever you feel shame in daily life.

- To begin, please bring to mind a situation where you feel mild shame. Just mild shame since you are learning this practice for the first time.

Mindfulness

- When you feel shame, try labeling the experience for yourself in a kind and gentle way, as you might for a good friend. For example, "Ahh . . . shame. This is shame. This is how shame feels." (*Pause*)
- And then drop your awareness inside your body and see if you can notice any *physical* sensations associated with shame, perhaps some tension or uneasiness. And can you identify where you feel shame *the most* in your body? (*Pause*)
- And to the best of your ability, try allowing your experience to be just as it is, perhaps by making just a *little more room* than usual for the experience of shame. (*Pause*)
- If you like, you can also give a label to what you are afraid that *others* might be thinking about you when you feel shame, or what you might be thinking about *yourself*. For example, you might be thinking, "I'm a mess" or "I'm stupid" or "I'm worthless." These are negative beliefs and they are part of shame, but they are only beliefs and not facts. If you have any such beliefs when you feel shame, see if you can name them for yourself as you might for a good friend, with kindness and understanding. (*Pause*)

(continued)

Common Humanity

- When you feel shame, you probably feel *isolated and alone*. That's the nature of shame. But you are not alone. Everyone feels shame. Shame is a universal emotion.
- Know that what you are experiencing now is *part of the human experience*. Many people would feel just as you do in the same situation.
- And also consider for a moment that you only feel this way because you, like all human beings, *wish to be loved*. There are other words for this pull to connect that we are all born with—the wish to *belong*, to be *appreciated*, *valued*, or *respected*. Is there is a word that captures for you the universal wish to connect? See if you can name that, too. (*Pause*)

Self-Kindness

- Now let's see if we can respond to shame in a new way. Can you give yourself some kindness simply *because* you're having a moment of shame?
- If you like, perhaps *placing a hand* on the part of your body that feels shame the most. (*Pause*) And if it feels comfortable, see if you can send kindness through your fingertips into that part of your body that is holding shame for you (*pause*) or gently massaging that part of your body. (*Pause*)
- And consider for a moment what you would most like to hear in a moment of shame—perhaps words of comfort, such as "I'm here for you," "I love you," or "You are a good person." (*Pause*)
- Or stronger language in response to a critical inner voice, such as "Not helpful, not now." (*Pause*)
- What words do you need to hear at a time like this? Please repeat those words for yourself, in your own mind, in your own way. (*Pause*)
- Continue offering yourself kindness in a way that feels just right for you, perhaps savoring compassionate touch or offering yourself words of kindness, or both, doing this just *because* you feel shame, not trying to change it or make it go away. (*Pause*)
- And now let's begin to release the practice, letting the practice settle. (*Pause*) Allowing the exercise be as it was for you, and allowing yourself to be, if only for this one moment, just as you are. (*Pause*)
- And when you're ready, please begin to slowly open your eyes.

PRACTICE M

Implementing Self-Compassion in the Treatment of Borderline Personality Disorder

Christian Stiglmayr (Chapter 14)

Practice M.1. How Would I Treat a Friend? (adapted from Germer & Neff, 2019)

- Begin by taking a few deep breaths to arrive at your place, in your body, at yourself.
- If you like, you can focus on your breathing for a few moments.
- Then I invite you to think of a time when a close friend was suffering in some way. Ask yourself how you typically respond to your friend. What do you say? What tone do you use? How is your posture? What nonverbal gestures do you use? And finally, what do you normally do in such a situation?
- Then think about a time when you were suffering in some way. Ask yourself how you typically respond to yourself in these situations. What do you say to yourself? What tone do you use? How is your posture? What nonverbal gestures do you use? And finally, what do you normally do in such a situation?
- Close the exercise by asking yourself if you have noticed any patterns of difference in how you respond to yourself and others?

Practice M.2. Self-Compassion Break (adapted from Germer & Neff, 2019)

Start

- Begin by taking a few deep breaths to arrive at your place, in your body, at yourself.
- If you like, you can focus on your breathing for a few moments.
- Then focus on the distress you are experiencing right in the moment.
- Where do you feel the distress in your body? Notice any discomfort or pain in your body. Try just to be present with the sensations as they arise in your body.

(continued)

Mindfulness

- Now try saying to yourself, "This is a moment of struggle and suffering."
- Recognize the struggle while struggling.
- Validate your feelings while experiencing stress and pain.

Common Humanity

- Now try saying to yourself, "Struggle and suffering are parts of life."
- Be aware that you are not alone; many other people struggle and suffer like you, exactly right in this moment.

Self-Kindness

- And now try saying to yourself, "I am here for me," "May I be kind to myself just because you have this moment of discomfort."
- Speak with a gentle voice to yourself, maybe as if you are speaking to a little child or little animal.
- Try to accept yourself as you are, for this moment.

End

- Are there any needs you have now? What needs are they?
- Is there anything you can do right now to satisfy your needs?
- Finish the exercise by taking a few deep breaths. If you like, place a hand over your heart or another comfortable place of your body and try to let yourself be as you are—at least for this moment.

Practice M.3. Being with Difficult Emotions (adapted from Germer & Neff, 2019)

Start

- Begin by taking a few deep breaths to arrive at your place, in your body, at yourself.
- If you like, you can focus on your breathing for a few moments.
- Be aware that there is nothing to achieve or accomplish in the following minutes.
- Then focus on the distress you are experiencing right in the moment.

(continued)

- Are there any emotions that arise within you? Can you name which emotions are involved? Can you focus on the strongest emotion?
- Where do you feel the emotion and the associated discomfort in your body most strongly? Allow yourself to experience the sensation directly, without changing anything.

Soften

- Now begin to soften into that location in your body. Let the muscles soften and relax, as if warm water is running over this part of your body.

Soothe

- If you want, place a hand over the part of your body that feels uncomfortable.
- If you wish, simply feel the warmth and gentle touch of your hand. If it feels right for you, you can also gently massage this part of your body.
- Are there some comforting words that you might wish to hear? Can you say these words to yourself?
- Soothe yourself because of this difficult situation.

Allow

- Finally, allow any remaining discomfort to be there, just as it is.
- Allow yourself to be just as you are, just like this, if only for this moment.

End

- Now expand your attention to your whole body. Allow yourself to feel whatever you feel, to be exactly as you are in this moment. Just leave yourself in peace for a moment.
- Finish the exercise by taking a few deep breaths. If you like, you can ask yourself if there are there any needs you have now. Is there anything you can do right now to satisfy your needs?

PRACTICE N

Adaptation of "How Would You Treat Your Friend?"

Lizabeth Roemer, Gerson F. Borrero, Molly Sawdy, and Jessica R. LoPresti (Chapter 15)

Here we include an adapted version of the "How Would You Treat Your Friend?" self-compassion exercise (Neff, 2012) to use with a client who is struggling with their anxious response to discrimination. (This can also be adapted for other struggles clients are feeling anxious about.)

- First, the clinician asks that the client imagine that a sibling, friend, or other loved one is experiencing an issue that the client is currently struggling with, such as instances of discrimination or internalized racism.
- Ask the client to describe (or write down in the form of a letter when outside of the session) how they would respond to a friend who was experiencing discrimination similar to their own experience.
- Ask the client to especially take note of and describe what their tone would be as they are supporting their friend.
- Then, ask the client to describe how they have been responding to themselves as they deal with instances of discrimination or internalized oppression, with an emphasis on the tone that they have been using.
- Ask the client if there are any differences in how they would respond to a friend as compared to how they have been responding to themselves.
- Ask the client to describe possible reasons for differences in how they respond.
- Finally, ask the client to imagine how they believe things might change for them if they responded to themselves the same way that they would respond to the chosen loved one.

PRACTICE O

The Process of Self-Compassion in Eating Disorder Recovery

Ann Saffi Biasetti (Chapter 16)

Practice O.1. Feet, Spine, and Seat: Welcoming the Body into the Room

Close your eyes (or keep them open with a soft, fixed gaze).

1. Take a breath in through your nose and out through your mouth (release breath)
2. Bring your attention down to your feet and press them into the ground deeply until you can feel all corners of your feet. Notice the sensations that begin to form around your feet and even into your ankles and legs. Notice how pressing firmly also engages your back body. See if you can feel sensations build in your lower back.
3. Follow those sensations now up the length of your spine, traveling up all the way to the crown of your head.
4. And now draw your attention back down to the chair beneath you, grounding your seat.
5. Repeat this awareness from your feet, up your spine, and back down to your seat a few times along with your breath.

Practice O.2. Body Forgiveness Practice

- For this practice, I invite you to take a comfortable sit, one that can support your body for the next 5–7 minutes of this practice.
- As you prepare your body, bringing it to support in whatever way you may need, I'll invite you to close your eyes, or you can keep them open to a relaxed fixed gaze.
- For this practice, you can either just rest your hand on your lap or you can place a hand or two to the space of your heart or any other area of your body that feels comforting and or soothing to you in any way.

(continued)

- And just begin to listen to the words, and see how the words land within your body as you hear them:

"May all pain be eased.
May all wounds be healed.
May all sorrows and regrets soften and dissipate.
May all faults and errors be forgiven.

May worry and frustration fall away.
May all pain be eased.
May all wounds be healed.
May all sorrows and regrets soften and dissipate.
May all faults and errors be forgiven.

May worry and frustration fall away.
May I forgive myself for the ways in which I have done or continue to do any harm to my body in any way through behaviors that have been unkind.
May I forgive myself for the ways in which I have done or continue to do any harm to my body in any way through behaviors that have been unkind.

May my body heal, balance, and repair as I continue to heal, balance, and repair.
May my body heal, balance, and repair as I continue to heal, balance, and repair.

If I am not yet ready to forgive myself, may I forgive myself for that, and offer compassion for what I am capable of today.

If I am not yet ready to forgive myself, may I forgive myself for that, and offer compassion for what I am capable of today.

For all the ways that I may harm, negate, doubt, belittle, judge, or be unkind to myself through my own confusions, may I learn to forgive myself.

For all the ways that I may harm, negate, doubt, belittle, judge, or be unkind to myself through my own confusions, may I learn to forgive myself.

May I now understand what my body has endured out in this world. The messages it has received. The beliefs it has held. The judgments and the shame.

May I now understand what my body has endured out in this world. The messages it has received. The beliefs it has held. The judgments and the shame.

(continued)

May I come to understand that due to these messages, it was easy, to belittle, to judge, and be unkind to my body.

May I come to understand that due to these messages, it was easy, to belittle, to judge, and be unkind to my body.

Through this understanding, may I begin to heal, balance, and repair as my body continues to heal, balance, and repair.

Through this understanding, may I begin to heal, balance, and repair as my body continues to heal, balance, and repair.

And if I am still not yet ready to forgive myself, may I forgive myself for that, and offer compassion for what I am capable of today.

If I am still not yet ready to forgive myself, may I forgive myself for that, and offer compassion for what I am capable of today.

And may I slowly and gently come to understand that my body never meant to cause me any harm and that it now needs me to be by its side.

May I slowly and gently come to understand that my body never meant to cause me any harm and that it now needs me to be by its side."

- Notice how the words land within, how they land in your body.
- Stay here as long as you need to offer the comfort that you may require at this moment, and when you are ready you can gently begin to take a deeper breath and then come to open your eyes.
- I encourage you to use this practice initially on a daily basis, even if you just listen to the words and then turn to it whenever you need a reminder to be gentle, compassionate, and kind to yourself and to your body.

PRACTICE P

Couple and Relationship Distress

Michelle Becker (Chapter 17)

A Note about Guiding Exercises

The following exercises are usually most effective when done for the first time in their entirety. Later, therapists may wish to ask just one of the questions or refer back to a specific part of the exercise. As always, therapists should use their own discretion as to what would work best with any particular patient/couple and how best to deliver the exercises.

Practice P.1. Exercise to Help Identify Relational Patterns

1. Call to mind a conflict or other distress in your relationship with your partner (or other relationship). Something that activates your threat/defense system, but not something traumatic. Choose a specific event.
2. Allow yourself to recall the situation and, letting go of the storyline, notice what happened for you and how that translated to how you interacted with your partner. Did you find yourself attacking them, or defending yourself? Or maybe you withdrew in an attempt to find safety? Sometimes we even go into placate mode where we tell our partner what we think will calm them down, even though it may not be true for us. See what happened for you.
3. Or maybe you found yourself recruiting the drive system in an effort to restore safety. Did you move into fix-it mode? Take control? Tell them how to do better?
4. What effect did that have on your partner?
5. Please know that this is our human wiring for survival that gets activated when we feel threatened, especially when we feel a threat to our closest relationships. Even though these responses can make the situation worse, we are just trying to restore safety and we are not alone in our unskillfulness. This is part of our shared human condition. (Adapted from Becker, 2023.)

(continued)

Practice P.2. Exercise to Help Foster Common Humanity—Just Like Me

1. Call to mind the same situation you worked with earlier.
2. Focusing now on your partner, what was happening for them? Might they also have been in their threat/defense system or their drive system?
3. What behavior did they exhibit? Attacking/defending, withdrawing/avoiding, or placating, for example? Or maybe they went into fix-it mode, took control, or told you how you were doing it wrong and could do it better.
4. Can you see that underneath their unskillful behavior was the pain of the threat/defense system and that their survival wiring was activated? Can you hold their unskillful behavior in the context of our shared human condition as well?
5. Now consider when you were caught in your unskillful behavior. Even though you may have been upset with them, angry with them, withdrew from them, judged their actions and their choices, did you still love them—even if you didn't feel loving in that moment? Even if you said otherwise, from your perspective now—safe in this present moment—do you care about them and want to be in a relationship with them?
6. Consider your partner, even if they blamed you or abandoned you, likely still loved and loves you too. Perhaps like you, they got caught in survival mode and didn't put their best foot forward.
7. What would it be like to see your partner's behavior as a reflection of their suffering, rather than view it through the lens of how much they do or don't care about you?
8. Does a desire to offer compassion arise? What would compassion look like in this situation?

Practice P.3. Self-Compassion Break (adapted from Germer & Neff, 2019)

1. Call to mind a situation you are in the midst of that is causing you some distress, especially in the context of a relationship. For this exercise, please choose a situation that does not involve your partner or a child. For example, maybe you are struggling with something a coworker said to you or a difficult interaction with your neighbor, or perhaps you're tired of being the only one to plan events with a friend.
2. Choose something that causes enough distress that you can feel it in your body but not something that is overwhelming: a 3–4 on a scale of distress where 10 is extremely stressful.

(continued)

3. When you settle on a situation, let yourself recall the situation. Who was or wasn't there? What was or wasn't said?
4. Letting go of the storyline now, take a moment to notice the distress it causes you. What kind of emotions are present, and what kind of physical sensations are present?
5. Acknowledging the reality of this difficulty. Perhaps say to yourself, "This is hard," or "This really hurts," or even "This is a moment of suffering." That's the mindfulness part, opening to the truth of how things are right now. (*Pause*)
6. Then remember that this is part of the shared human condition. Relationships have their ups and downs, it's painful when situations like this arise. Perhaps say to yourself, "This is how it feels when things like this come up in relationships—I'm not alone" or "Everyone makes mistakes, I'm only human" or "Anyone would feel the way I do in this situation." (*Pause*)
7. If there is a place in your body where you feel distress most easily, place a hand over that place with the intention of bringing kindness to that part of the body. Perhaps letting the hand fill with kindness and the kindness seep from the hand into the body, if that feels okay. You can even give that part a pat or rub if it feels good to do so. (*Pause*)
8. And are there any kind words you need to hear? Perhaps something like "It wasn't your fault" or "You're lovable just as you are" or "I'll be here for you, even when others let you down." See what it is for you and offer yourself your own kind words. (*Pause*)
9. If you are having trouble finding kind words to offer yourself, you can imagine what you would say to a dear friend in the same situation, or what someone you love and trust would say to you in this situation. Then try saying those words to yourself, in a kind and understanding voice. (*Pause*)
10. Then, let go of the practice and take a moment to notice the effects of this practice. As best you can, accepting yourself and your practice just like this, even if only for this moment. And thanking yourself for showing up, caring, and being willing to try something new.

Practice P.4. Exercise to Foster Kindness

1. Call to mind the situation you were working with, or various situations with your partner.
2. What is it you long for from them when you are having a hard time? Comforting words? Validation? Some kind of touch or reassurance, a hug or pat on the leg? Do you want them to just hear you? Maybe you want to go for a walk together without talking about it? See what it is for you.

(continued)

3. Now consider what your partner wants when they are distressed. What do they long for from you? Do they just want to be heard? Do they want some sort of physical comfort—a hug, for example? Or maybe they want you to do something together—like go for a bike ride. See what it is for them.
4. Do you tend to offer your partner what you need or what they need?
5. Is there a way for both of you to get what you need, even if it is sequential rather than simultaneous? What typically makes your relationships stronger?

PRACTICE Q

Holding Your Own Hand Practice (A Modified Soothing Touch)

Lisa Shetler and Lorraine Hobbs (Chapter 18)

- Let's begin by sitting comfortably anywhere you would like. And when you are ready, take a nice deep inhalation and just let the breath out slowly. You might want to take a couple of easy breaths to follow.
- Let's begin by experimenting with ways that you can "hold your own hand" and the purpose of this is to bring kindness and comfort to yourself maybe when things are a little rough, there is a little stress, or you encounter some sort of challenge.
- You might begin just by interlocking your fingers, or one hand resting on top of the other, just see what it feels like for you. The idea is to bring kindness to yourself, so setting the intention that this is a way you want to meet whatever situation you are experiencing in this moment.
- Just noticing what is it like to support yourself this way.
- You might notice the warmth of your hands, you might notice if it feels warm anywhere else in your body, and if it is comforting in any way.
- And then if you like, you could try a few other ways to soothe and comfort yourself. Here are just a few that might be comforting when things are uncomfortable. Just to keep in mind that there is a physiological reason that this practice works. When we make physical contact through a soothing gesture, even with ourselves or with others, even patting your dog, we release a hormone called oxytocin. This hormone, commonly called "the feel-good chemical," can elicit feelings of trust, relaxation, and reduced stress responses.
- So you might want to explore when on your body right now you might want to feel supported and might want to try and offer yourself a simple gesture of kindness through touch.
- So this can begin with something as simple as touching your fingertips together, and noticing how that feels. Sometimes we want to begin slowly because we are bringing a very different intention—bringing an intention of kindness and compassion to ourselves.

(continued)

- If you like, you can put one hand on your cheek, or both hands, one hand on each cheek. As if you are cradling your face. Notice how that feels. Is it soothing? Is it warm? And then take your hands, bring them across your chest, and hold your opposite upper arm, as if you are crossing your arms but you are actually placing the palms of your hands on the other bicep area. You might want to rub that arm a little bit. Give a gentle squeeze, notice how that feels.
- If you like, you can put one hand on your chest, just over your heart area, and one hand on your belly. Feeling the rise and fall of your chest, the rise and fall of your belly, or to your heart beating and your whole body breathing.
- Then if you like, you can bring your second hand up to your chest and give that area of the body just a little more pressure, just to let yourself know that you are here, connecting to yourself. Offering yourself a little bit of kindness.
- Go ahead and bring those hands to your belly so that both hands are resting on your belly and see how that feels. That might be more inviting or reassuring or comforting. And if you like, you can simply rest your hands, one palm in the other on your lap and just see if this is comforting, maybe more relaxing, again remembering that the intention is just to be kind to yourself.
- All of these different ways of offering support to yourself can release that hormone oxytocin.
- This is a modified version called "Holding Your Hand" practice and it's all about a mindful soothing touch, a compassionate soothing touch, and a comforting soothing touch.
- Thank you so much for participating in this practice with me.

PRACTICE R

Mindfulness and Self-Compassion for Chronic Pain

Ronald D. Seigel (Chapter 19)

Practice R.1. Mindfulness of Pain-Related Thoughts and Feelings

- Find a comfortable, relaxed, and alert posture. If sitting, you might imagine a string tied to the top of your head pulling upward, gently elongating the spine. If you're lying down, perhaps place a pillow under your knees to help straighten your back. Begin by choosing a sensory object of awareness that's comfortable and easy to attend to. This might be the cycles of the breath, the sounds around you, or another sensation.
- As you gently attend to the sensations, it would not be unusual for thoughts to arise. That's okay, they're our friends. Each time that you notice that the attention has wandered away from sensations and into the thought stream, just gently and lovingly bring it back to your chosen sensations.
- As you continue this practice, be on the lookout for pain-related thoughts or feelings. These could be worries spurred by pain at this moment, memories of pain, or anticipation of future pain. Also, notice any sensations of anxiety or tension arising in the body in response to these thoughts. There's no need to control these, just notice when concerns about pain enter the thought stream, and gently return your attention to the sensations of the moment. See if you might approach the whole experience with kindness and understanding, perhaps soothing yourself with kind, caring words, such as "Of course, I'm frightened, pain is so scary."

Practice R.2. Separating Pain from Aversion[1]

Begin by finding a comfortable and alert posture, attending to the breath wherever it's most clearly felt in the body. Notice the texture and contour of each inhalation and exhalation. See if you can be with all of these sensations with an attitude of interest, curiosity, and acceptance for about 10 minutes.

(continued)

[1] A variation of this practice, called "Separating the Two Arrows," is available free of charge in audio at *DrRonSiegel.com*.

Now begin to shift your focus to wherever you feel discomfort or pain. Allow the breath to settle into the background and bring your attention to the uncomfortable sensations. See if you can attend to the general area of the pain. Relax and settle into the physical sensations. Carefully observe their nature—whether burning, tight, piercing, dull, or sharp.

Next, imagine having a wise, compassionate friend by your side offering loving support. Talk to yourself as they might speak to you. For example, they might say, "I'm so sorry this is difficult. Pain is really hard." Imagine that they are soothing you, perhaps holding your hand, massaging the area that hurts, or otherwise giving you whatever care you need.

Now zero in on the spot in your body that particularly hurts. You're not trying to change it, but rather to just experience it clearly, with care and love. Notice how the sensations vary subtly from moment to moment. Perhaps one second they throb, while the next they burn or ache. See if you can observe that "pain" is actually a series of momentary sensations strung together like frames in a movie, creating an illusion of continuity. See if you can also relax into feeling loved and supported by your imaginary companion.

Should the pain become particularly intense, and the mind recoil from it, notice the form that recoiling takes. Does the body tense? Do aversive thoughts arise, such as "I hate this!" "When will it ever end?" See if you might give those thoughts labels, such as "fearing, hating, worrying," and return loving attention to the painful area.

If these aversion responses become too difficult to bear, you can experiment with bringing your attention back to the general area of the pain or even back to the breath for a while. Be kind to yourself as you see the effects of shifting your attention. See if you might also ramp up the love and self-soothing: "Of course, this is hard. Nobody likes pain." Continue trying to lovingly be with the discomfort, and the mind and body's reactions to it, for the next 10 minutes or so.

Practice R.3. Compassionate Urge Surfing for Pain[2]

Close your eyes if you're comfortable doing so, find a relaxed and alert upright posture, and bring your attention to the cycles of your breath for a few minutes. Allow yourself to open to any pain sensations that might arise, attending to them with loving curiosity and interest. See how they change from moment to moment.

Should the discomfort become intense and you feel an urge to get up, see if you can notice exactly where in your body you feel this urge. Does it involve

(continued)

[2]A variation of this practice, called "Urge Surfing for Pain," is available free of charge in audio at *DrRonSiegel.com.*

tension in the chest? Elsewhere? Bring your full attention to the urge, noticing its location, intensity, and texture. See if you can notice how the urge to get up is actually distinct from the pain sensations.

Now consider how hard it is to be a human being, and how our ancestors, as well as everyone else on the planet today, have had the urge to escape pain. Imagine that you're a wise, compassionate being, soothing both yourself and the countless other people struggling with discomfort at this very moment.

Finally, return your attention partially to your breath. Using your breath as a surfboard, ride each wave of urgency to get up from its beginning as a small wavelet to the point where it crests. Allow each wave to rise up as high as it wants, trusting that it will reach a crescendo and then subside again.

PRACTICE S

Integrating Self-Compassion into Acceptance and Commitment Therapy and Other Third-Wave Cognitive-Behavioral Therapies

Benjamin Weinstein (Chapter 20)

Practice S.1. Kind Coach

This practice helps clients develop their capacity to self-compassionately connect with core values that can guide their actions while encouraging and motivating themselves with kindness (rather than with self-criticism). "Kind Coach" focuses on building the motivating element of fierce self-compassion. From an acceptance and commitment therapy (ACT) perspective, it focuses on providing empowering motivation to engage with valued directions and behaviors. The exercise builds on and extends the practice of "Motivating Ourselves with Compassion" (Germer & Neff, 2019). It can be practiced as a guided visualization or can be approached as a dialogue between the therapist and the client.

Steps

1. Invite the client to bring into mind a specific behavior they would like to change or a specific situation/context in which they would like more motivation and encouragement. Invite the client to begin to visualize themselves in this situation.
2. For some clients, self-judgment, self-blame, and self-criticism begin to arise. This is particularly true when clients have a long history with this behavior or context. Support clients to notice, name, acknowledge, and respond compassionately to any self-criticism that arises. You can help the client to observe the way their mind works as spontaneous and automatic, arising from past conditioning. That doesn't have to govern the client's choices in the present moment. This step must be sensitively adapted to fit with each client's history and experiences. Some clients may wish to acknowledge and thank the inner critic for good intentions to help the client grow or improve. Other clients, whose self-criticism originates in trauma and abuse, may wish to commit to developing their ability to heal by turning away from the

(continued)

harsh inner critic and gradually relating to themselves in a kinder way, little by little.

3. The therapist emphasizes our common humanity; facing challenges or wanting to change are natural and shared experiences. Carrying around our learning history within us, which can be triggered at any moment, is also simply part of being human, not a defect or a weakness. When we practice self-compassion or ACT, we recognize our common humanity and use our resources to be there for ourselves in the same way we would support a good friend.
4. Invite the client to visualize a "kind coach"—whatever that means to them. This can be any figure, real or imaginary, that symbolizes the qualities of kind encouragement and persistence to this client. Encourage the client for their kind coach to take whatever form feels right for them. (*Pause*)
5. Tell the client that the kind coach also wants to support the client to try to make a change or face this moment in accord with what matters to them. The kind coach cares about them and wants the best for them. The kind coach understands the client and knows what matters to the client. The client can imagine that their kind coach is smiling at them and encouraging them to do what's possible at this moment, even just one small step toward what matters to them. The kind coach knows that the past can't be changed and believes in the client's ability to stand up and take a small step today, a small step that moves in the direction that matters to the client. (*Pause for client reflection*)
6. Ask the client to imagine what this kind of coach might say to them and how they might say it. Provide some pauses for reflection. The therapist can offer examples like "I believe in you and want you to live well"; "You don't have to be perfect, just try what's possible today"; or "I support what matters to you and I want to help you live that today by taking just one small step in that direction"; or "I don't want you to hurt yourself—I want you to grow and be your best you for today"; and so on. These can also be adapted to fit what you already know about the client and their values. Allow the client enough time to reflect on what their kind coach might say. For some clients, it can be useful to write down the words they imagine.

Some clients may wish to finish this exercise with a written reflection to record and consolidate the images or messages they experienced. Follow the exercise with a dialogue to explore the client's experience. Focus on what is connected for the client in the exercise, particularly their felt experience, before focusing on the obstacles that may have arisen. Emphasize that whatever the client experiences is part of the clients themselves. This is a resource they're always carrying within and can learn to access when they need it. Invite the

(continued)

client to consider how to use this in the context of their own daily life and make a plan for how they'll do that (i.e., homework).

Practice S.2. Suggestions for Working with Fears of Compassion and Backdraft in ACT

Fears and doubts frequently arise and having effective clinical dialogues about this is a key element to effectively integrating self-compassion into therapy. Self-compassion-informed therapists use three primary techniques for dealing with milder fears and doubts that arise about self-compassion (Germer & Neff, 2019; Steindl et al., 2023):

1. *Psychoeducation:* Sharing with clients the research evidence (Germer & Neff, 2019) that (a) doubts, initial discomfort, and mild fears about self-compassion are so common as to be universal; and (b) the research shows that these doubts and mild fears just aren't true. This is less ACT-consistent than the next two options.
2. *Inviting a flexible, playful perspective:* Inviting the client to notice how, when we offer kindness and compassion to people we care about, we don't have doubts and fears that our kindness might harm or be bad for them. The mind only generates these doubts when we do this new, unfamiliar thing—directing kindness to ourselves. Invite the client to smile at or even tease their mind for this double standard!
3. *Emphasizing common humanity (destigmatizing):* Highlighting the universality of these fears can help clients understand them as a product of our brain's response to the discomfort of unfamiliarity.

The therapist support in identifying and resolving backdraft is essential for clients to fully benefit from self-compassion. The experience of backdraft is quite variable; for a full treatment of this topic, refer to Germer and Neff (2019). Several core guidelines for working with backdraft are:

1. Recognize and name the experience.
2. Emphasize the common humanity of backdraft.
3. Taking care of the backdraft becomes the focus: (a) if they choose, the client can slow down or stop completely; (b) notice whatever form backdraft is taking and move into asking themselves what they need to cope with the pains of backdraft in the current moment; and (c) explore and experiment with responses that help the client manage it in a way aligned with their values. The client might wish to "dip" in and out of the backdraft, alternating between the experience of the

(continued)

backdraft and another coping skill. Since backdraft tends to look like whatever other forms of dysregulation the client is vulnerable to, other coping skills that are useful in helping the client regulate may help with backdraft as well.

4. Empower client choice. The client decides how best to work with their backdraft.
5. Integrate backdraft in the "passengers on the bus" metaphor. ACT therapists use a wide variety of metaphors that help clients visualize private experiences (affects and cognitions) as passengers in a car, bus, or boat. Backdraft can be easily integrated into this framework to allow a helpful dialogue about the different elements of the client's backdraft experience.

PRACTICE T

Self-Compassion and Teens

Lisa Shetler and Lorraine Hobbs (Chapter 18)

The following two exercises are of a different nature from the rest of the Appendix. Given the specific style and needs of adolescents, we include guidelines for how to offer practices to teen clients.

Exercise T.1. Mindfulness through Music

Mindfulness through music is a great way to invite adolescent clients to practice the skill of noticing, using a medium that they are comfortable and connected to, such as their favorite music. It provides flexibility in pendulating between an internal and external focus, which may be a safer starting place for teens who struggle to stay present with the felt experience of the body.

- I'd like to talk you through how I invite an adolescent client to participate in a mindfulness through music practice. I like to begin by inviting the client to choose a piece of music that they feel connected to in some way. This could be an instrumental piece or something with lyrics that speak to them.
- To begin with, play through the song, listening to it together and invite the client to tune into their body and notice how they're feeling as the song plays out. We might then listen to the track again, paying particular attention to the lyrics, the melody, the beat, tuning into individual instruments, before broadening our awareness and listening to the song as a whole again.
- Sometimes it might be nice to experiment with listening to different versions of a song. Perhaps listening to an instrumental version of a song and acoustic version or a remix and tuning into the way that may change the client's relationship to the song, the felt experience as they're listening to what arises for them, or if it changes the meaning of the song.
- Throughout this practice, I like to gently invite the client to tune into the thoughts and their felt experience, noticing what's arising for them as they listen to the track. This could be a really lovely and gentle way of inviting an adolescent client to experience mindfulness through a medium that they feel comfortable and connected to, and that also can give you some flexibility

(continued)

between tuning into the body and tuning into something more external, for clients who might find it hard to stay present with the body for extended periods of time.

Exercise T.2. Modified "Compassionate Friend" Practice

This modified "Compassionate Friend" practice is a gentle way of helping a teen client discover or connect with their compassionate voice and begin to experiment with offering themselves kindness in the midst of suffering.

- I'd like to talk you through how I invite an adolescent client to participate in the compassionate friend meditation. You may notice that this is a condensed version of the standard practice. The practice has been intentionally shortened to give our teen client the opportunity to have a taste of this experience, without leaving them sitting in the practice for too long where we run the risk of them disengaging or becoming too activated by the practice.
- I like to begin by inviting my adolescent client to choose a posture that feels really natural and comfortable for them, one that allows them to be at ease but still alert. That might be sitting on a chair, that might be sitting or lying down on the floor, that might be using a pillow or a blanket to help them find a posture that's really comfortable for them to be in.
- I then like to invite them to call to mind a time recently when they've felt stressed or upset. I'm careful to include some instruction around choosing something that's happened in the past week or two that would be only rate as a 2 or 3 on a 0 to 10 scale of distress. We don't want them picking the most difficult thing that they're experiencing right now because we want to make sure that they stay in the "safe zone," where they can learn and practice without becoming overwhelmed or activated by a distressing thought or memory.
- Once they indicate that they've identified a small stress that they feel comfortable working with, I invite them to imagine a wise or kind figure that could come and support them during this difficult time. Particularly with teenagers, I make sure to include some instruction here that this doesn't have to be a real person that they know. It could, indeed, be a fictional character, somebody from a movie or a book, it could be somebody that's no longer present in their lives, or it could be a pet or an animal that they feel could offer them comfort during a difficult time.
- I then invite them to take the next few moments to imagine what this might say or do that would help to bring them some comfort or some guidance in relation to this difficult situation.

(continued)

- If I get the sense that maybe my client is struggling to think of what a kind or compassionate gesture might be, I might offer them some suggestions. Offering them words like "This is really tough, but we're going to figure this out" or "It doesn't feel good what you're going through right now, but you've been through hard times before and you're going to come through this one okay."
- I invite them to just notice what it feels like to receive this comfort to hear these words from someone who really deeply cares about them. Then gently bring to their attention the fact that this wisdom, this kindness, this source of comfort has come from within them, that it actually already exists and is something that they can access whenever they need it. It can sometimes be surprising to our adolescent clients who maybe felt that they didn't know how to be kind to themselves.
- After inviting the client to reorient to the room, to open their eyes if they were closed, we might take a moment to talk about what that experience was like for them, what they noticed, and for some clients, it might be appropriate to invite them to journal some of those kind or wise words, or to create a compassionate figure that they can connect with again in the future.

Index

Note. *f* following a page number indicates a figure

D

J

K

L

M

N

Q

R

S

T

LIST OF AUDIO FILES

Scan the QR code to access the audio files.

Track	Title	Run Time
1	Self-Compassion Break (Chapter 1)	05:54
2	Giving and Receiving Compassion (Chapter 1)	21:20
3	Compassion Practice Sequences to Aid Cultivating Compassion Brain, Body, and Mind States (Chapters 2 and 13)	21:25
4	Self-Compassion Practice for My Social and Cultural Identities (Chapter 4)	11:23
5	Soften, Calm, Allow (Chapter 5)	16:09
6	Embodied Presence Practice: Core Body Centering (Chapter 6)	05:28
7	Sitting Compassion Meditation Practice (Chapter 8)	07:36
8	The Practice of Self-Compassion with Equanimity (Chapter 8)	14:38
9	Anchoring Safely in the Body Practice (Chapter 9)	02:42
10	Self-Compassion Break for Shame (Chapter 11)	07:49
11	Body Forgiveness Practice (Chapter 16)	09:22
12	Exercise to Help Identify Relational Patterns (Chapter 17)	04:17
13	Holding Your Own Hand Practice (A Modified Soothing Touch) (Chapter 18)	07:16
14	Separating Pain from Aversion (Chapter 19)	07:07
15	The Kind Coach (Chapter 20)	08:47
16	Mindfulness through Music (Chapter 18)	02:09
17	Modified "Compassionate Friend" Practice (Chapter 18)	04:29